Cardiovascular Intensive Care

Editors

UMESH K. GIDWANI
SAMIN K. SHARMA
ANNAPOORNA S. KINI

CARDIOLOGY CLINICS

www.cardiology.theclinics.com

Consulting Editors

ROSARIO FREEMAN
JORDAN M. PRUTKIN
DAVID M. SHAVELLE
AUDREY H. WU

November 2013 • Volume 31 • Number 4

ELSEVIER

1600 John F. Kennedy Boulevard • Suite 1800 • Philadelphia, Pennsylvania, 19103-2899

http://www.theclinics.com

CARDIOLOGY CLINICS Volume 31, Number 4

November 2013 ISSN 0733-8651, ISBN-13: 978-0-323-24217-2

Editor: Barbara Cohen-Kligerman

Cardiology Clinics (ISSN 0733-8651) is published quarterly by Elsevier Inc., 360 Park Avenue South, New York, NY 10010-1710. Months of issue are February, May, August, and November. Business and Editorial Offices: 1600 John F. Kennedy Blvd., Ste. 1800, Philadelphia, PA 19103-2899. Customer Service Office: 3251 Riverport Lane, Maryland Heights, MO 63043. Periodicals post-age paid at New York, NY and additional mailing offices. Subscription prices are $320.00 per year for US individuals, $530.00 per year for US institutions, $155.00 per year for US students and residents, $390.00 per year for Canadian individuals, $665.00 per year for Canadian institutions, $455.00 per year for international individuals, $665.00 per year for international institutions and $220.00 per year for Canadian and international students/residents. To receive student/resident rate, orders must be accompanied by name of affiliated institution, data of term, and the *signature* of program/residency coordinator on institution letterhead. Orders will be billed at individual rate until proof of status is received. Foreign air speed delivery is included in all *Clinics* subscription prices. All prices are subject to change without notice. **POSTMASTER:** Send address changes to *Cardiology Clinics*, Elsevier Health Sciences Division, Subscription Customer Service, 3251 Riverport Lane, Maryland Heights, MO 63043. **Customer Service: 1-800-654-2452 (U.S. and Canada); 314-447-8871 (outside U.S. and Canada). Fax: 314-447-8029. E-mail: journalscustomerservice-usa@ elsevier.com (for print support); journalsonlinesupport-usa@elsevier.com (for online support).**

Reprints. For copies of 100 or more, of articles in this publication, please contact the Commercial Reprints Department, Elsevier Inc., 360 Park Avenue South, New York, NY 10010-1710. Tel.: 212-633-3874; Fax: 212-633-3820; E-mail: reprints@elsevier.com.

Cardiology Clinics is also published in Spanish by McGraw-Hill Interamericana Editores S. A., P.O. Box 5-237, 06500, Mexico D. F., Mexico; in Portuguese by Reichmann and Alfonso Editores Rio de Janeiro, Brazil; and in Greek by Dimitrios P. Lagos, 8 Pondon Street, GR115-28 Ilissia, Greece.

Cardiology Clinics is covered in *MEDLINE/PubMed (Index Medicus)*, *Excerpta Medica*, *The Cumulative Index to Nursing and Allied Health Literature* (CINAHL).

Printed and bound by CPI Group (UK) Ltd, Croydon, CR0 4YY

Transferred to digital print 2012

Contributors

IVAN ROCHA FERREIRA DA SILVA, MD
Neurocritical Care Unit and Stroke
Department, Hospital Copa D'Or,
Rio de Janeiro, Brazil

JENNIFER ANN FRONTERA, MD
Associate Professor of Medicine (Neurology),
Cerebrovascular Center, Neurological Institute,
Cleveland Clinic Lerner College of Medicine,
Cleveland, Ohio

VAANI PANSE GARG, MD
Department of Medicine, The Cardiovascular
Institute, Mount Sinai Medical Center, Icahn
School of Medicine at Mount Sinai, New York,
New York

UMESH K. GIDWANI, MD, FCCP, FCCM
Chief, Cardiac Critical Care, The Zena and
Michael A. Weiner Cardiovascular Institute,
Mount Sinai Hospital; Assistant Professor,
Cardiology, Pulmonary, Critical Care and Sleep
Medicine, Icahn School of Medicine at Mount
Sinai, New York, New York

JONATHAN L. HALPERIN, MD
Department of Medicine, The Cardiovascular
Institute, Mount Sinai Medical Center, Icahn
School of Medicine at Mount Sinai, New York,
New York

SIAN I. JAGGAR, CertMedEd, MD, FRCA
Anaesthesia and Critical Care Department,
Royal Brompton Hospital, London,
United Kingdom

**NICOLA JONES, MA, BM BCh, MRCP,
FRCA, FFICM**
Department of Cardiothoracic Intensive Care,
Papworth Hospital, University of Cambridge,
Cambridge, United Kingdom

ANNAPOORNA S. KINI, MD, MRCP, FACC
Professor of Medicine and Cardiology, The
Zena and Michael A. Wiener Cardiovascular
Institute, Mount Sinai Hospital, The Icahn
School of Medicine at Mount Sinai, New York,
New York

RAMESH S. KUTTY, MBBS, MRCS
Department of Cardiothoracic Surgery,
Papworth Hospital, University of Cambridge,
Cambridge, United Kingdom

ANURADHA LALA, MD
Division of Cardiology, Department of
Medicine, Brigham and Women's Hospital,
Harvard Medical School, Boston,
Massachusetts

JACK Z. LI, MD, MBA
Department of Internal Medicine, University
of Michigan Medical School, University of
Michigan Health System, Ann Arbor, Michigan

J. KEITH MANSEL, MD, FACCP
Section of Palliative Medicine, Division of
General Internal Medicine, Department of
Medicine; Assistant Professor of Medicine,
Program in Professionalism and Ethics, Mayo
Clinic College of Medicine, Mayo Clinic,
Rochester, Minnesota

MANDEEP R. MEHRA, MD
Professor of Medicine, Division of Cardiology,
Department of Medicine, Harvard Medical
School; Executive Director, Center for
Advanced Heart Disease, Brigham and
Women's Hospital, Boston, Massachusetts

BIBHU MOHANTY, MD
Fellow, Zena and Michael A. Weiner
Cardiovascular Institute, Mount Sinai Hospital,
New York, New York

**NARAIN MOORJANI, MB ChB, MRCS, MD,
FRCS (C-Th)**
Department of Cardiothoracic Surgery,
Papworth Hospital, University of Cambridge,
Cambridge, United Kingdom

JULIO A. PANZA, MD
Chief, Division of Cardiology, Westchester
Medical Center, Valhalla, New York

**SUSANNA PRICE, MD, PhD, MRCP, EDICM,
FFICM, FESC**
Department of Intensive Care, Royal Brompton
Hospital, Imperial College, University of
London, London, United Kingdom

J. WILLIAM SCHLEIFER, MD
Division of Cardiovascular Diseases, Mayo
Clinic Arizona, Scottsdale, Arizona

SAMIN K. SHARMA, MD, FSCAI, FACC
Director of Clinical and Interventional
Cardiology, The Zena and Michael A. Wiener
Cardiovascular Institute, Mount Sinai Hospital,
The Icahn School of Medicine at Mount Sinai,
New York, New York

KOMANDOOR SRIVATHSAN, MD
Division of Cardiovascular Diseases, Mayo Clinic Hospital, Mayo Clinic Arizona, Phoenix, Arizona

KEITH M. SWETZ, MD, MA, FACP, FAAHPM
Section of Palliative Medicine, Division of General Internal Medicine, Department of Medicine; Associate Professor of Medicine, Program in Professionalism and Ethics, Mayo Clinic College of Medicine, Mayo Clinic, Rochester, Minnesota

MATTHEW I. TOMEY, MD
Chief Fellow, The Zena and Michael A. Wiener Cardiovascular Institute, The Icahn School of Medicine at Mount Sinai, New York, New York

PRASHANT VAISHNAVA, MD
Department of Internal Medicine, Cardiovascular Center, University of Michigan Medical School, University of Michigan Health System, Ann Arbor, Michigan

KOMANDOOR SRINATHASAN, MD
Division of Cardiovascular Diseases, Mayo Clinic Hospital, Mayo Clinic Arizona, Phoenix, Arizona

KEITH M. SWETZ, MD, MA, FACP, FAAHPM
Section of Palliative Medicine, Division of General Internal Medicine, Department of Medicine; Associate Professor of Medicine, Program in Professionalism and Ethics, Mayo Clinic College of Medicine, Mayo Clinic, Rochester, Minnesota

MATTHEW I. TOMEY, MD
Chief Fellow, The Zena and Michael A. Wiener Cardiovascular Institute, The Icahn School of Medicine at Mount Sinai, New York, New York

PRASHANT VAISHNAVA, MD
Department of Internal Medicine, Cardiovascular Center, University of Michigan Medical School, University of Michigan Health System, Ann Arbor, Michigan

Contents

This article presents an overview of the evolution of cardiac critical care in the past half century. It tracks the rapid advances in the management of cardiovascular disease and how the intensive care area has kept pace, improving outcomes and incorporating successive innovations. The current multidisciplinary, evidence-based unit is vastly different from the early days and is expected to evolve further in keeping with the concept of "hybrid" care areas where care is delivered by the "heart team".

Acute aortic syndromes are among the most lethal of the cardiovascular diseases. Delays in recognition, diagnosis, and treatment are associated with increases in mortality. Signs and symptoms are sometimes subtle and atypical, and a high index of suspicion is useful to guide the diagnostic evaluation. Uncontrolled hypertension remains the most significant treatable risk factor. Immediate management involves blood pressure reduction. β-Blockers are the first drugs of choice. Although future directions should involve the evolution of operative and endovascular techniques and the development of sophisticated risk prediction tools, risk factor modification by addressing the burden of uncontrolled hypertension cannot be overlooked.

Massive pulmonary embolism (PE) is a potentially lethal condition, with death usually caused by right ventricular (RV) failure and cardiogenic shock. Systemic thrombolysis (unless contraindicated) is recommended as the first-line treatment of massive PE to decrease the thromboembolic burden on the RV and increase pulmonary perfusion. Surgical pulmonary embolectomy or catheter-directed thrombectomy should be considered in patients with contraindications to fibrinolysis, or those with persistent hemodynamic compromise or RV dysfunction despite fibrinolytic therapy. Critical care management predominantly involves supporting the RV, by optimizing preload, RV contractility, and coronary perfusion pressure and minimizing afterload. Despite these interventions, mortality remains high.

Acute myocardial infarction (AMI) can result in ischemic, mechanical, arrhythmic, embolic, or inflammatory complications. The development of mechanical complications following AMI is associated with a significantly reduced short-term and long-term survival. Since the introduction of primary percutaneous coronary intervention as the principal reperfusion strategy following acute ST-elevation myocardial infarction, the incidence of mechanical complications, including rupture of the left ventricular free wall, papillary muscle, and ventricular septum, has reduced significantly to less than 1%. Despite high operative mortality, the lack of an effective medical alternative makes surgical repair the mainstay of current management for these patients.

Novel Antiplatelet and Anticoagulant Agents in the Cardiac Care Unit   533

Vaani Panse Garg and Jonathan L. Halperin

This article reviews the pivotal studies of several novel antiplatelet (prasugrel and ticagrelor) and anticoagulant (dabigatran, rivaroxaban, and apixaban) agents. The clinical use of these drugs in cardiac intensive care is discussed, focusing on the management of acute coronary syndromes, ischemic stroke, atrial fibrillation, and venous thromboembolism.

The Pulmonary Artery Catheter: A Critical Reappraisal   545

Umesh K. Gidwani, Bibhu Mohanty, and Kanu Chatterjee

Balloon floatation pulmonary artery catheters (PACs) have been used for hemodynamic monitoring in cardiac, medical, and surgical intensive care units since the 1970s. With the availability of newer noninvasive diagnostic modalities, particularly echocardiography, the frequency of diagnostic pulmonary artery catheterization has declined. In this review, the evolution of PACs, the results of nonrandomized and randomized studies in various clinical conditions, the uses and abuses of bedside hemodynamic monitoring, and current indications for pulmonary artery catheterization are discussed.

Cardiogenic Shock   567

Howard A. Cooper and Julio A. Panza

Cardiogenic shock (CS) is a condition in which a marked reduction in cardiac output and inadequate end-organ perfusion results from an array of cardiac insults, the most common of which is acute myocardial infarction. CS is a systemic disease involving a vicious cycle of inflammation, ischemia, and progressive myocardial dysfunction, which often results in death. This life-threatening emergency requires intensive monitoring accompanied by aggressive hemodynamic support; other therapies are tailored to the specific pathophysiology. The development of novel therapeutic strategies is urgently required to reduce the unacceptably high mortality rates currently associated with CS.

Durable Mechanical Circulatory Support in Advanced Heart Failure: A Critical Care Cardiology Perspective   581

Anuradha Lala and Mandeep R. Mehra

Though cardiac transplantation for advanced heart disease patients remains definitive therapy for patients with advanced heart failure, it is challenged by inadequate donor supply, causing durable mechanical circulatory support (MCS) to slowly become a new primary standard. Selecting appropriate patients for MCS involves meeting a number of prespecifications as is required in evaluation for cardiac transplant candidacy. As technology evolves to bring forth more durable smaller devices, selection criteria for appropriate MCS recipients will likely expand to encompass a broader, less sick population. The "Holy Grail" for MCS will be a focus on clinical recovery and explantation of devices rather than the currently more narrowly defined indications of bridge to transplantation or lifetime device therapy.

The management of ventricular tachycardia and ventricular fibrillation in the cardiac intensive care unit can be complex. These arrhythmias have many triggers, including ischemia, sympathetic stimulation, and medication toxicities, as well as many different substrates, ranging from ischemic and nonischemic cardiomyopathies to rare genetic conditions such as Brugada syndrome and long QT syndrome. Different settings, such as congenital heart disease, postoperative ventricular arrhythmias, and ventricular assist devices, increase the complexity of management. This article reviews the variety of situations and cardiac conditions that give rise to ventricular arrhythmias, focusing on inpatient management strategies.

Transcatheter aortic valve replacement (TAVR) is a new therapy for severe aortic stenosis now available in the United States. Initial patients eligible for TAVR are defined by high operative risk, with advanced age and multiple comorbidities. Following TAVR, patients experience acute hemodynamic changes and several possible complications, including hypotension, vascular injury, anemia, stroke, new-onset atrial fibrillation, conduction disturbances and kidney injury, requiring an acute phase of intensive care. Alongside improvements in TAVR technology and technique, improvements in care after TAVR may contribute to improved outcomes. This review presents an approach to post-TAVR critical care and identifies directions for future research.

Patients admitted to the Cardiac Intensive Care Unit (CICU) are of increasing complexity and often require ventilatory support. A deep understanding of respiratory physiology and the interactions between the cardiovascular and respiratory systems is essential. Ventilatory support should be tailored to the specific patient condition, ensuring effective minute ventilation, reducing work of breathing and minimizing adverse hemodynamic effects. The weaning process can stress the cardiovascular system and cardiac failure is a common cause of failure to wean. Identification of patients likely to fail and prompt pre-emptive intervention is crucial for successful weaning and avoiding complications related to prolonged mechanical ventilation.

Mild therapeutic hypothermia (MTH) results in a significant decrease in mortality and improvement of neurologic outcomes in cardiac arrest (CA) survivors. Cardiologists and intensivists must be acquainted with the indications and technique because MTH is the only proven neuroprotective therapy for CA survivors. CA involves reinstituting meaningful cardiac activity and minimizing secondary neurologic injuries. This article focuses on MTH as the main strategy for post-CA care.

Medical advances over the past 50 years have helped countless patients with advanced cardiac disease or who are critically ill in the intensive care unit (ICU), but have added to the ethical complexity of the care provided by clinicians, particularly at the end of life. Palliative care has the primary aim of improving symptom burden, quality of life, and the congruence of the medical plan with a patient's goals of care. This article explores ethical issues encountered in the cardiac ICU, discusses key analyses of these issues, and addresses how palliative care might assist medical teams in approaching these challenges.

CARDIOLOGY CLINICS

FORTHCOMING ISSUES

February 2014
Heart Failure
Howard Eisen, *Editor*

May 2014
Pacemakers and ICDs
Theofanie Mela, *Editor*

August 2014
Coronary Artery Disease
David Shavelle, *Editor*

RECENT ISSUES

August 2013
**Catheter Interventions for
Structural Heart Disease**
Ray Matthews, *Editor*

May 2013
**Echocardiography in Diagnosis and
Management of Mitral Valve Disease**
Judy W. Hung and Timothy C. Tan, *Editors*

February 2013
Syncope
Robert Sheldon, *Editor*

ISSUES OF RELATED INTEREST

Interventional Cardiology Clinics, October 2013 (Vol. 2, No. 4)
Interventional Pharmacology
George D. Dangas *Editor*
Available at http://www.interventional.theclinics.com/

Heart Failure Clinics, October 2013 (Vol. 9, No. 4)
Atrial Fibrillation and Heart Failure
Andrew A. Grace, Sanjiv M. Narayan, and Mark D. O'Neill, *Editors*
Available at http://www.heartfailure.theclinics.com/

**DOWNLOAD
Free App!**

Review Articles
THE CLINICS

NOW AVAILABLE FOR YOUR iPhone and iPad

Preface

CARDIOLOGY CLINICS

Preface
Cardiovascular Intensive Care

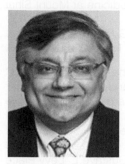

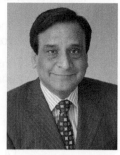

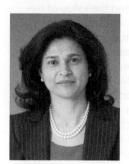

Umesh K. Gidwani,
MD, FCCP, FCCM

Samin K. Sharma, MD,
FSCAI, FACC

Annapoorna S. Kini,
MD, MRCP, FACC

Editors

This monograph on cardiac intensive care arrives six years after the last such endeavor in a sister publication, *Critical Care Clinics*. The timing is propitious; in the intervening period a lot has changed, and there is much new material to review.

The nomenclature, epidemiology, and philosophy of the critical care of cardiac patients have undergone a radical transformation. This accelerated evolution is reviewed in the article that opens this issue. The interventional management of structural heart disease has undergone an even more abbreviated growth phase and learning curve. What only five years ago was undergoing trials has now become widespread practice not only in tertiary university centers but also in regional community hospitals. Our protocols for the CICU management of transcatheter aortic valve replacement (TAVR) patients are reviewed herein. Similarly, as we become more successful in reducing mortality from acute myocardial infarction, we see a growing population of patients living with a significant heart failure burden. While the number of patients with heart transplants has not increased dramatically, the number of patients on mechanical circulatory support has. A state-of-the-art review of the management of heart failure, including circulatory support devices, is presented here. Similar advances in the management of cardiogenic shock ventricular arrhythmias, and hypertensive and acute aortic syndromes are reported comprehensively. The past decade has seen a proliferation of new oral antiplatelet and anticoagulant agents. Even as we continually refine indications for these agents and characterize their behavior, their development continues apace. We not only focus on such newfangled advances but also review the old enemies that continue to bedevil our ICUs such as pulmonary embolism and respiratory failure requiring mechanical ventilation. These topics as well as an update on mechanical complications of acute myocardial infarction are addressed by our British colleagues.

It is a personal honor to serve as a coauthor with Dr Kanu Chatterjee in our review of the pulmonary artery catheter (PAC) and its place in the modern firmament. Dr Chatterjee is a legend who was "present at the creation" around the development of PACs and who was recruited by Dr Swan in 1971, a few short months after having described his first-generation PAC in the *New England Journal of Medicine*. Dr Chatterjee arrived from England to run the Myocardial Infarction Research Unit at the Cedars-Sinai Hospital and to improve and modify the PAC. The PAC has described a trajectory of unbridled overutilization followed by the inevitable backlash and its near-extinction. It seems to have settled into its niche in cardiac and transplantation critical care, which now serve as the repository of knowledge about and expertise with the PAC.

Cardiol Clin 31 (2013) xiii–xiv
http://dx.doi.org/10.1016/j.ccl.2013.09.001
0733-8651/13/$ – see front matter © 2013 Elsevier Inc. All rights reserved.

Five decades after Dr Peter Safar presciently recommended in 1964 that "hypothermia should be started within 30 minutes if there is no sign of CNS recovery" after CPR, the first two randomized controlled trials in 2002 confirmed the value of hypothermia for neuroprotection after resuscitation for cardiac arrest. Dr Safar wrote the accompanying editorial comment on these landmark trials. A review of this topic is presented by our Cleveland Clinic colleagues. Finally, the Mayo team reviews the treacherous landscape of advanced heart failure and palliative approaches to the worsening symptoms and the myriad technologies used to support such patients as they approach the end of life. These ethical quandaries will surely multiply as will the number of patients and complexity of interventions with advanced heart failure.

The goal of this monograph was never intended to be comprehensive. In fact, the subspecialty has developed so vastly that it would be impossible to discuss all but a few brief topics. We hope that our selection of topics spans the most relevant of these areas and begins to unravel the complexity of modern cardiovascular intensive care. We would like to thank the accomplished authors for this contemporary overview of a rapidly evolving area. We would also like to thank Barbara Cohen-Kligerman and Elsevier for their support of this work and Dr Valentin Fuster and Dr Jagat Narula for their encouragement and inspiration.

Umesh K. Gidwani, MD, FCCP, FCCM
The Zena and Michael A. Weiner
Cardiovascular Institute
Mount Sinai Hospital
Icahn School of Medicine at Mount Sinai
Box 1030
One Gustave L. Levy Place
New York, NY 10029-6754, USA

Samin K. Sharma, MD, FSCAI, FACC
The Zena and Michael A. Weiner
Cardiovascular Institute
Mount Sinai Hospital
Icahn School of Medicine at Mount Sinai
Box 1030
One Gustave L. Levy Place
New York, NY 10029-6754, USA

Annapoorna S. Kini, MD, MRCP, FACC
The Zena and Michael A. Weiner
Cardiovascular Institute
Mount Sinai Hospital
Icahn School of Medicine at Mount Sinai
Box 1030
One Gustave L. Levy Place
New York, NY 10029-6574, USA

E-mail addresses:
Umesh.Gidwani@mountsinai.org (U.K. Gidwani)
Samin.Sharma@mountsinai.org (S.K. Sharma)
Annapoorna.Kini@mountsinai.org (A.S. Kini)

From the Coronary Care Unit to the Cardiovascular Intensive Care Unit
The Evolution of Cardiac Critical Care

Umesh K. Gidwani, MD, FCCP, FCCM*,
Annapoorna S. Kini, MD, MRCP

KEYWORDS

- Cardiac critical care • Cardiovascular intensive care • Multidisciplinary heart care

KEY POINTS

- In the 1960s, patients with acute myocardial infarction were sent to the coronary care unit primarily for close monitoring and management of arrhythmias.
- Contemporary cardiovascular intensive care units have adopted the evidence based and multidisciplinary care principles that were the hallmark of general ICUs and had lead to improvements in patient safety and outcomes.
- Modern cardiac critical care will surely evolve as the concept of 'hybrid' cardiac care areas where care is delivered by the 'heart team' becomes standard, and will present opportunities for new areas of research and further improvement in patient outcomes.

The Times They Are a-Changin'
— Bob Dylan, 1963

THE EARLY YEARS

Around the time that Bob Dylan penned this song, Hughes Day published a paper "Preliminary Studies of an Acute Coronary Care Area" in the Lancet[1] in February 1963. This article described his experience with 17 acute myocardial infarction (AMI) patients admitted to the first area specifically designed to treat patients with AMI at Bethany Hospital in Kansas City, Kansas. In May 1962, Day had established a monitored area that contained 4 private rooms adjacent to the intensive care unit (ICU). The concept was similar to what was described by Wilburne in an abstract[2] published in the United States in 1961, simultaneous with the publication of Julian's article[3] in the United Kingdom. Both had realized at about the same time that post-AMI ventricular arrhythmias carried significant mortality and that with continuous monitoring in a unit equipped with monitors with alarms, supervision by trained personnel, and the availability of a defibrillator ("AC 440 V or more!")[4] and other appropriate equipment and medications, it was possible to reduce mortality by initiating prompt cardiopulmonary resuscitation (CPR). Such a rapid diffusion of technology was replicated in the 1970s with the enthusiastic adoption of Swan-Ganz catheterization, which originated at the same institution where Wilburne practiced, Cedars of Lebanon Hospital.

Besides improving survival, the coronary care unit (CCU) concept served to fundamentally change how inpatient medicine was practiced in the United States. Up to that point, American

The Zena and Michael A. Wiener Cardiovascular Institute, The Icahn School of Medicine at Mount Sinai, One Gustave L. Levy Place, New York, NY 10029, USA
* Corresponding author. One Gustave L. Levy Place, Box 1030, New York, NY 10029.
E-mail address: umesh.gidwani@mountsinai.org

Cardiol Clin 31 (2013) 485–492
http://dx.doi.org/10.1016/j.ccl.2013.07.012
0733-8651/13/$ – see front matter © 2013 Elsevier Inc. All rights reserved.

medicine had established a strict hierarchy, where the doctor dealt with all events and emergencies, outpatient or inpatient, issuing orders for the nurse to follow. However, in the case of life-threatening arrhythmias, like those complicating AMI, there was no time to track down the attending doctor for medical orders. Nurses were empowered to initiate treatment, such as defibrillation and CPR, without waiting for the doctor to enter the unit.

This growth in the CCU model was championed by Corday, also from Cedars of Lebanon Hospital, when he became president of American College of Cardiology in 1965. He helped push legislation in Congress that funded the growth of CCUs as a way to advance care of patients with heart disease.[5] Corday had heard Day speak in Los Angeles in 1962 and became convinced that this was an effective way of reducing mortality in AMI. By 1966 there were more than 200 CCUs in operation in United States. In 1967, Lown published his work, in which he described how he moved myocardial infarction (MI) care from reactive care (defibrillation and CPR) to the prevention and treatment of arrhythmias in his CCU.[6]

THE MIDDLE AGES

Of course, times kept on changing, and before long there were new, more definitive therapies for myocardial ischemia. As early as 1933, the fibrinolytic activity of hemolytic streptococci had been known,[7] and streptokinase had been used for thrombolysis previously. However, it was not until the publication of the first Gruppo Italiano per lo Studio della Sopravvivenza nell'Infarto Miocardico study in 1986 that thrombolysis became standard for the management of AMI.[8] In 1993, the Global Utilization of Streptokinase and t-PA for Occluded Coronary Arteries investigators showed that an accelerated tissue plasminogen activator (tPA) protocol was superior to standard thrombolytic regimens.[9] A quickening of the pulse was palpable; "time is muscle" was the mantra, and "door-to-needle time" entered the lexicon. There were public health programs educating patients to report to the nearest emergency room heralding symptoms of myocardial ischemia. While more people were identified and treated earlier, they were managed in the CCU prior to as well as after coronary angiography.

Even before the concept of the CCU was described, Sones, a pediatrician who was experimenting with catheter techniques, inadvertently injected the coronary artery and performed the first reported cine coronary arteriography in 1959.[10]

Dotter and Judkins published their report of transluminal angioplasty of the superficial femoral artery (SFA) in 1964.[11] They were able to dilate the SFA by threading successive coaxial catheters into a stenosed SFA. Gruentzig[12] modified the Dotter catheter by adding a balloon at the tip and successfully dilated the iliac artery in 1975. In 1977, he performed the first coronary balloon angioplasty on a severe proximal left anterior descending artery (LAD) stenosis of a 38-year-old insurance salesman in Zurich with a positive stress test. Around this time, US surgeons were opposed to this technology, and in Europe, the management of peripheral vascular disease was the domain of the nonsurgeons. Consequently, catheter techniques were researched and advanced by nonsurgeons, primarily radiologists and cardiologists.[13]

With the increasing utilization of balloon angioplasty, the high rates of abrupt vessel closure and restenosis became apparent. This led to the development of catheter-delivered stents and administration of dual antiplatelet therapy. In the 19th century, an English dentist, Charles Stent, developed a mold to make an impression of the teeth and gums.[14] Thus it came to pass that his name became associated with a device that provided a support for tubular structures and now with the endovascular scaffolding that prevents stenoses. Alexis Carrell, a French surgeon who pioneered vascular suturing techniques, first showed that stenting of a canine aorta with a glass tube did not necessarily lead to thrombosis. Carrell received the Nobel Prize in Medicine for his work in 1912. Dotter built on his previous work and experimented with metal springs/coils to maintain the patency of the vessels that he had succeeded in opening and in 1983 reported on transluminal placement of expandable nitinol coil stents.[15] In 1987, Sigwart and Puel reported on the results of implantation of 24 stents in 19 patients for the management of restenosis, acute closure, and venous bypass grafts.[16] With this, the era of interventional cardiology had arrived, and the further development of future generations of stents continued apace.

In 1997, the GUSTO investigators reported that primary angioplasty provided superior outcomes when compared with thrombolysis for ST elevation MIs (STEMIs).[9] However short-, medium-, and long-term closure and restenosis remained significant problems. By 2003, Andersen and colleagues[17] reported that primary angioplasty with stenting was superior to fibrinolysis in acute STEMIs, especially when delivered within 2 hours. The era of "door-to-balloon time" had arrived. The management of AMI evolved into a hub and spoke type of public health delivery, where patients with a STEMI were transported to the local percutaneous coronary intervention (PCI)-capable hospital, preferably within 90 minutes of onset of symptoms. CCUs at these PCI-capable hospitals saw more STEMIs and comorbidities and complications that came with the sicker STEMI patients. The heat was being turned up, with catheter laboratory teams that could respond within minutes and high-acuity patients transferred to the CCU at all hours of the day and night.

THE CONTEMPORARY CICU

The hectic pace of innovation radically changed the function and acuity of the CCU. It had evolved from managing AMIs with monitoring and defibrillation/CPR in the event of ventricular tachycardia (VT)/ventricular fibrillation (VF) to actively managing relatively acute and unstable patients with active hemodynamic, cardiovascular, and respiratory complications. In the first 30 or so years, remarkable improvements in survival were noted, as close monitoring and early resuscitation became ubiquitous. Killip reported that the mortality in MI in his CCU decreased from 26% to 7% over a 2-year period from January 1965 to 1967.[18] Patients were no longer dying from sudden arrhythmias but from pump failure. However, the low hanging fruit had been picked. In their remarkable review of the changing epidemiology in their CCU[19] over a 17-year period from 1989 to 2006, Katz and colleagues were unable to replicate this reduction in mortality. At the same time that rapid advancements in technology were leading to a decrease in AMI mortality, the burden of patients with ischemic cardiomyopathy and advanced heart failure was increasing. This was reflected in the increase in such patients in their CCU. To manage these patients, improved therapies, both pharmacologic as well as mechanical circulatory support, were being increasingly utilized. These patients were older and sicker and had many more comorbid medical conditions requiring a broader knowledge and experience base and a wider therapeutic armamentarium. This was clearly shown in Katz's study of the changing trends in pathophysiology of CCU patients. He documented a pattern of increasing patient complexity, evolving critical illness, and accelerated resource utilization. Over the 17-year period, he noted a significant decrease in patients with STEMI, and a significant increase in patients with non-STEMI (NSTEMI) and cardiogenic shock. There was a significant increase in the number of patients with pneumonia, sepsis and septic shock, acute and chronic

kidney failure, acute and chronic respiratory failure, and prolonged ventilation. More invasive procedures such as central venous catheterization, gastrointestinal endoscopy, bronchoscopy, and renal replacement therapies were performed. Interestingly, despite the increased case mix and Charlson comorbidity indices, there was no significant increase in CCU length of stay or unadjusted in-hospital and CCU mortality. This was attributed to a better understanding and prophylaxis of potential complications of ongoing critical care.

Practitioners at Mount Sinai have noted a similar increase in severity of illness in the CCU. Most PCI patients today are discharged the same day, and those who are admitted go to a step-down monitored unit. Increasingly the CCU of today is becoming more like a general ICU with a focus on cardiac patients. **Table 1** highlights this severity and complexity in 1370 admissions in 2012.

The coronary care units of the 1970s have evolved into the cardiovascular ICUs (CICUs) of the 21st century and this evolution will certainly continue. As the modern CICU develops, it must follow the trends that have been evolving in the more organized general critical care realm. The principles of the approach to intensive care are evidence-based and can be examined in the context of 3 domains, which will be discussed in the next sections.

Table 1
The distribution of 1370 consecutive admissions to Mount Sinai CCU, from Jan. 1, 2012 to Dec. 1, 2012

Primary Reason	Number of Patients
PCI	624
Structural interventions	167
EP interventions	220
Heart failure	
Acute heart failure	133
Cardiogenic shock	30
LVAD	6
Peripheral vascular interventions	11
Carotid artery interventions	15
Other	
Hypothermia for cardiac arrest	11
Miscellaneous (sepsis, gastrointestinal bleed, and others)	153
Total	1370

Quality, Safety, and Resource Utilization

The modern patient safety movement began with the Harvard Medical Practice Study (MPS), which was published in 1991 and found that 3.7% of hospitalized patients suffered an adverse event, of which 69% were preventable, and 14% were fatal.[20] Although this study also ran as a front-page article in the New York Times, it was essentially ignored. Only in 1996 did the American Medical Association (AMA) join the Joint Commission on the Accreditation of Healthcare Organizations (JCAHO), the American Academy of Arts and Sciences, and the Annenberg Foundation to host the first ever conference on medical errors in California.[21] The patient safety movement gathered further steam after the 1999 Institute of Medicine report "To Err is Human," which estimated that medical errors were the cause of up to 98,000 preventable deaths per year.[22] The focus also shifted from a culture of blame to a problem of defective processes and systems. Since then, various agencies have established organizations focused on increasing patient safety and improving the quality of care. Some of these agencies are the Centers for Medicare and Medicaid Services (CMS), the National Quality Forum (NQF), JCAHO, the Agency for Healthcare Research and Quality (AHRQ), the AMA, through its National Patient Safety Foundation, and the Institute for Healthcare Improvement (IHI). The Society of Critical Care Medicine (SCCM) collaborates with most of these organizations to promote evidence-based care in the ICU. The SCCM also collaborates with the National Institutes of Health's (NIH) United States Critical Illness and Injury Trial (USCIIT) Group, to study organizational structure, processes of care, use of protocols, and outcomes in ICUs and determine which of these structures and processes of care and other factors might be associated with patient outcomes.[23] To date, more than 200 USCIIT Group investigators have enrolled more than 10,000 patients from more than 30 academic and community hospitals in studies during the last 3 years.[24]

The modern CICU must be cognizant of and incorporate these structures and processes into daily work flow. These processes will be discussed briefly.

The Centers for Disease Control and Prevention (CDC), The Joint Commission (TJC), the IHI, and several state departments of health all have rigorous protocols for the prevention and monitoring of central line-associated blood stream infections (CLABSIs). Similar protocols and requirements exist for the prevention of catheter-associated urinary tract infections (CAUTIs), *Clostridium difficile*-associated diarrhea (CDAD), ventilator-associated pneumonia (VAP), and coronary artery bypass grafting (CABG) surgical site infections.

The IHI promotes comprehensive protocols such as the ventilator bundle, central line bundle, and methicillin-resistant Staphylococcus aureus (MRSA) prevention and best practices to reduce patient harm from sedation, immobility, and delirium. All of these are germane to the practice of modern cardiac critical care.

TJC and the CMS collaborate to monitor core measure sets that standardize the use of evidence-based interventions to maximize patient safety and outcomes. Some of the core measure sets relevant to cardiac critical care include

1. Venous thromboembolism
2. Heart failure
3. Surgical care improvement project
4. Tobacco treatment
5. Pneumonia and influenza vaccination
6. Acute Myocardial Infarction
7. Stroke

On its Web site www.medicare.gov/hospital compare, CMS posts various data points relating to care delivered to its Medicare recipients. Some of these are

1. Hospital Consumer Assessment of Health Care Providers and Systems (HCAHPS), which collects patient feedback on 10 important hospital quality topics in recently discharged hospitalized Medicare patients
2. Measures of timely care such as for heart attack, heart failure, pneumonia, and surgical management
3. 30-day mortality and readmission rates
4. Medicare payment

The CMS also has the authority to deny payment to hospitals for hospital-acquired conditions (HACs, also known as "not present on admission"), which obviously has implications for resource management for the hospital and its ICUs. For 2013, there are 14 HACs for which CMS can deny payment (http://www.cms.gov/Medicare/ Medicare-Fee-for-Service-Payment/ HospitalAcqCond/Downloads/ FY_2013_ Final_ HACsCodeList.pdf). Those relevant to cardiac critical care are

1. Foreign object retained after surgery
2. Air embolism
3. Blood incompatibility
4. Stage 3 and 4 pressure ulcers
5. Falls and trauma

6. Manifestations of poor glycemic control
7. Catheter-associated urinary tract infection
8. Central line-associated blood stream infection
9. Deep vein thrombosis/pulmonary embolism
10. Iatrogenic pneumothorax
11. Surgical site infection and mediastinitis following CABG
12. Surgical site infection following implantable cardiac electronic device

THE MULTIDISCIPLINARY APPROACH TO INCREASINGLY COMPLEX PATIENTS

The first steps toward multidisciplinary care were taken in the earliest CCUs with the empowerment of specially trained nurses to initiate emergency protocols for medical care. As complexity has increased and CCUs have come to resemble general ICUs, the importance of multidisciplinary care has become evident. The increasing complexity of pharmacotherapy and attention to adverse drug events and drug–drug interactions mean that pharmacists must become an integral part of the multidisciplinary critical care team.[25] Similarly, the focus on maintaining optimal nutritional status, specific blood glucose targets, and the use of complex nutritional products make dieticians a valuable part of the team as well.[26] Respiratory therapists who ensure daily sedation interruption and daily evaluation for early liberation from mechanical ventilation and the emerging evidence for early mobilization and rehabilitation make the role of physical therapists critical to the multidisciplinary team.[27,28] Social workers contribute to ensuring that the patient's and family's social situations are assessed and social needs met, to promote early and appropriate progression through the next continuum of care and decrease length of stay.[29]

Human Resource Management

Special skills

While the early CCUs essentially required personnel to be trained for rhythm monitoring, defibrillation and initiation of CPR, the skill sets required today are significantly more complex. The modern CICU should be staffed by people who are comfortable and trained to manage

- Respiratory support devices such as invasive and noninvasive positive pressure ventilation
- Insertion of central venous and pulmonary artery catheters, intra-arterial lines, and devices
- Cardiac support with percutaneous devices (eg, Intra-Aortic Balloon Pump, Impella, Tandem Heart) and implanted devices (LVADs, Syncardia Total Artificial Heart)

- Cardiopulmonary support with extracorporeal membrane oxygenation (ECMO), Cardiohealth, Centrimag
- Neurologic support, including sedation monitoring and interruption, delirium management, hypothermia devices, and continuous electroencephalogram (EEG) monitors
- Renal support with various hemodialysis and ultrafiltration protocols
- Multiple vasoactive, sedative–hypnotic and paralytic agents delivered by intravenous drip
- Bedside imaging with vascular ultrasound and transthoracic and transesophageal echocardiography

Similarly, skill and staffing levels should be sufficient to competently manage patients who have undergone complex PCI, complex electrophysiology, and structural heart interventions or are in various shock states.

Personnel skill should also extend to a competent understanding of palliative and end-of-life issues, as many of these patients have complex and advanced multiorgan illnesses.[30] Familiarity with standardized approaches such as the Improving Palliative Care in the ICU tools and specific CICU issues such as deactivation of implantable cardioverter-defibrillator (ICDs) and LVADs is essential.[31]

Finally, CICU professionals must realize that research in this growing subspecialty is integral to promoting both patient outcomes and the body of knowledge. The interested reader is referred to a "call to action" article by van Diepen and colleagues,[32] in which areas of, and solutions to CICU research are identified (**Table 2**).

Staffing requirements

The preceding paragraphs lay out a landscape that demands patient management by an experienced multidisciplinary team led by a clinician who has significant training or experience in both intensive care and cardiovascular medicine. This marriage of skills is unlikely to be present in a person who is not practicing such medicine for the majority of his or her time and is not based in the CICU. Morrow and colleagues[33] address this issue in great detail in an AHA scientific statement. How one trains such physicians has moved beyond the debate stage; at least 1 large academic center in New York is adding an additional year to enable either a cardiology or critical care fellowship trained physician to seek further training and expertise (V. Kvetan, MD, personal communication, 2013) in this area.

The Leapfrog Group, a group of large purchasers of health care services, seeks to promote

Table 2 Urgent areas for cardiac critical care research	
Shock in the Cardiac Patient	• Defining the best fluid and vasoactive pharmacologic management strategies in cardiogenic shock • Managing septic shock and inflammatory response syndromes in patients with heart failure
Cardio-renal Syndrome	• Timing preventive and therapeutic interventions for cardio-renal syndromes
Cardiac Arrest Care	• Improving systems of care and identifying therapies beyond hypothermia that can improve postcardiac arrest neurologic outcomes and survival
Delivery of Care	• Evaluating whether institutional or physician volumes and regionally centralized care affect the outcomes of critically ill cardiac patients • Evaluating whether electronic medical record systems and clinical decision support systems can reduce errors and improve safety • Examining the role of cardiology and intensive care cross-training
Measurement	• Establishing standardized definitions, processes of care, and outcome measures for patients with advanced cardiac disease and critical illness through registry platforms and databases
Palliative Care	• Enhancing support of patients and families to ensure optimal decision making about end-of-life care, including admiration, withholding or withdrawal of advanced cardiac and other critical care technologies, and integrating palliative care into both the in-patient and out-patient settings
Training	• Cross-fertilizing in clinical practice and clinical research for cardiology and critical care trainees

From van Diepen Cook DJ, Jacka M, Granger CB. Critical care cardiology research: a call to action. Circ Cardiovasc Qual Outcomes 2013;6(2):238; with permission.

high-value health care through its purchasing power and has recommendations on ICU physician staffing as one of its initiatives. The Leapfrog Group's benchmark is that the ICU be managed or comanaged by intensivists who are present during clinical hours and provide clinical care exclusively in the ICU, and when not present be available at least 95% of the time within 5 minutes. Given the well-recognized shortage of dedicated intensivists, this is an unrealistic goal for all CICUs to meet in the short term.[34] In the authors' experience, collaboration between an intensivist and a cardiologist to serve as physician leadership of the CICU makes sense as the CICU becomes populated by patients with increasingly complex cardiovascular and multiorgan illness. The authors' CICU is best described as a transitional unit, in which 1 of 4 subspecialty (interventional, EP, heart failure/transplant, or cardiac intensivist) physicians is the primary attending for the CICU patients, and a cardiac intensivist is present. Morrow's article discusses in detail both the physician staffing paradigms as well as a proposal for categorization of CICUs. Finally given the duty hour regulations and increasing primary care focus of house staff training programs, the presence of

physician extenders in ICUs is growing and is a welcome trend.

SUMMARY

There has been a remarkable transformation of cardiac intensive care. Gone are the days when patients suffering from AMI were sent to the CCU primarily for close monitoring. The incredible progress made in patient care in the past 50 years has dramatically changed the landscape. The CICU patient of the modern era is admitted for a wide variety of reasons, ranging from well-defined pathologies such as decompensated heart failure, AMI or ventricular arrhythmias, to newer indications such as complications from modern percutaneous procedures, therapeutic hypothermia for neuroprotection after cardiac arrest, or the advanced management of cardiogenic shock. Cardiovascular pathologies are now seen as a part of a spectrum of illness, including all other comorbidities from which the patient suffers. This has put new demands on health care delivery, resource utilization, clinician training, and physician staffing in the CICU. Clearly this trend toward increasing complexity, and subspecialty expertise with emerging technologies will continue. Clinicians should be prepared to address the issues that will arise.

REFERENCES

1. Day HW. Preliminary studies of an acute coronary care area. J Lancet 1963;83:53–5.

2. Wilburne M. Coronary care unit: new approach to treatment of acute coronary occlusion [abstract]. Circulation 1961;24:1071.

3. Julian D. Treatment of cardiac arrest in acute myocardial ischemia and infarction. Lancet 1961;2: 840–4.

4. Wilburne M, Fields J. Cardiac resuscitation in coronary artery disease: a central coronary care unit. JAMA 1963;184(6):453–7.

5. Fye WB. Resuscitating a circulation abstract to celebrate the 50th anniversary of the coronary care unit concept. Circulation 2011;124(17):1886–93.

6. Lown B, Fakhro AM, Hood WB Jr, et al. The coronary care unit: new perspectives and directions. JAMA 1967;199(3):188–98.

7. Tillett WS, Garner RL. The fibrinolytic activity of hemolytic streptococci. J Exp Med 1933;58(4): 485–502.

8. Effectiveness of intravenous thrombolytic treatment in acute myocardial infarction. Gruppo Italiano per lo Studio della Streptochinasi nell'Infarto Miocardico (GISSI). Lancet 1986;1(8478):397–402.

9. The GUSTO Investigators. An international randomized trial comparing four thrombolytic strategies for acute myocardial infarction. N Engl J Med 1993; 329(10):673–82.

10. Sones FM Jr, Shirey EK, Proudfit WL, et al. Cine coronary arteriography [abstract]. Circulation 1959;20:773.

11. Dotter CT, Judkins MP. Transluminal treatment of arteriosclerotic obstruction: description of a new technic and a preliminary report of its application. Circulation 1964;30(5):654–70.

12. Gruentzig A, Myler R, Hanna R, et al. Coronary transluminal angioplasty [abstract]. Circulation 1977;56:84.

13. King SB. Angioplasty from bench to bedside to bench. Circulation 1996;93(9):1621–9.

14. Ruygrok PN, Serruys PW. Intracoronary stenting: from concept to custom. Circulation 1996;94(5):882–90.

15. Dotter CT, Buschmann RW, McKinney MK, et al. Transluminal expandable nitinol coil stent grafting: preliminary report. Radiology 1983;147(1):259–60.

16. Sigwart U, Puel J, Mirkovitch V, et al. Intravascular stents to prevent occlusion and restenosis after transluminal angioplasty. N Engl J Med 1987; 316(12):701–6.

17. Andersen HR, Nielsen TT, Rasmussen K, et al. A comparison of coronary angioplasty with fibrinolytic therapy in acute myocardial infarction. N Engl J Med 2003;349(8):733–42.

18. Killip T, Kimball JT. Treatment of myocardial infarction in a coronary care unit: a two year experience with 250 patients. Am J Cardiol 1967;20(4): 457–64.

19. Katz JN, Shah BR, Volz EM, et al. Evolution of the coronary care unit: clinical characteristics and temporal trends in healthcare delivery and outcomes. Crit Care Med 2010;38(2):375–81.

20. Brennan TA, Leape LL, Laird NM, et al. Incidence of adverse events and negligence in hospitalized patients. N Engl J Med 1991;324(6):370–6.

21. Leape LL. Scope of problem and history of patient safety. Obstet Gynecol Clin North Am 2008;35(1): 1–10.

22. Kohn LT, Corrigan JM, Donaldson MS, editors. To err is human: building a safer health system. Washington, DC: National Academy Press; 1999.

23. Cobb JP, Cairns CB, Bulger E, et al. The United States critical illness and injury trials group: an introduction. J Trauma 2009;67(Suppl 2):S159–60.

24. Blum JM, Morris PE, Martin GS, et al. United states critical illness and injury trials group. Chest 2013; 143(3):808–13.

25. Horn E, Jacobi J. The critical care clinical pharmacist: evolution of an essential team member. Crit Care Med 2006;34(3):S46–51.

26. Roberts SR, Kennerly DA, Keane D, et al. Nutrition support in the intensive care: unit adequacy, timeliness, and outcomes. Crit Care Nurse 2003;23(6): 49–57.

27. Morris PE, Goad A, Thompson C, et al. Early intensive care unit mobility therapy in the treatment of acute respiratory failure. Crit Care Med 2008;36(8): 2238–43.

28. Truong AD. Bench-to-bedside review: mobilizing patients in the intensive care unit—from pathophysiology to clinical trials. Crit Care 2009; 13(4):216.

29. Carr DD. Building collaborative partnerships in critical care: the RN case manager/social work dyad in critical care. Prof Case Manag 2009; 14(3):121–32 [quiz: 133–4].

30. Penrod JD, Pronovost PJ, Livote EE, et al. Meeting standards of high-quality intensive care unit palliative care: clinical performance and predictors. Crit Care Med 2012;40(4):1105–12.

31. Allen LA, Stevenson LW, Grady KL, et al. Decision making in advanced heart failure: a scientific statement from the American Heart Association. Circulation 2012;125(15):1928–52.

32. van Diepen S, Cook DJ, Jacka M, et al. Critical care cardiology research: a call to action. Circ Cardiovasc Qual Outcomes 2013;6(2):237–42.

33. Morrow DA, Fang JC, Fintel DJ, et al. Evolution of critical care cardiology: transformation of the

cardiovascular intensive care unit and the emerging need for new medical staffing and training models: a scientific statement from the American Heart Association. Circulation 2012;126(11):1408–28.

34. Angus DC, Shorr AF, White A, et al. Critical care delivery in the United States: distribution of services and compliance with Leapfrog recommendations. Crit Care Med 2006;34(4):1016–24.

Hypertensive and Acute Aortic Syndromes

Jack Z. Li, MD, MBA[a], Kim A. Eagle, MD, MACC[b],
Prashant Vaishnava, MD[b],*

KEYWORDS

- Management and treatment of acute aortic syndromes • Type A aortic dissection
- Type B aortic dissection

KEY POINTS

- Delays in recognition, diagnosis, and treatment of acute aortic syndromes are associated with unacceptable increases in mortality.
- Signs and symptoms are sometimes subtle and atypical, and a high index of clinical suspicion is useful to guide the diagnostic evaluation.
- Uncontrolled hypertension is the most significant treatable risk factor for acute aortic syndrome.
- Immediate management involves blood pressure reduction; β-blockers are the first drugs of choice.
- Multidisciplinary evaluation should be a common thread in the management of both type A aortic dissection (TAAD) and type B aortic dissection (TBAD), with early surgical consultation. TAAD is managed surgically, whereas patients with uncomplicated TBAD should be treated with medical therapy.
- Operative techniques in the management of TAAD include selective cerebral perfusion, aortic valve–sparing procedures, and thoracic endovascular repair (TEVAR) as part of a complex hybrid procedure when there is involvement of the descending aorta.
- When feasible, TEVAR is considered the first-line treatment of complicated TBAD.

INTRODUCTION

Acute aortic syndromes are preventable but life-threatening conditions with particularly high case-fatality rates, despite evolving treatment guidelines. Management of these conditions relies on accurate diagnosis and prompt, evidence-based decision making. Acute aortic dissection (AAD) can be further subdivided into 2 types per the Stanford classification[1]: type A aortic dissection (TAAD) involves the ascending aorta with or without the descending aorta including the aortic root up to the proximal brachiocephalic artery, whereas type B aortic dissection (TBAD) involves only the descending aorta. Pathophysiology of a dissection involves the separation of the tunica intima from the tunica media with subsequent penetration of blood. The incidence of AAD is estimated at 16.3 per 100,000 people/y in men and 9.1 per 100,000 people/y in women.[2] In-hospital mortality of patients with type A dissection receiving surgical or medical therapy is estimated at 26.6% and 55.9% respectively.[3] Type B dissection carries less overall in-hospital mortality risk at 13% compared with TAAD, but is nonetheless associated with significant morbidity.

Disclosures: The authors have nothing to disclose.
[a] Department of Internal Medicine, University of Michigan Medical School, University of Michigan Health System, 1500 E. Medical Center Drive, Ann Arbor, MI 48109, USA; [b] Department of Internal Medicine, Cardiovascular Center, University of Michigan Medical School, University of Michigan Health System, 1500 E. Medical Center Drive, Ann Arbor, MI 48109, USA
* Corresponding author.
E-mail address: pvaishna@umich.edu

Cardiol Clin 31 (2013) 493–501
http://dx.doi.org/10.1016/j.ccl.2013.07.011
0733-8651/13/$ – see front matter © 2013 Elsevier Inc. All rights reserved.

The diagnosis of AAD may require a high index of clinical suspicion, because the presenting signs and symptoms may be subtle and atypical. Nonetheless, early diagnosis is critical to potentially avert incremental morbidity and mortality. Immediate and initial management of both TAAD and TBAD is directed at the reduction of aortic wall stress through lowering of both heart rate and blood pressure. Management of TAAD requires immediate surgical treatment; patients with uncomplicated TBAD are best treated medically. This article reviews the initial evaluation of, and pharmacologic management for, AAD. Options and indications for surgical and endovascular interventions for both TAAD and complicated TBAD are discussed.

INITIAL EVALUATION: RISK FACTORS, CLINICAL PRESENTATION, AND DIAGNOSIS

Diagnosis of AAD is paramount in the early stages of evaluation because mortality is correlated with symptom onset, and each hour of symptom presentation is associated with a 1% to 2% increase in risk of mortality in TAAD.[4] Risk factors for acute aortic syndrome include conditions that increase stress on the aortic wall, such as chronic uncontrolled hypertension, blunt trauma, pheochromocytoma, cocaine or other stimulant use, and deceleration or torsional injury.[1,3,5] Connective tissue disorders like Marfan syndrome, Ehlers-Danlos syndrome type IV (vascular form), and Loeys-Dietz syndrome may result in aortopathic changes, weakening the aortic wall and rendering it susceptible to aortic dissection.[6,7] Congenital bicuspid aortic valve morphology and pregnancy are additional predisposing factors that should not be overlooked.

In the first prospective population-based study of acute aortic disease, Howard and colleagues[8] recently showed that uncontrolled hypertension was the most significant treatable risk factor for AAD in a population of nearly 100,000 individuals participating in the Oxford Vascular Study (OXVASC). Premorbid control of blood pressure was often poor even though 67.3% of patients were prescribed antihypertensive medications. Review of primary care records in this analysis showed that nearly half of all patients had at least one systolic blood pressure reading greater than or equal to 180 mm Hg in the 5 years preceding their acute aortic event. Findings from OXVASC are a confirmation of the robust association between hypertension and AAD and are a call to action to better manage this treatable risk factor.

The diagnosis of AAD may be challenging to make because of the diverse and sometimes subtle symptoms with which patients may present and the overlap between signs and symptoms of acute aortic syndromes and those of other disorders like acute myocardial infarction. Nonetheless, sudden onset of severe chest pain that radiates to the neck or jaw in ascending dissection, and to the back in descending dissection, are classic presentations. Atypical symptoms such as neurologic deficits or cramping abdominal pain are also observed.[9] Symptoms of heart failure may be secondary to aortic valve regurgitation (generally from aortic leaflet prolapse or distortion of leaflet alignment by the dissection flap) or dilation of the aortic root. Patients may also present with tamponade, myocardial infarction, or shock. In addition, patients may experience hoarseness, stridor, dyspnea, or dysphagia caused by compression from an expanding aorta. End-organ effects such as embolization of atherosclerotic debris into the kidneys or distal extremities may be seen. Hypertension may or may not be seen with AAD, and with some patients hypotension may portend a worse outcome.[10]

Cardiovascular examination should be focused on the assessment of signs of cardiac tamponade, including jugular venous distension, pulsus paradoxus, changes in pulse pressure, and distant heart sounds on auscultation. Extremities should be examined for perfusion deficits, including diminished or absent pulses, and limb ischemia. Neurologic complications may occur, with syncope seen in 9% of AADs and secondary to tamponade, aortic rupture, cerebral vessel obstruction, or activation of cerebral baroreceptors.[6] Positive likelihood predictors on examination suggestive of AAD are suddenness of chest pain, tearing or ripping quality with migration, history of hypertension, focal neurologic deficits, and a pulse deficit.[11] Three independent clinical factors can be used in a prediction model: chest pain, mediastinal widening, and pulse/blood pressure differentials. Probability of dissection was 7% in the absence of these factors, 31% with isolated finding of aortic pain, 39% with isolated finding of mediastinal widening, and greater than 83% blood pressure/pulse differential with any combination of the other factors.[12]

Imaging is essential in establishing the diagnosis of AAD. Chest radiograph should be performed on low-risk and intermediate-risk patients as a precursor to more advanced imaging.[10] High-risk patients need definitive aortic imaging during initial evaluation. Computed tomography (CT) is especially useful for detecting descending aortic aneurysm or dissection and is the preferred modality for urgent evaluation given its ability to be performed quickly. The sensitivity of CT for identifying type A and B AAD exceeds 90%.[13] Transesophageal echocardiography is particularly useful in offering dynamic information about the aortic valve, including the presence and severity of aortic regurgitation. Magnetic resonance imaging can be considered but is used less in practice, comprising less than 1% of the total number of initial imaging studies ordered, limited largely by the time needed for image acquisition.[3] All three modalities have comparable sensitivity and specificity for diagnosing or ruling out AAD.[14]

The excessive mortality associated with AAD makes the need for timely, accurate diagnosis critical. However, variability in presentation, as discussed, may delay definitive imaging and diagnosis. A serum biomarker (if widely available, cost-effective, and adequately sensitive and specific) could facilitate the diagnosis, counter some of the clinical uncertainty associated with presentation, and avoid delays in imaging and treatment.[9] D-dimer is the most promising biomarker for risk stratification in suspected AAD and is available for use at the point of care. A cutoff level of 500 ng/mL has been confirmed in multiple studies to rule out AAD.[10] An even more stringent D-dimer level of less than 100 ng/mL is thought to achieve a negative predictive value of 100%.[15] The largest study on the use of D-dimer in AAD showed a sensitivity and specificity of 95.7% (95% confidence interval [CI], 78.1–99.9) and 61.3% (95% CI, 42.2–78.2), respectively, at a cutoff level of 500 ng/mL, within the first 6 hours of presentation of AAD.[16] This study also showed that AAD could be ruled in using a cutoff of 1600 ng/mL in the initial 6 hours. **Fig. 1** shows how D-dimer testing could be used to rule in or rule out aortic dissection in the appropriately selected patient presenting with chest pain.

INITIAL THERAPY

Once the diagnosis has been established, initial management in both type A and B AAD is directed at hemodynamic stabilization, achieving stringent blood pressure control and limiting end-organ damage. Efforts directed at minimizing the exposure of the aortic wall to sheer stress and stopping the propagation of dissection are foremost. Surgical consultation should be sought in all patients with AAD.[10] Common themes for management of both type A and B AAD include invasive hemodynamic monitoring, achieving hemodynamic stability, and pain relief. Blood pressure should be regulated between 100 and 120 mm Hg systolic and less than or equal to 60 to 70 mm Hg diastolic. Refractory hypotension should be managed with rapid volume expansion in combination with vasopressors (such as norepinephrine or phenylephrine) to maintain organ perfusion in anticipation of definitive surgical repair.

First-line pharmacologic therapy for AAD is beta-blockade, generally in rapid-acting intravenous formulations of esmolol, labetalol, or propranolol. The short half-lives of these agents, combined with their capacity for quick titration, make them ideally suited to blunt the 3 components that contribute to aortic wall stress: velocity of ventricular contraction, rate of ventricular contraction, and blood pressure. Beta-blockade should be used cautiously in the setting of aortic regurgitation because it may compromise compensatory tachycardia. In an analysis of 1301 patients with AAD in the International Registry for Acute Dissection (IRAD) global registry database and followed for less than or equal to 5 years to analyze the impact of medications on mortality,

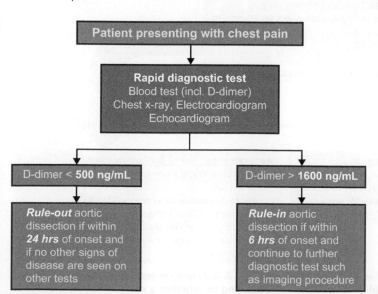

Fig. 1. D-dimer is the most promising biomarker for risk stratification in suspected AAD and is available for use at the point of care. A cutoff level of 500 ng/mL has been confirmed in multiple studies to rule out AAD. AAD could be ruled in using a cutoff of 1600 ng/mL in the initial 6 hours. (*Data from* Suzuki T, Distante A, Zizza A, et al. Diagnosis of acute aortic dissection by D-dimer: the International Registry of Acute Aortic Dissection Substudy on Biomarkers (IRAD-Bio) experience. Circulation 2009;119(20):2702–7.)

Suzuki and colleagues[17] showed that beta-blockade was associated with improved survival in all patients (P = .03), in patients with TAAD overall (P = .02), and in patients with TAAD who received surgery (P = .006).

Multiple antihypertensive agents are often required to achieve target blood pressure acutely. Sodium nitroprusside can be used as an adjunct for blood pressure control. Its use as a sole agent should be avoided, because the vasodilating effect can lead to a reflex tachycardia and an increased force of left ventricular contraction. Sodium nitroprusside is therefore generally coadministered with beta-blockade and once adequate heart rate control has been achieved. Infusion periods of sodium nitroprusside should be as short as possible to minimize the risk of thiocyanate and cyanide toxicity.

Nondihydropyridine calcium channel blockers, such as verapamil or diltiazem, may be used in patients intolerant of beta-blockade or in whom inadequate heart rate control is achieved with beta-blockade alone. In the aforementioned analysis of the IRAD global registry database to analyze the impact of medications on survival, Suzuki and colleagues[17] showed that calcium channel blockers

are associated with improved survival in patients with TBAD overall (P = .02) and in those with TBAD receiving medical management (P = .03).

Although not associated with a survival advantage in the acute setting,[17] angiotensin-converting enzyme inhibitors have a role acutely when the patient with an acute aortic event remains hypertensive, and may also reduce long-term aortic events in medically treated TBAD.[18] Renal insufficiency and hyperkalemia may limit the use of angiotensin-converting enzyme inhibitors, and pregnancy and angioedema on previous therapy are absolute contraindications. Hydralazine is generally contraindicated in the management of AAD unless the heart rate has been well controlled and the risk for reflex tachycardia has been mitigated.

Once hemodynamic stability is established, treatment strategies between type A and B dissections diverge. With TAAD, the mainstay of therapy is emergent surgical repair, if possible. With type B dissection, aggressive medical management with surveillance imaging is the standard for uncomplicated disease and represents the best strategy to date carrying the lowest mortality compared with endovascular repair and open surgery.[19] **Fig. 2**

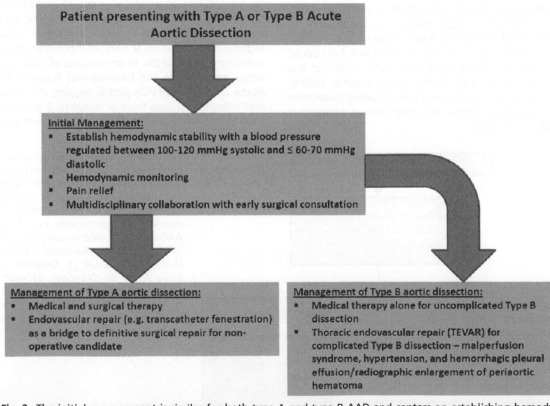

Fig. 2. The initial management is similar for both type A and type B AAD and centers on establishing hemodynamic stability. The management paradigm then diverges depending on whether a patient has TAAD or TBAD.

shows a summary of the principles of treatment of both TAAD and TBAD.

SURGICAL MANAGEMENT OF TYPE A AAD

Patients with TAAD require emergent surgical repair. Operative management involves resection of the intimal tear to the proximal extent of the dissection when possible, elimination of entry into the false lumen proximally and distally, and interposition graft replacement of the aorta. Resuspension or replacement of the aortic valve is required when dissection involves the aortic root and compromises the function of the aortic valve. When the function of the aortic valve is preserved, patients may be treated with valve-sparing procedures such as the David or Yacoub technique, but these surgeries are generally technically demanding and should be performed at high-volume centers with specialized expertise.[20,21] If the dissection involves the aortic valve, aortic root, and ascending aorta, a Bentall procedure may be performed through which a composite graft is used to replace all of the affected components with reimplantation of the coronary arteries into the graft. The elephant trunk technique, which necessitates a staged operation, may offer reduced patency of the false lumen.[22] When extensive tears in the aortic arch are present (as in 15%–20% of all patients with TAAD), as well as in the presence of arch aneurysm, complex arch dissection, or connective tissue disease, total arch replacement should be considered and supra-aortic vessels may be reimplanted separately or with the use of the island technique.[23,24]

Postoperative mortality ranges from 10% to 35%.[25] Medical management alone is associated with incrementally greater risks, with a mortality of 20% at 24 hours following presentation, 30% at 48 hours after presentation, and greater than 50% more than 1 month following presentation.[1] Nonetheless, for extremely ill patients, operative intervention may not be offered because mortality is highly likely with or without surgery. Although surgical mortality increases with age, the relative benefits of surgery outweigh the risks of medical management alone for TAAD until at least the age of 80 years and decision making about risks and benefits of operative management should be individualized. In the German Registry for Acute Aortic Dissection Type A (GERAADA), septuagenarians had a 30-day postoperatively mortality of 16% (n = 60 of 381), compared with 35% (n = 29 of 83) among octogenarians.[26] Stroke remains an important postsurgical complication of open thoracic surgical repair, developing in 4% to 8% of patients. A brain-protective strategy to prevent stroke is a cornerstone of the surgical, anesthetic, and perfusion techniques used during open surgical repair, and selective cerebral perfusion may be a useful strategy during complex repair of the aortic arch.[10,27]

Although surgical repair is the standard of care for the appropriate operative candidate with TAAD, endovascular repair may offer a second option for those who are not surgical candidates or who refuse surgical repair, or as a bridge to definitive surgical repair. Among patients with TAAD, endovascular procedures (eg, transcatheter fenestration) relieve malperfusion by decompressing the false lumen (equalizing pressures between the true and false lumens) and facilitating reexpansion of the true lumen. Stent placement in the true lumen may redirect flow into the true lumen and facilitate closure of the entry tear into the false lumen. When transcatheter fenestration is performed, complimentary aortic branch stenting may be used as adjunct to manage malperfusion.[28,29] Total endovascular treatment of TAAD remains an experimental procedure, but has been successfully performed and reported.[30]

Hybrid procedures are not routinely performed, but may have a role at high-volume centers with specialized expertise and for patients considered unsuitable for open surgical repair. The limited data on outcomes from hybrid repair of the aortic arch and such information, derived primarily from a heterogeneous collection of case series and retrospective studies, indicate that this procedure is associated with considerable perioperative morbidity and mortality. In a systematic review of 50 studies involving hybrid aortic arch procedures from 2002 to 2011, Cao and colleagues[31] showed pooled rates of mortality of 9.8% (95% CI, 7.7–12.4); perioperative stroke, 4.3% (95% CI, 3.0–6.3); and spinal cord ischemia, 5.8% (95% CI, 4.2–7.9).

Although TAAD is overall a highly lethal condition, a recent analysis drew attention to the potential added lethality of TAAD complicated by mesenteric malperfusion, in particular. In a retrospective analysis of nearly 2000 consecutive patients with TAAD enrolled at 18 institutions between December 1995 and August 2010 in the IRAD, mesenteric malperfusion was detected in 68 (3.7%) of 1809 patients. Overall in-hospital mortality was 63.2% (43 of 68) and 23.8% (414 of 1741) in patients with and without mesenteric malperfusion, respectively ($P<.001$).[32] In-hospital mortality of patients with mesenteric malperfusion receiving medical, endovascular, and surgical/hybrid therapy was 95.2% (20 of 21), 72.7% (8 of 11), and 41.7% (15 of 36), respectively ($P<.001$). Patients with mesenteric malperfusion were less likely to undergo surgical/hybrid treatment (52.9% vs 87.9%; P<.001) and more likely to receive medical (30.9% vs 11.6%; P<.001) or endovascular (16.2% vs 0.5%, P<.001) management, compared with patients without mesenteric malperfusion. Although this analysis was not able to establish the best therapeutic option for the management of TAAD complicated by mesenteric ischemia, it does call attention to the potential underuse of the therapeutic strategy that may be associated with the best outcomes in this particularly vulnerable population.[32]

MANAGEMENT OF TYPE B AAD

The management of TBAD involves 3 key principles: medical management of uncomplicated TBAD, accurate definition and characterization of a complicated event, and endovascular treatment of complicated TBAD to achieve optimal outcomes.[19] Patients with uncomplicated TBAD should be managed with aggressive medical therapy. An analysis from the IRAD database established an in-hospital mortality of 13% among those with acute TBAD, with most deaths occurring in the first week following the acute aortic event.[33] Furthermore, among patients with uncomplicated TBAD, 90% of patients survive hospitalization with adequate antihypertensive therapy.

At present, thoracic endovascular repair (TEVAR) has failed to show outcomes that are superior to medical management alone among patients with uncomplicated TBAD. The INSTEAD (Investigation of Stent Grafts in Patients with Type B Aortic Dissection) trial did not show a survival advantage of patients with subacute or chronic uncomplicated TBAD treated with TEVAR compared with medical management,[34] and the 1-year results of the ADSORB (A European Study on Medical Management vs TAG Device plus Medical Management for Acute Uncomplicated Type B Dissection) trial showed more frequent false lumen thrombosis and aortic remodeling in those patients with acute TBAD treated with TEVAR compared with those managed medically.[35] In the absence of long-term outcome data, medical treatment is therefore the preferred management paradigm for uncomplicated TBAD. Although outcomes following medical management of uncomplicated TBAD may be favorable, aneurysmal evolution and eventual rupture may occur, sometimes without warning symptoms. Accordingly and initially, surveillance with CT or magnetic resonance imaging is indicated at admission, 7 days, discharge, and within 6 weeks.[10]

The management of complicated TBAD begins with identification of a complicated acute aortic event, for which there are no uniform criteria. Approximately 25% of patients presenting with TBAD are complicated at admission by malperfusion syndrome or hemodynamic instability, justifying a more aggressive approach.[36] A recent Interdisciplinary Expert Consensus Document on Management of Type B Aortic Dissection[19] established the following as the definition for complicated TBAD: (1) malperfusion, (2) refractory hypertension, and (3) increase in periaortic hematoma and hemorrhagic pleural effusion in 2 subsequent CT examinations. Malperfusion syndrome, reported in 10% of patients with TBAD, may lead to a variety of signs and symptoms depending on the aortic branches that are involved. Paraparesis or paraplegia may signify involvement of the spinal arteries; lower limb ischemia, the iliac arteries; and abdominal pain, nausea, and diarrhea, the visceral arteries. Organ malperfusion may be corroborated by laboratory markers, as with bilirubin, amylase, and hepatic enzymes associated with mesenteric and celiac artery malperfusion. Refractory hypertension constitutes hypertension persisting despite 3 or more different classes of antihypertensive therapy at maximal recommended or maximal tolerated doses and not having been present before the onset of dissection. The inclusion of refractory hypertension in the definition of complicated TBAD is partly informed by data from IRAD, in which in-hospital mortality among patients with medically managed TBAD was significantly greater in those with refractory hypertension, compared with those without (35.6% vs 1.5%, P = .0003).[37]

Once the patient with complicated TBAD is identified, TEVAR, when feasible, should be considered the first-line treatment.[19,38] Open surgery should be reserved for patients in whom endovascular techniques are not feasible or have failed. Midterm results after endovascular treatment of acute, complicated TBAD from the Talent Thoracic Registry are favorable.[39] In this registry of 29 patients with acute complicated TBAD, freedom from treatment failure (defined as reintervention; aortic rupture; device-related complications; aortic-related death; or sudden, unexplained late death) at 1 year and 5 years was 82% and 77%, respectively.

Overall, TEVAR is associated with in-hospital mortality between 2.6% and 9.8% and neurologic complications between 0.6% and 3.1%.[40,41] Stroke, paraplegia and paraparesis, incidental occlusion of the left subclavian artery, and inadequate placement of the graft are all significant complications of TEVAR.[42] Paraplegia is among the most feared complications of descending thoracic aortic repair. As a spinal-protective strategy, cerebrospinal fluid drainage is an option during open and endovascular thoracic aortic repair for patients at high risk for spinal cord ischemic injury.[10]

SUMMARY

Acute aortic syndromes are among the most lethal of the cardiovascular diseases. Delays in recognition, diagnosis, and treatment are associated with unacceptable increases in mortality. Signs and symptoms are sometimes subtle and atypical and a high index of clinical suspicion is useful to guide the diagnostic evaluation. Although underlying connective tissue diseases, pregnancy, and aortopathy associated with congenital bicuspid aortic valve morphology should not be overlooked as predisposing conditions, uncontrolled hypertension remains the most significant treatable risk factor. Immediate management involves blood pressure reduction. β-Blockers are the first drugs of choice. Multidisciplinary evaluation should be a common thread in the management of both TAAD and TBAD, with early surgical consultation. TAAD is managed surgically, whereas patients with uncomplicated TBAD should be treated with medical therapy. Operative techniques in the management of TAAD have evolved and include selective cerebral perfusion, aortic valve–sparing procedures, and TEVAR as part of a complex hybrid procedure when there is involvement of the descending aorta. Complicated TBAD, characterized by malperfusion, refractory hypertension, and/or radiographic evidence of an enlarging periaortic hematoma or hemorrhagic pleural effusion on serial imaging, requires more aggressive therapy. When feasible, TEVAR is considered the first-line treatment of complicated TBAD. False lumen expansion is the main complication of chronic type B dissection and mandates appropriate surveillance. Although future directions should involve the evolution of operative and endovascular techniques and the development of sophisticated risk prediction tools, risk factor modification by addressing the burden imposed by uncontrolled hypertension cannot be overlooked.

REFERENCES

1. Ramanath VS, Oh JK, Sundt TM III, et al. Acute aortic syndromes and thoracic aortic aneurysm. Mayo Clin Proc 2009;84(5):465–81.
2. Olsson C, Thelin S, Stahle E, et al. Thoracic aortic aneurysm and dissection: increasing prevalence and improved outcomes reported in a nationwide population-based study of more than 14,000 cases from 1987 to 2002. Circulation 2006;114(24):2611–8.
3. Tsai TT, Trimarchi S, Nienaber CA. Acute aortic dissection: perspectives from the International Registry of Acute Aortic Dissection (IRAD). Eur J Vasc Endovasc Surg 2009;37(2):149–59.
4. Hirst AE Jr, Johns VJ Jr, Kime SW Jr. Dissecting aneurysm of the aorta: a review of 505 cases. Medicine 1958;37(3):217–79.
5. Eagle KA, Isselbacher EM, DeSanctis RW, International Registry for Aortic Dissection Investigators. Cocaine-related aortic dissection in perspective. Circulation 2002;105(13):1529–30.
6. Braverman AC. Acute aortic dissection: clinician update. Circulation 2010;122:184–8.
7. Loeys BL, Schwarze U, Holm T, et al. Aneurysm syndromes caused by mutations in the TGF-beta receptor. N Engl J Med 2006;355(8):788–98.
8. Howard DP, Banerjee A, Fairhead JF, et al. Population-based study of incidence and outcome of acute aortic dissection and pre-morbid risk-factor control: 10-year results from the Oxford Vascular Study. Circulation 2013;127(20):2031–7.
9. Suzuki T, Bossone E, Sawaki D, et al. Biomarkers of aortic diseases. Am Heart J 2013;165(1):15–25.
10. Hiratzka LF, Bakris GL, Beckman JA, et al. 2010 ACCF/AHA/AATS/ACR/ASA/SCA/SCAI/SIR/STS/SVM Guidelines for the diagnosis and management of patients with thoracic aortic disease. A Report of the American College of Cardiology Foundation/American Heart Association Task Force on Practice Guidelines, American Association for Thoracic Surgery, American College of Radiology, American Stroke Association, Society of Cardiovascular Anesthesiologists, Society for Cardiovascular Angiography and Interventions, Society of Interventional Radiology, Society of Thoracic Surgeons, and Society for Vascular Medicine. J Am Coll Cardiol 2010;55(14):e27–129.
11. Klompas M. Does this patient have an acute thoracic aortic dissection? JAMA 2002;287(17):2262–72.
12. von Kodolitsch Y, Schwartz AG, Nienaber CA. Clinical prediction of acute aortic dissection. Arch Intern Med 2000;160(19):2977–82.
13. Moore AG, Eagle KA, Bruckman D, et al. Choice of computed tomography, transesophageal echocardiography, magnetic resonance imaging, and aortography in acute aortic dissection: International Registry of Acute Aortic Dissection (IRAD). Am J Cardiol 2002;89(10):1235–8.
14. Shiga T, Wajima Z, Apfel CC, et al. Diagnostic accuracy of transesophageal echocardiography, helical computed tomography, and magnetic resonance imaging for suspected thoracic aortic dissection: systematic review and meta-analysis. Arch Intern Med 2006;166(13):1350–6.

15. Sodeck G, Domanovits H, Schillinger M, et al. D-dimer in ruling out acute aortic dissection: a systematic review and prospective cohort study. Eur Heart J 2007;28(24):3067–75.

16. Suzuki T, Distante A, Zizza A, et al. Diagnosis of acute aortic dissection by D-dimer: the International Registry of Acute Aortic Dissection Substudy on Biomarkers (IRAD-Bio) experience. Circulation 2009; 119(20):2702–7.

17. Suzuki T, Isselbacher EM, Nienaber CA, et al. Type-selective benefits of medications in the treatment of acute aortic dissection (from the International Registry of Acute Aortic Dissection [IRAD]). Am J Cardiol 2012;109(1):122–7.

18. Takeshita S, Sakamoto S, Kitada S, et al. Angiotensin-converting enzyme inhibitors reduce long-term aortic events in patients with acute type B aortic dissection. Circ J 2008;72(11):1758–61.

19. Fattori R, Cao P, De Rango P, et al. Interdisciplinary expert consensus document on management of type B aortic dissection. J Am Coll Cardiol 2013; 61(16):1661–78.

20. David TE. The aortic valve-sparing operation. J Thorac Cardiovasc Surg 2011;141(3):613–5.

21. Yacoub MH, Gehle P, Chandrasekaran V, et al. Late results of a valve-preserving operation in patients with aneurysms of the ascending aorta and root. J Thorac Cardiovasc Surg 1998;115(5):1080–90.

22. Milewski RK, Szeto WY, Pochettino A, et al. Have hybrid procedures replaced open aortic arch reconstruction in high-risk patients? A comparative study of elective open arch debranching with endovascular stent graft placement and conventional elective open total and distal aortic arch reconstruction. J Thorac Cardiovasc Surg 2010;140(3): 590–7.

23. Patel HJ, Nguyen C, Diener AC, et al. Open arch reconstruction in the endovascular era: analysis of 721 patients over 17 years. J Thorac Cardiovasc Surg 2011;141(6):1417–23.

24. Sundt TM III, Orszulak TA, Cook DJ, et al. Improving results of open arch replacement. Ann Thorac Surg 2008;86(3):787–96.

25. Nienaber CA, Eagle KA. Aortic dissection: new frontiers in diagnosis and management, part II: therapeutic management and follow-up. Circulation 2003;108(6):772–8.

26. Rylski B, Suedkamp M, Beyersdorf F, et al. Outcome after surgery for acute aortic dissection type A in patients over 70 years: data analysis from the German Registry for Acute Aortic Dissection Type A (GERAADA). Eur J Cardiothorac Surg 2011; 40(2):435–40.

27. Kazui T, Kimura N, Komatsu S. Surgical treatment of aortic arch aneurysms using selective cerebral perfusion. Experience with 100 patients. Eur J Cardiothorac Surg 1995;9(9):491–5.

28. Barnes DM, Williams DM, Dasika NL, et al. A single-center experience treating renal malperfusion after aortic dissection with central aortic fenestration and renal artery stenting. J Vasc Surg 2008;47(5): 903–10.

29. Beregi JP, Haulon S, Otal P, et al. Endovascular treatment of acute complications associated with aortic dissection: midterm results from a multicenter study. J Endovasc Ther 2003;10(3):486–93.

30. Metcalfe MJ, Karthikesalingam A, Black SA, et al. The first endovascular repair of an acute type A dissection using an endograft designed for the ascending aorta. J Vasc Surg 2012;55(1):220–2.

31. Cao P, De RP, Czerny M, et al. Systematic review of clinical outcomes in hybrid procedures for aortic arch dissections and other arch diseases. J Thorac Cardiovasc Surg 2012;144(6):1286–300.

32. Di Eusanio M, Trimarchi S, Patel HJ, et al. Clinical presentation, management, and short-term outcome of patients with type A acute dissection complicated by mesenteric malperfusion: observations from the International Registry of Acute Aortic Dissection. J Thorac Cardiovasc Surg 2013;145:385–90.

33. Suzuki T, Mehta RH, Ince H, et al. Clinical profiles and outcomes of acute type B aortic dissection in the current era: lessons from the International Registry of Aortic Dissection (IRAD). Circulation 2003; 108(Suppl 1):II312–7.

34. Nienaber CA. Influence and critique of the INSTEAD Trial (TEVAR versus medical treatment for uncomplicated type B aortic dissection). Semin Vasc Surg 2011;24(3):167–71.

35. Brunkwall J, Lammer J, Verhoeven E, et al. ADSORB: a study on the efficacy of endovascular grafting in uncomplicated acute dissection of the descending aorta. Eur J Vasc Endovasc Surg 2012;44(1):31–6.

36. Tsai TT, Fattori R, Trimarchi S, et al, International Registry of Acute Aortic Dissection. Long-term survival in patients presenting with type B acute aortic dissection: insights from the International Registry of Acute Aortic Dissection. Circulation 2006;114: 2226–31.

37. Trimarchi S, Eagle KA, Nienaber CA, et al, International Registry of Acute Aortic Dissection (IRAD) Investigators. Importance of refractory pain and hypertension in acute type B aortic dissection: insights from the International Registry of Acute Aortic Dissection (IRAD). Circulation 2010;122:1283–9.

38. Cheng D, Martin J, Shennib H, et al. Endovascular aortic repair versus open surgical repair for descending thoracic aortic disease a systematic review and meta-analysis of comparative studies. J Am Coll Cardiol 2010;55(10):986–1001.

39. Ehrlich MP, Rousseau H, Heijmen R, et al. Midterm results after endovascular treatment of acute, complicated type B aortic dissection: the Talent

Thoracic Registry. J Thorac Cardiovasc Surg 2013; 145(1):159–65.

40. Eggebrecht H, Nienaber CA, Neuhauser M, et al. Endovascular stent-graft placement in aortic dissection: a meta-analysis. Eur Heart J 2006;27(4): 489–98.

41. Xiong J, Jiang B, Guo W, et al. Endovascular stent graft placement in patients with type B aortic dissection: a meta-analysis in China. J Thorac Cardiovasc Surg 2009;138(4):865–72.

42. Buth J, Harris PL, Hobo R, et al. Neurologic complications associated with endovascular repair of thoracic aortic pathology: incidence and risk factors. A study from the European Collaborators on Stent/Graft Techniques for Aortic Aneurysm Repair (EUROSTAR) registry. J Vasc Surg 2007;46(6):1103–10.

Massive Pulmonary Embolism

Narain Moorjani, MB ChB, MRCS, MD, FRCS (C-Th)[a],*,
Susanna Price, MD, PhD, MRCP, EDICM, FFICM, FESC[b]

KEYWORDS

- Pulmonary embolism • Thrombolysis • Pulmonary embolectomy • Anticoagulation
- Right ventricular dysfunction

KEY POINTS

- The presentation of pulmonary embolism (PE) is frequently nonspecific and scoring systems may aid the diagnosis and risk stratification of patients.
- The main cause of mortality is obstructive shock and associated right ventricular (RV) failure.
- Systemic thrombolysis (unless contraindicated) is recommended as the first-line treatment of patients with massive PE to decrease the thromboembolic burden on the RV and increase pulmonary perfusion.
- Surgical pulmonary embolectomy or catheter-directed thrombectomy should be considered in those with contraindications to fibrinolysis, or those who have persistent hemodynamic compromise or RV dysfunction despite fibrinolytic therapy.
- Critical care management predominantly involves supporting the right ventricle, by optimizing preload, RV contractility, and coronary perfusion pressure and minimizing afterload.

INTRODUCTION

Acute pulmonary embolism (PE) represents the sudden obstruction of part of the pulmonary arterial vasculature, which is usually caused by embolization of thrombus from the deep veins within the lower limbs and pelvis. It may also be caused by air, fat, or amniotic fluid. PE is the third commonest cause of cardiovascular death (after coronary artery disease and stroke) and more than 600,000 cases are believed to occur in the United States annually.[1] PE was found in 18% of autopsies and in most (70%) of these was considered to be the main or a contributory cause of death.[2] The incidence increases exponentially with age, with the mean age at presentation of 62 years,[2,3] affecting men and women equally.[4]

Although no predisposing factors are identified in approximately 20% of patients (idiopathic or unprovoked PE),[5] most patients have either patient-related or setting-related attributable risk factors (secondary or provoked PE). Patient-related factors include advanced age, previous venous thromboembolism, active cancer, underlying coagulopathy (including factor V Leiden and prothrombin mutations), smoking, hormone replacement therapy, and the oral contraceptive pill.[6,7] Medical conditions associated with an increased risk of PE include heart failure, stroke, respiratory failure, sepsis, and inflammatory bowel disease.[8] Setting-related risk factors include protracted immobility secondary to major general/orthopedic surgery, major fracture, air travel, pregnancy, chemotherapy, or the presence of a central venous line.[9] Commonly, more than 1 risk factor is present.

Historically, PE was classified according to the anatomic burden of the thrombus in the pulmonary vasculature.[10] However, the outcome of these patients is more dependent on the hemodynamic compromise induced by the PE, such as the presence of circulatory arrest, hypotension, or right

Disclosures: The authors have nothing to disclose.
[a] Department of Cardiothoracic Surgery, Papworth Hospital, University of Cambridge, Cambridge CB23 3RE, UK; [b] Department of Intensive Care, Royal Brompton Hospital, Imperial College, University of London, London SW3 6NP, UK
* Corresponding author.
E-mail address: narain.moorjani@papworth.nhs.uk

Cardiol Clin 31 (2013) 503–518
http://dx.doi.org/10.1016/j.ccl.2013.07.005

ventricular (RV) dysfunction.[5] PE has therefore been reclassified into 3 different prognostic categories by the European Society of Cardiology and American Heart Association (**Box 1**).[11,12]

Data from the International Cooperative Pulmonary Embolism Registry (ICOPER) reported 90-day mortality for patients with massive PE of 52% compared with 15% for those with submassive and nonmassive PE.[5] Similarly, data from the Management Strategy and Prognosis of Pulmonary Embolism Registry (MAPPET) reported 65% in-hospital mortality for patients with acute PE requiring cardiopulmonary resuscitation, compared with 25% for those presenting with cardiogenic shock, and 8% for hemodynamically stable patients.[13] The presence of RV dysfunction is associated with a 2-fold increase in 90-day mortality.[14]

PATHOPHYSIOLOGY

Obstruction of flow through the main pulmonary arteries results in increased afterload on the RV. In addition to mechanical obstruction of the RV, release of vasoactive mediators, such as thromboxane A_2 and serotonin, result in pulmonary vasoconstriction and increased pulmonary vascular resistance.[15] The resultant increase in RV wall tension results in displacement of the interventricular septum to the left and impaired left ventricular (LV) filling.[16] If untreated, the RV outflow obstruction also results in reduced preload on the LV, reduced cardiac output, and circulatory collapse and shock.[17] Younger patients with otherwise normal underlying cardiac function may tolerate the hemodynamic stress placed by a large PE without developing RV dysfunction or shock. However, in patients with compromised cardiac function, the onset of RV failure and circulatory collapse may be more rapid. In addition, hypoxia may result from the low cardiac output entering the pulmonary circulation, ventilation-perfusion mismatch, and the presence of a right-to-left shunt (through a patent foramen ovale, opened by the increased right-sided pressure).[18]

CLINICAL PRESENTATION

The clinical presentation of PE varies widely. Patients with massive PE may present with severe dyspnea at rest, syncope, or even cardiac arrest, whereas those with nonmassive PE may be asymptomatic or have limited symptoms. Their past medical history may include some of the risk factors for venous thromboembolism. Physical signs include tachycardia, tachypnea, systemic hypotension, and cyanosis. Evidence of RV dysfunction includes distended neck veins, parasternal heave, accentuated pulmonary component of the second heart sound, and a systolic murmur consistent with tricuspid regurgitation. An RV gallop rhythm may also be heard. The presence of a pleural rub, in association with pleuritic chest pain, may be secondary to pleural irritation caused by pulmonary infarction. Use of a scoring system, such as the Wells criteria or Geneva score, may aid

---

> **Box 1**
> **Classification of PE into prognostic categories by the European Society of Cardiology and American Heart Association**
>
> 1. High-risk (massive) PE (20%), which is a life-threatening condition and defined as PE in the presence of
>
>   a. Arterial hypotension (systolic blood pressure <90 mm Hg or a decrease of >40 mm Hg) for more than 15 minutes or requiring inotropic support, which is not caused by a new-onset arrhythmia
>
>   b. Cardiogenic shock (oliguria, lactic acidosis, cool extremities, or altered level of consciousness)
>
>   c. Circulatory collapse, in patients with syncope or undergoing cardiopulmonary resuscitation
>
> 2. Intermediate-risk (submassive) PE (32%), which is defined as PE with a systolic blood pressure greater than 90 mm Hg but echocardiographic evidence of RV dysfunction or pulmonary hypertension, or the presence of increased markers of myocardial injury (such as troponin)
>
> 3. Low-risk (nonmassive) PE (48%), which is defined as PE with a systolic blood pressure greater than 90 mm Hg and no evidence of RV dysfunction, pulmonary hypertension, or increased markers of myocardial injury.
>
> *Data from* Torbicki A, Perrier A, Konstantinides S, et al. ESC Committee for Practice Guidelines (CPG). Guidelines on the diagnosis and management of acute pulmonary embolism: the Task Force for the Diagnosis and Management of Acute Pulmonary Embolism of the European Society of Cardiology (ESC). Eur Heart J 2008;29(18):2282; and Jaff MR, McMurtry MS, Archer SL, et al, American Heart Association Council on Cardiopulmonary, Critical Care, Perioperative and Resuscitation, American Heart Association Council on Peripheral Vascular Disease, American Heart Association Council on Arteriosclerosis, Thrombosis and Vascular Biology. Management of massive and submassive pulmonary embolism, iliofemoral deep vein thrombosis, and chronic thromboembolic pulmonary hypertension: a scientific statement from the American Heart Association. Circulation 2011;123(16):1789–93.

the clinical diagnosis and risk stratification of the patient.[19,20]

DIAGNOSIS AND RISK STRATIFICATION

The combination of clinical features and predisposing risk factors has been incorporated into clinical scoring systems that are used to predict the likelihood of PE and determining which investigations to perform. These investigations include the Wells score, simplified Geneva score and Pulmonary Embolism Severity Index (PESI) (**Tables 1–3**).[19–21] The most extensively validated and widely used clinical scoring system is the Wells score.[22]

The chest radiograph is usually abnormal in patients with acute PE.[23,24] Although the features are mainly nonspecific, such as atelectasis or pleural effusion, it can be used to exclude other causes of dyspnea or chest pain, such as pneumonia or pleural effusion. Arterial blood gas analysis usually shows hypoxemia (Pao_2 <80 mm Hg), with hypocapnia and respiratory alkalosis.[25] In up to 20%

Table 1
Wells score

Variable	Points
Predisposing factors	
Previous DVT or PE	1.5
Recent surgery or immobilization	1.5
Cancer	1
Symptoms	
Hemoptysis	1
Clinical signs	
Heart rate >100 bpm	1.5
Clinical signs of DVT	3
Clinical judgment	
Alternative diagnosis less likely than PE	3
	Total
Clinical probability (3 levels)	
Low	0–1
Intermediate	2–6
High	≥7
Clinical probability (2 levels)	
PE unlikely	0–4
PE likely	>4

Abbreviation: DVT, deep venous thrombosis.
Data from Wells PS, Anderson DR, Rodger M, et al. Derivation of a simple clinical model to categorize patients probability of pulmonary embolism: increasing the models utility with the SimpliRED D-dimer. Thromb Haemost 2000;83(3):418.

Table 2
Simplified Geneva score

Variable	Points
Predisposing factors	
Age >65 y	1
Previous DVT or PE	1
Surgery or fracture within 1 mo	1
Active malignancy	1
Symptoms	
Unilateral lower limb pain	1
Hemoptysis	1
Clinical signs	
Pain on deep palpation of lower limb and unilateral edema	1
Heart rate 75–94 bpm	1
Heart rate >94 bpm	2
Clinical Probability	**Total**
PE unlikely	0–2
PE likely	>2

Abbreviation: DVT, deep venous thrombosis.
Data from Le Gal G, Righini M, Roy PM, et al. Prediction of pulmonary embolism in the emergency department: the revised Geneva score. Ann Intern Med 2006;144:165–71.

of patients, a normal Pao_2 and alveolar-arterial gradient may be found. Alternatively, hypercapnia with respiratory and metabolic acidosis may be seen in patients with massive PE requiring cardiopulmonary resuscitation. After assessment of the clinical and hemodynamic status of the patient using a clinical scoring system, the patients are subdivided into different probabilities of PE.

If the patient has a high clinical probability of PE, as determined by the clinical scoring systems, then multidetector computed tomography pulmonary angiography (CTPA) is required to determine the presence of thrombus within the pulmonary arterial vasculature.[11] CTPA has become the imaging of choice in patients with suspected PE, because of its speed of scanning, widespread availability, and high sensitivity and specificity (>90%).[26] It provides excellent visualization of the pulmonary arterial vasculature, including the main, lobar, and segmental pulmonary arteries, evidence of RV strain, characterization of extravascular structures, and for the detection of venous thrombosis (**Fig. 1**). However, in hemodynamically unstable patients, who cannot be transferred for CTPA, echocardiography may be required. An alternative imaging modality, such as VQ scintigraphy, may also be required in

Table 3 PESI	
Variable	**Points**
Age	1 per y
Male gender	10
Cancer (active or past history)	30
Heart failure	10
Chronic lung disease	10
Heart rate >110 bpm	20
Systolic blood pressure <100 mm Hg	30
Respiratory rate >30 bpm	20
Temperature <36°C	20
Altered mental status (disorientation, lethargy, stupor, or coma)	60
Oxygen saturation <90% on room air	20
Clinical Interpretation (Mortality at 30 d)	
Class 1: very low mortality risk (0%–1.6%)	<66
Class 2: low mortality risk (1.7%–3.5%)	<86
Class 3: moderate mortality risk (3.2%–7.1%)	<106
Class 4: high mortality risk (4.0%–11.4%)	<126
Class 5: very high mortality risk (10.0%–24.5%)	>126

Data from Aujesky D, Obrosky DS, Stone RA, et al. Derivation and validation of a prognostic model for pulmonary embolism. Am J Respir Crit Care Med 2005;172(8):1041–6.

patients with a contraindication to CTPA, such as those with renal failure or contrast allergy.[27]

If the patient has been classified as a low or intermediate clinical probability of PE, a D-dimer enzyme-linked immunosorbent assay (ELISA) should be performed as the first-line investigation (sensitivity 96% and specificity 39%).[28] Serum D-dimer is a degradation product of cross-linked fibrin and acts as an indirect marker for coagulation and subsequent fibrinolysis. Because the D-dimer ELISA has a high negative predictive value, its absence effectively rules out acute PE, and an alternative diagnosis should be sought.[29] However, the positive predictive value of increased serum D-dimer levels is low, because although D-dimer is specific for fibrin, fibrin can be produced in a wide variety of conditions, including aortic dissection, cancer, inflammation, and infection.[30,31] Hence, if the D-dimer ELISA is positive, the patient should undergo CTPA.[11]

Once the diagnosis of acute PE has been made, the patients are stratified into low-risk (nonmassive), intermediate-risk (submassive) and high-risk (massive) groups, according to the presence of hypotension, shock, or RV dysfunction. The clinical status of the patient differentiates the high-risk (massive) PE from patients with non–high-risk PE. Echocardiography can then be used to further delineate patients with non–high-risk PE into intermediate-risk PE (with evidence of RV dysfunction) or low-risk PE (with no RV dysfunction) groups.[32] Surrogate markers of RV dysfunction include RV dilatation (RV end diastolic dimension >30 mm), interventricular septal flattening with paradoxic motion, increased RV/LV

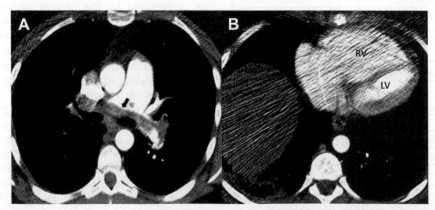

Fig. 1. Contrast-enhanced CTPA axial images showing (*A*) a large saddle embolus at the pulmonary artery bifurcation (*arrow*) with extension into both the left and right pulmonary arteries, and (*B*) evidence of right heart strain shown by enlarged right heart chambers, an RV/LV ratio greater than 1.5, and displacement of the interventricular septum. (*Courtesy of* Dr Deepa Gopalan, Cambridge, United Kingdom.)

ratio (>0.9), RV hypokinesis, pulmonary hypertension (pulmonary artery systolic pressure >30 mm Hg), and increased tricuspid regurgitation jet velocity (>2.6 m/s), which are found in approximately 25% of patients with acute PE (**Fig. 2**).[33,34] Echocardiography can also be used to exclude other important causes of acute circulatory collapse, including acute myocardial infarction, pericardial tamponade, or type A aortic dissection. The absence of RV dysfunction on echocardiography in a patient with shock or hypotension virtually rules out acute PE as a cause of the hemodynamic instability.[32] Transesophageal echocardiography can provide excellent imaging of the RV and proximal pulmonary vasculature to identify thrombus, as well as assessing RV function and size.[35] In patients with suspected PE with evidence of RV dysfunction, it has a sensitivity of 80% and specificity of 97%.[35]

Biomarkers, including serum troponin I or T and brain natriuretic peptide (BNP), may also be useful in detecting evidence of RV dysfunction in patients with acute PE.[36] Troponin levels, including troponin I and troponin T, are increased in the presence of PE, secondary to increased RV wall tension and end-diastolic pressure, reduced right coronary artery flow, increased RV myocardial oxygen demand, RV myocardial ischemia (even in the presence of normal coronary arteries) and subsequent leakage of the enzymes from the RV myocytes into the bloodstream.[37] They can be used to risk stratify patients with non–high-risk PE into intermediate-risk PE (with increased troponin levels) or low-risk PE (normal troponin levels), because increased troponin levels are used as a surrogate of RV dysfunction.[38] Similarly, plasma B-type natriuretic peptide (BNP) is released from the RV in response to increased pressure and stretch and has been shown to correlate with the presence of RV dysfunction.[39] Increased levels of both troponin and BNP have been shown to be associated with adverse prognosis and short-term outcomes in patients with acute PE.[40,41] However, increased levels of both troponin and BNP are not specific to PE.

Electrocardiography (ECG) is normal in up to 30% of patients[42] but often shows nonspecific changes, such as sinus tachycardia, atrial fibrillation, or ST/T wave changes.[43,44] Despite having a low sensitivity and specificity, the ECG may be useful in showing evidence of right heart strain, such as T-wave inversion in V_{1-4}, P pulmonale, right axis deviation, incomplete or complete right bundle branch block, or the combination of a prominent S wave in lead I, Q wave in lead III, and T-wave inversion in lead III (classic $S_1Q_3T_3$ pattern, which is present in only 2%–15% of patients with PE).[45]

Because massive PE has a high mortality in the first 6 hours after the onset of symptoms, early diagnosis is paramount in order to instigate timely management. The diagnosis is frequently first made at autopsy.[46,47]

MANAGEMENT

The primary cause of death in patients with massive PE is low cardiac output. Massive PE should be suspected in patients with major hemodynamic instability accompanied by an increased central venous pressure, which is not otherwise explained by pericardial tamponade, acute myocardial infarction, or tension pneumothorax. Because the short-term mortality increases depending on the degree of hemodynamic insult caused by the obstruction to RV outflow, the choice of initial therapy also depends on the severity of the hemodynamic insult.

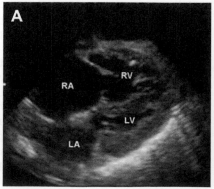 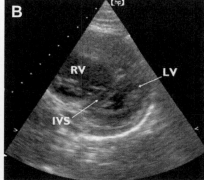

Fig. 2. Transthoracic echocardiography images in a patient with massive PE, with (A) subcostal long axis view showing acute right heart dilatation, with the RV larger than the LV and (B) parasternal short axis view showing a small compressed LV, which is D-shaped with a flattened IVS, and a dilated RV. IVS, interventricular septum; LA, left atrium; RA, right atrium.

ANTICOAGULATION

Unless there is a strong contraindication, parenteral anticoagulation should be commenced immediately in all patients in whom acute PE is believed to be the diagnosis.[12] Options include low-molecular-weight heparin (LMWH), intravenous unfractionated heparin (UFH), or subcutaneous fondaparinux (a selective factor Xa inhibitor). Subcutaneous LMWH or fondaparinux are preferred for most patients, because they are associated with a lower incidence of thromboembolic events, heparin-induced thrombocytopenia, and major bleeding (LMWH 1.3% vs UFH 2.1%) and do not require monitoring.[48,49] Fondaparinux can be given in weight-adjusted doses without monitoring as a once-daily subcutaneous injection, because it has a half-life of 15 to 20 hours.[50] UFH is indicated in patients with an increased risk of bleeding or in those in whom thrombolysis is being considered, because its short-acting effects can be directly reversed with protamine.[51] Intravenous UFH should also be used in patients with high-risk (massive) PE, because the effectiveness of LMWH and fondaparinux has not been investigated in this patient population.[48] UFH is also preferred in patients with severe renal impairment (because LMWH and fondaparinux are excreted by the kidney) and in patients with extreme obesity (in whom dosing of LMWH is unpredictable).[11] It is administered intravenously with a bolus of 80 U/kg followed by a continuous infusion of 18 U/kg per hour, which is subsequently adjusted to achieve an activated partial thromboplastin time ratio (aPTTR) between 2.0 and 2.5. The aPTTR is measured 4 to 6 hours after the initial dose, 3 hours after each dose adjustment, and then once daily when the therapeutic aPTTR has been achieved. Anticoagulation with heparin (UFH, LMWH, or fondaparinux) should be continued for at least 5 days.[52] For patients with heparin-induced thrombocytopenia, an alternative non–heparin-based anticoagulant, such as lepirudin, argatroban, or bivalirudin, can be used.[53]

FIBRINOLYSIS

In contrast to the passive action of heparin, fibrinolytic drugs (including urokinase, streptokinase, tenecteplase, and tissue plasminogen activator) actively promote thrombus lysis by hydrolysis of fibrin molecules. These drugs are enzymes that convert circulating inactive plasminogen into its active analogue plasmin. Plasmin is a serine protease enzyme that cleaves fibrin, releasing fibrin degradation products, including D-dimer molecules.[54] These agents are therefore able to induce a more rapid regression of the obstructive thrombotic burden to RV outflow compared with heparin alone.[55,56] However, the benefits of adding fibrinolytic therapy to heparin need to be balanced by the potential side effects, including the increased risk of major hemorrhage and increased blood transfusion requirement.[57]

Fibrinolytic therapy should ideally be initiated within 48 hours of symptoms onset for the greatest benefit but has been shown to have some efficacy up to 14 days.[58,59] Absolute contraindications to thrombolysis include recent major surgery, bleeding, trauma (within 2 weeks), intracranial hemorrhage, recent stroke (within 2 months), any hemorrhagic stroke, or significant coagulopathy. Relative contraindications include pregnancy, thrombocytopenia, and prolonged cardiopulmonary resuscitation.[12] Of the 478 patients who received fibrinolysis in MAPPET, over 40% (n = 193) had at least 1 relative contraindication.[13] These patients require high-dependency or intensive care monitoring for observation of the complications of acute PE and identification of the hemorrhagic complications of thrombolytic therapy.

The role of thrombolytic therapy for patients with intermediate-risk (submassive) PE remains controversial. The effects of thrombolysis in this patient group have been examined in 2 prospective randomized, placebo-controlled trials.[55,60] The Management Strategies and Prognosis of Pulmonary Embolism-3 Trial randomly assigned 256 patients with acute PE and RV dysfunction but without arterial hypotension or shock to heparin plus 100 mg of alteplase (n = 118) or heparin plus placebo (n = 138).[60] The primary end point, which was defined as in-hospital death or clinical deterioration requiring an escalation of treatment (including catecholamine infusion, secondary thrombolysis, endotracheal intubation, cardiopulmonary resuscitation, emergency surgical embolectomy, or thrombus fragmentation by catheter), was significantly higher in the placebo group compared with the alteplase group, especially the need for emergency escalation of treatment (24.6% vs 10.2%, P = .004). However, there was no difference in mortality between the 2 groups (placebo 2.2% vs alteplase 3.4%, P = .71). There were no episodes of fatal bleeding or cerebral bleeding in patients receiving heparin plus alteplase. In the second study, 200 patients were randomly allocated intravenous tissue plasminogen activator plus heparin or heparin alone to determine the incidence of pulmonary hypertension after intermediate-risk (submassive) PE.[55] Patients treated with tissue plasminogen activator had a significant reduction in median pulmonary artery systolic pressure compared with those treated with heparin alone (22 vs 2 mm Hg, P<.05). At 6 months, 27% of the patients treated with heparin alone developed increased pulmonary artery systolic pressure, suggesting an increased risk of developing long-term chronic thromboembolic pulmonary hypertension.

In a meta-analysis assessing patients with intermediate-risk PE,[61] there was no difference in mortality between those receiving heparin plus thrombolysis compared with heparin alone. The potential benefits of thrombolysis in patients with intermediate-risk PE needs to be balanced with the risk of bleeding, especially in patients with absolute and relative contraindications to systemic fibrinolysis. Even in carefully selected patients without absolute contraindications to thrombolysis, the rate of major hemorrhage and hemorrhagic stroke approaches 20% and 3%, respectively.[5] Hence, the clinical benefit of thrombolysis may be present only in a subgroup of patients with intermediate-risk PE, especially in those patients without an increased risk of bleeding. To further risk stratify patients in this group, the prospective, international, multicenter, randomized, double-blind PIETHO (Pulmonary Embolism Thrombolysis) trial has been initiated.[62] The trial will compare thrombolysis with tenecteplase plus heparin versus placebo plus heparin in 1000 normotensive patients with confirmed PE, RV dysfunction, and increased troponin levels. Until the results of this trial are available, the current guidelines suggest managing stable patients with intermediate-risk (submassive) PE using therapeutic heparin alone, in a similar manner to low-risk (nonmassive) patients.[12]

However, in hemodynamically unstable patients (high-risk PE), systemic thrombolysis (unless contraindicated) is recommended as the first-line treatment to decrease the thromboembolic burden on the RV and increase pulmonary perfusion.[51] This recommendation is supported by evidence from a prospective randomized controlled trial, in which patients with cardiogenic shock, RV dysfunction, and acute PE were randomized to either streptokinase (1,500,000 IU) followed by intravenous UFH or intravenous UFH alone.[63] The study was stopped early, because the 4 patients randomized to streptokinase improved in the first hour after treatment, survived and at 2-year follow-up were all without pulmonary arterial hypertension, whereas the 4 patients in the heparin-alone group all died within 1 to 3 hours of arrival in the emergency room. These results were confirmed in a meta-analysis of 5 trials with 254 patients[57] that investigated the effectiveness of thrombolysis in patients with high-risk (massive)

PE and cardiogenic shock. It showed a significant reduction in recurrent PE or death (9.4% vs 19.0%; odds ratio 0.45, 95% confidence interval [CI] 0.22–0.92) with the number needed to treat being 10. However, retrospective data from ICOPER showed that thrombolytic therapy did not significantly reduce 90-day mortality (46.3% vs 55.1%; hazard ratio 0.79; 95% CI, 0.44–1.43) in patients with acute PE and cardiogenic shock (n = 108).[5]

Systemic thrombolysis has also been shown to improve hemodynamic parameters in patients with high-risk PE, compared with heparin alone, including a 12% decrease in vascular obstruction, 30% reduction in mean pulmonary arterial pressure, 15% increase in cardiac index, faster improvement in pulmonary blood flow, and improved reduction in the total perfusion defect.[55,64,65] The potential therapeutic benefit of thrombolysis in these patients needs to be balanced with the risk of bleeding. The risk of nonmajor bleeding is significantly increased and major bleeding nonsignificantly increased in patients receiving thrombolysis compared with heparin. Of the 304 patients who received fibrinolysis in ICOPER, 22% had major bleeding complications and 3% had intracranial bleeding.[5,66]

The guidelines suggest that thrombolytic therapy should be considered for patients with high-risk (massive) PE and an acceptable risk of bleeding complications.[12] Fibrinolysis may be considered for patients with submassive acute PE judged to have clinical evidence of adverse prognosis (new hemodynamic instability, worsening respiratory insufficiency, severe RV dysfunction, or major myocardial necrosis) and low risk of bleeding complications. However, this strategy needs to be balanced with the increasing the risk of bleeding. Thrombolytic therapy should be not used in patients with low-risk (nonmassive) PE or stable patients with intermediate-risk (submassive) PE.

PULMONARY EMBOLECTOMY

Current indications for surgical embolectomy include patients with massive central PE with contraindications to fibrinolysis or those who have persistent hemodynamic compromise or RV dysfunction despite fibrinolytic therapy.[12] In addition, patients with free-floating thrombus within the right atrium or RV or with impending paradoxic embolism through a patent foramen ovale should also undergo surgical intervention.[18,67] Before embarking on surgical embolectomy, it is important to radiologically show a centrally accessible PE, within the main pulmonary trunk, or left or right main pulmonary artery, because patients with most thrombus burden located peripherally do not benefit from surgery.

Standard surgical technique involves a median sternotomy and institution of cardiopulmonary bypass (CPB), usually with bicaval venous cannulation. This technique allows careful inspection of the right atrium, interatrial septum, and the RV. In cases in which thrombus is visible in the right atrium on echocardiography, cannulation of the femoral vein and superior vena cava can be used. To minimize myocardial ischemia, the procedure may be performed using normothermic CPB on a beating heart without cross-clamping the aorta. Access to the thrombus is gained via a curved incision in the main pulmonary artery extending into the left pulmonary artery. An additional incision in the right pulmonary artery (between the ascending aorta and superior vena cava) may also be required. Adequate exposure is gained using CPB suction and short episodes of reduced CPB flow. In some patients, cardioplegic arrest with or without systemic hypothermia is required, for greater periods of circulatory arrest and better visualization during removal of the thrombus; if a patent foramen ovale is present; or if intracardiac thrombi are present.[68,69] A combination of curved forceps, Fogarty catheter, suction catheter, and manual compression of the lungs is used to extract the thrombus from the pulmonary arteries. It is important to extract only visible thrombus, which can be achieved up to the level of the segmental pulmonary arteries, and to avoid blind instrumentation of the fragile pulmonary arteries. Intraoperative transesophageal echocardiography can be used to aid thrombus location and extraction.[70] In these patients, protracted weaning of CPB may be necessary, especially in patients with RV dysfunction. Bleeding may also be a problem, especially in those who have had preoperative thrombolysis. Heparin is started 6 hours after surgery and continued until warfarin is therapeutic. In patients with persistent RV failure after embolectomy, temporary mechanical support using an RV assist device or extracorporeal membrane oxygenation (ECMO) may also be required.[71]

Compared with medical therapy, surgical embolectomy has been shown to have improved outcomes in patients with massive PE. In a nonrandomized study comparing pulmonary embolectomy versus thrombolysis and best medical therapy, patients in the surgical group had reduced mortality and recurrence of PE.[72] In view of this finding, some centers have taken a more aggressive approach and extended the indications to also include patients with anatomically extensive PE with RV dysfunction but in the absence of circulatory shock (intermediate-risk PE).[73]

Previously, outcomes after surgical embolectomy were associated with high in-hospital mortality.[74] With improved surgical techniques and early intervention, current mortality is reported as low as 3.6%.[75] Predictors of early mortality after pulmonary embolectomy include patients with cardiac arrest or undergoing cardiopulmonary resuscitation and those with clot extending peripherally into and beyond the subsegmental arteries.[76] Hemodynamically stable patients who undergo surgical intervention have excellent long-term results, with a recent study reporting 83% 3-year survival.[71] The recurrence rate of PE after surgical embolectomy can be as high as 5%.[77]

Surgical embolectomy provides an excellent therapeutic option for patients with high-risk (massive) PE, with comparable early mortality and significantly fewer bleeding complications than thrombolysis.[72] However, results are worse for those who undergo surgical intervention after cardiopulmonary resuscitation or failed thrombolysis.[75]

CATHETER-DIRECTED THROMBECTOMY

Catheter-directed thrombectomy is an alternative therapeutic strategy that can be used for the treatment of acute PE. It is usually performed in patients with acute high-risk (massive) PE, in whom thrombolysis is contraindicated or has failed, and in whom surgical intervention is not available or contraindicated.[11] However, catheter-directed thrombectomy is not recommended for patients with low-risk PE or patients with intermediate-risk PE, in the absence of hemodynamic instability.[12]

The principal aim of catheter-directed thrombectomy is to achieve rapid debulking of a large central occlusive thrombus to reduce the afterload and strain on the RV, thereby increasing pulmonary and systemic perfusion. However, the fragmentation process redistributes the thrombus into multiple smaller branches further downstream. The hemodynamic consequence of multiple smaller thrombi in a large volume of the peripheral arterial tree is believed to be less significant than that of a central thrombus in the main PA.[78] Furthermore, by breaking up the large central thrombus into smaller fragments, it increases the surface area for exposure of the fibrinolytic agent or intrinsic thrombolytic enzymes to cause thrombus dissolution.[79] Using access via the femoral vein, catheter-directed thrombectomy involves either rheolytic or rotational techniques to disrupt the thrombus, in combination with aspiration of the thrombus fragments. Rheolytic techniques use a high-pressured jet system infusing saline to mechanically disrupt the thrombus.[80] In combination, ultrasound energy can be used to dissociate the fibrin bonds within the thrombus to increase clot permeability and increase the number of plasminogen activation receptor sites for fibrinolysis.[81,82] Rotational techniques involve using a specifically designed thrombectomy catheter, with a covered, high-speed spiral fragmentation tip that rotates at up to 40,000 rpm and also aspirates thrombus fragments.[83]

Complications include distal thrombus embolization, perforation or dissection of the pulmonary artery, injury to the RV, arrhythmia, pulmonary hemorrhage, pericardial tamponade, and femoral venous injury. To reduce the risk of perforation, only pulmonary artery branches greater than 6 mm should be treated, and the procedure should be stopped once the hemodynamic status of the patient improves, irrespective of the angiographic result.[84]

Catheter-directed thrombolysis can be used as an adjunct to catheter-directed thrombectomy.[79] It involves delivering the fibrinolytic agent directly into the pulmonary embolus via a catheter with multiple side holes under fluoroscopic guidance. In combination with catheter-directed thrombectomy, local administration of fibrinolytic agents allows lower doses to be used, because it is delivered directly and the mechanical thrombectomy has increased the surface area of the thrombus available to the drug. The fibrinolytic agent should be injected directly into the thrombus, because any drug injected proximal to the obstructing thrombus is washed out by the local eddy currents into the nonobstructed pulmonary arteries, thereby reducing its therapeutic efficacy.[85] Results of catheter-directed thrombolysis in patients with acute high-risk (massive) PE were examined in a meta-analysis, which described the procedural success of hemodynamic improvement in 86% of patients.[86] However, a prospective, randomized trial failed to show any improvement in PA flow or pressures after local administration of the fibrinolytic agent, compared with systemic administration.[87] In view of this finding, catheter-directed thrombolysis is not recommended in the current guidelines.[12] Although no studies have compared the therapeutic efficacy of surgery and catheter-directed techniques, the PERFECT (Pulmonary Embolism Response to Fragmentation, Embolectomy and Catheter Thrombolysis) registry has been set up to identify the role of catheter-directed therapies in patients with acute PE.

ICU MANAGEMENT

The main cause of death in patients with massive PE is cardiogenic shock related to RV dysfunction.[14] Thus, in addition to standard treatment of the critically ill patient, intensive care management in PE demands consideration of the physiologic role of the RV, knowledge of the mechanisms of RV failure, and the pharmacologic and mechanical options available to the intensivist.

The principal roles of the RV are to act as a conduit for blood flow between the systemic venous return and the lungs; to provide adequate pulmonary flow at an appropriate pressure to allow gas exchange; to maintain low filling pressures and avoid venous congestion and maintain cardiac output; to interact with the pericardium and left heart; and neurohormonal control of the circulation.[88] The right heart has important physiologic differences when compared with the left, which become increasingly important when there is an increase in afterload. It has a lower oxygen requirement (lower myocardial mass, preload, and afterload), greater extraction reserve, and receives perfusion in both systole and diastole.[89] Thus, as afterload increases, there is a high risk of ischemia with perfusion limited to diastole, and more chronically, an increase in myocardial mass. The principles of management of RV failure in the context of increased afterload therefore include ensuring optimal preload, maximizing RV contractility, reducing the pulmonary vascular resistance, and achieving adequate aortic root pressure to maintain right coronary artery perfusion.[90]

OPTIMIZATION OF RV PRELOAD

Although stroke volume from the RV is highly preload-dependent under normal circumstances, in pulmonary hypertension both underfilling and overfilling of the right heart may be deleterious.[91] Measured cardiac output may not be an accurate indicator of potential organ damage caused by RV failure, because the combination of venous hypertension with only a modest reduction in output may be associated with significant organ dysfunction.[92] Fluid studies in animal models of PE are controversial, with some showing volume loading increasing cardiac index but others showing worsening of shock by induction of RV ischemia or reduction in LV filling.[93–95] In the context of massive PE with acute RV failure, a volume challenge may initially increase cardiac output, but continued fluid challenges without careful monitoring may result in RV volume overload, venous hypertension, and a progressive decrease in cardiac output.[96] This situation should be suspected if there is an increase in serum lactate, increase in hepatic enzymes, an abnormal prothrombin time, oliguria, or gastrointestinal dysfunction. Hemodynamic parameters include an increasing V wave on the central venous pressure trace from increasing tricuspid regurgitation and progressive RV dilatation. In such circumstances, reduction in afterload, removal of volume, and escalation of RV support are indicated, including the use of inotropy and mechanical circulatory support.

RV CONTRACTILITY

RV systolic function can be increased with the use of positive inotropic agents or inodilators. Several studies have been conducted in patients with pulmonary hypertension, but no high-quality evidence supports the use of any single vasoactive drug in the context of PE.[97] The most extensively studied inotropic agent is dobutamine.[98] Although low-dose dobutamine (up to 10 μg/kg/min) improves RV contractility in patients with pulmonary vascular dysfunction, it may demand coadministration of pressor agents. Phosphodiesterase 3 inhibitors increase RV contractility and in addition reduce pulmonary vascular resistance, but, again, their effects on the systemic vascular resistance generally require concomitant administration of pressor agents.[99] The novel agent levosimendan has been shown to reduce pulmonary vascular resistance and increase RV contractility in patients with biventricular dysfunction.[100] Although it has been proposed to improve RV-pulmonary artery coupling in patients with PE, evidence for its use is limited. The proarrhythmogenic effects of dopamine significantly limit its use in these patients.

RV AFTERLOAD

The RV is exquisitely sensitive to increases in afterload. Thus, in addition to the pharmacologic, catheter-based, and surgical techniques described to reduce thrombus burden, manipulation of the pulmonary circulation, modification of ventilatory strategies, maintenance of normocarbia, and avoidance of hypoxia may also improve RV function.

Systemic administration of pulmonary vasodilators frequently results in a decrease in systemic blood pressure, with the potential to exacerbate RV ischemia and reduce preload. Administration of inhaled pulmonary vasodilators, including nitric oxide, adenosine, prostanoids, phosphodiesterase 5 inhibitors, milrinone, nigoglycerin, and nitroprusside, may avoid these systemic effects and act to reduce hypoxic vasoconstriction and improve ventilation-perfusion mismatch.[101] There have been reports of inhaled nitric oxide (iNO) effectively reducing pulmonary vascular resistance and increasing cardiac output in patients with PE, most commonly after surgical embolectomy.[102–104] A recent case series reported rapid

and dramatic improvement in hemodynamic parameters and oxygenation in patients with massive PE treated with iNO, suggesting that it should be considered as a temporizing agent pending initiation of definitive treatment (thrombolysis, surgery, or catheter-directed thrombectomy) until pulmonary dynamics have normalized.[105]

Positive pressure ventilation increases RV afterload, and in adult respiratory distress syndrome, high ventilatory pressures have been associated with increased acute cor pulmonale and increased mortality.[106] This potentially adverse effect has to be balanced against the effects of hypoxia and hypercarbia on the pulmonary circulation, when they act to increase pulmonary vascular resistance and hence RV afterload. When ventilation is unavoidable in the context of RV dysfunction, pressures (in particular positive end expiratory and plateau pressures) should be limited as far as possible, and the inspiratory time should be minimized, in particular in patients with restrictive RV physiology.[107]

CORONARY PERFUSION PRESSURE

In the context of pulmonary hypertension, when pulmonary vascular resistance exceeds systemic vascular resistance, right coronary artery filling occurs only in diastole. In this scenario, it is therefore essential to maintain aortic diastolic pressure, to enable coronary perfusion and avoid ischemia. Although augmentation of aortic root pressure with vasopressors is well established, the beneficial effects must be balanced against potentially detrimental pulmonary vasoconstriction. Sympathomimetic agents include the catecholaminergic pressor norepinephrine and the noncatecholaminergic pressor phenylephrine. The effects on the pulmonary vasculature are complex, relating to the dose-dependent α-adrenoreceptor and β-adrenoreceptor stimulation plus the severity of RV dysfunction.[17] Although arginine vasopressin, acting via the V_1 receptor, is a pulmonary vasodilator at low dose, it may cause bradycardia and dose-related myocardial dysfunction at higher doses. However, there is some evidence that low-dose arginine vasopressin may be of use in cases that are resistant to the usual treatments.[108]

MECHANICAL SUPPORT

A range of devices may be considered to maintain cardiac output on the ICU, including optimization of pacing, ventricular assist devices (VAD) and ECMO. In the critically ill patient with RV dysfunction, atrial arrhythmias are poorly tolerated. Therapeutic options should be to restore and maintain sinus rhythm, optimization of fluid and electrolyte balance, treatment of potential triggers (including sepsis), and institution of pharmacotherapy (amiodarone or digoxin).[109] Ensuring optimal electromechanical activity of the heart can be important but complex and must be individualized to each patient.[110] A restrictive right heart that is failing may have a limited stroke volume, requiring a relatively high heart rate to maintain cardiac output. However, patients with pulmonary hypertension may have a long duration of systole (indicated by the duration of tricuspid regurgitation on echocardiography), which limits cardiac filling if the heart rate is excessive. Echocardiography can be used to optimize the heart rate and atrioventricular delay in these patients. When cardiogenic shock is present despite all interventions, patients may be considered for advanced mechanical circulatory support. Several case series have been published using venoarterial ECMO (VA-ECMO), as a bridge to treatment or recovery in patients with massive PE.[111] Potential advantages over VAD include speed of initiation of therapy, normalization of blood oxygen levels, and bypassing the pulmonary bed, thereby avoiding the potential further increase of pulmonary pressures.[112] For patients in cardiogenic shock as a result of massive PE, VA-ECMO can be successful if extracorporeal support is initiated early. Over 48 to 72 hours, emboli generally either resolve or migrate more distally, allowing patients to be weaned from the mechanical support. VA-ECMO and VAD have in addition been reported as a successful bridge to recovery in patients who have undergone pulmonary thrombectomy with CPB support.[113]

INFERIOR VENA CAVA FILTER

An inferior vena cava (IVC) filter should be considered in patients with a contraindication to anticoagulation, major bleeding complication during anticoagulation, recurrent embolism while receiving therapeutic anticoagulation, and usually in patients who have required ECMO after PE.[11,114] The filters are usually placed in the infrarenal IVC (**Fig. 3**) but can be placed in a suprarenal position if thrombus exists just below the renal veins. The filters can be permanent, or retrievable if the patient no longer requires caval interruption.[115] Early complications of IVC filter deployment include device malposition, pneumothorax, hematoma, air embolism, inadvertent carotid artery puncture, and arteriovenous fistula.[116]

The PREPIC trial (Prevention du Risque d'embolie Pulmonaire par Interruption Cave), which randomized 400 patients with proximal deep venous thrombosis at high risk for PE, showed that

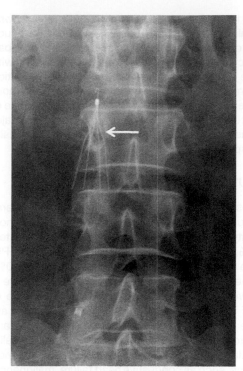

Fig. 3. Fluoroscopic image of a temporary caval filter (*arrow*) positioned in the infrarenal vena cava. (*Courtesy of* Dr Deepa Gopalan, Cambridge, United Kingdom.)

placement of an IVC filter significantly reduced the incidence of recurrent PE at 12 days (1.1% vs 4.8%, P = .03) and at 8 years (6.2% vs 15.1%, P = .008).[117] However, IVC filters were associated with an increased incidence of recurrent deep venous thrombosis (DVT) at 2 years (20.8% vs 11.6%, P = .02) and postthrombotic syndrome (40%). Because the beneficial effects of implanting an IVC filter in reducing the risk of recurrent PE are accompanied by an increased incidence of recurrent DVT with no effect on overall mortality, the use of an IVC filter in patients with acute PE is not routinely recommended.[12]

LONG-TERM ANTICOAGULATION

The long-term treatment of patients after PE is aimed at preventing extension of the thrombus and recurrent venous thromboembolism.[118] This goal is achieved with oral anticoagulation using a vitamin K analogue, such as warfarin, aiming for a target international normalized ratio of 2.5 (range 2.0–3.0). The treatment duration is determined by a balance between the risk of recurrence and risk of anticoagulation-related major bleeding. Anticoagulation is recommended for 3 months after a provoked PE, 6 months for an unprovoked PE, and as long as the cancer is active for patients with malignancy.[119] Newer oral anticoagulants, such as dabigatran (factor IIa inhibitor) and rivaroxaban (factor Xa inhibitor), have been introduced, with the advantage that neither requires dose titration or monitoring.[51] Both have been shown to be non-inferior to warfarin, with respect to the incidence of recurrent venous thromboembolism or major bleeding, in the RECOVER and EINSTEIN trials, respectively.[120,121]

OUTCOMES

Despite the improvement in diagnostic and thera-peutic modalities, contemporary in-hospital mor-tality for patients with PE is still approximately 7%.[5,122] For patients with high-risk (massive) PE, the mortality ranges between 25% and 50%, whereas patients with non–high-risk PE have a lower mortality of 3% to 15%. The presence of RV dysfunction and hemodynamic instability are the most significant predictors of a poor early outcome. Long-term predictors of mortality include age and the presence of comorbid condi-tions, such as congestive heart failure, malignancy, or chronic lung disease. Long-term follow-up of patients after acute PE is required to monitor for the development of chronic thromboembolic pul-monary hypertension.[123]

SUMMARY

PE is common and potentially lethal, with death usually caused by cardiogenic shock from RV fail-ure. Challenges in diagnosis provided by the often nonspecific symptoms and signs may lead to delay in institution of definitive treatment. Despite the availability of pharmacologic, catheter-based, and surgical interventions, mortality remains high. Strategies to avoid DVT and PE in patients judged to be at risk remain pivotal in reducing PE-associated mortality.

ACKNOWLEDGMENTS

We would like to thank Dr Deepa Gopalan, Consultant Radiologist, Papworth Hospital, Uni-versity of Cambridge, UK for the radiology images.

REFERENCES

1. Dalen JE, Alpert JS. Natural history of pulmonary embolism. Prog Cardiovasc Dis 1975;17:259–70.
2. Nordstrom M, Lindblad B. Autopsy-verified venous thromboembolism within a defined urban popula-tion–the city of Malmo, Sweden. APMIS 1998;106: 378–84.
3. Oger E. Incidence of venous thromboembolism: a community-based study in Western France. EPI-GETBP Study Group. Groupe d'Etude de la Throm-bose de Bretagne Occidentale. Thromb Haemost 2000;83:657–60.
4. Silverstein MD, Heit JA, Mohr DN, et al. Trends in the incidence of deep vein thrombosis and pulmo-nary embolism: a 25-year population-based study. Arch Intern Med 1998;158:585–93.
5. Goldhaber SZ, Visani L, De Rosa M. Acute pulmo-nary embolism: clinical outcomes in the Interna-tional Cooperative Pulmonary Embolism Registry (ICOPER). Lancet 1999;353(9162):1386–9.
6. Heit JA, O'Fallon WM, Petterson TM, et al. Relative impact of risk factors for deep vein thrombosis and pulmonary embolism: a population-based study. Arch Intern Med 2002;162:1245–8.
7. Koster T, Rosendaal FR, de Ronde H, et al. Venous thrombosis due to poor anticoagulant response to activated protein C: Leiden Thrombophilia Study. Lancet 1993;342:1503–6.
8. Spencer FA, Emery C, Lessard D, et al. The Worcester Venous Thromboembolism study: a population-based study of the clinical epidemi-ology of venous thromboembolism. J Gen Intern Med 2006;21:722–7.
9. White RH, Zhou H, Romano PS. Incidence of symp-tomatic venous thromboembolism after different elective or urgent surgical procedures. Thromb Haemost 2003;90:446–55.
10. Miller GA, Sutton GC, Kerr IH, et al. Comparison of streptokinase and heparin in treatment of isolated acute massive pulmonary embolism. Br Med J 1971;2:681–4.
11. Torbicki A, Perrier A, Konstantinides S, et al, ESC Committee for Practice Guidelines (CPG). Guide-lines on the diagnosis and management of acute pulmonary embolism: the Task Force for the Diag-nosis and Management of Acute Pulmonary Embo-lism of the European Society of Cardiology (ESC). Eur Heart J 2008;29(18):2276–315.
12. Jaff MR, McMurtry MS, Archer SL, et al, American Heart Association Council on Cardiopulmonary, Crit-ical Care, Perioperative and Resuscitation, American Heart Association Council on Peripheral Vascular Disease, American Heart Association Council on Arteriosclerosis, Thrombosis and Vascular Biology. Management of massive and submassive pulmo-nary embolism, iliofemoral deep vein thrombosis, and chronic thromboembolic pulmonary hyperten-sion: a scientific statement from the American Heart Association. Circulation 2011;123(16):1788–830.
13. Kasper W, Konstantinides S, Geibel A, et al. Man-agement strategies and determinates of outcome in acute major pulmonary embolism: results of a multi-center registry. J Am Coll Cardiol 1997;30: 1165–71.

14. Ten Wolde M, Sohne M, Quak E, et al. Prognostic value of echocardiographically assessed right ventricular dysfunction in patients with pulmonary embolism. Arch Intern Med 2004;164:1685–9.

15. Smulders YM. Pathophysiology and treatment of haemodynamic instability in acute pulmonary embolism: the pivotal role of pulmonary vasoconstriction. Cardiovasc Res 2000;48:23–33.

16. Jardin F, Dubourg O, Bourdarias JP. Echocardiographic pattern of acute cor pulmonale. Chest 1997;111:209–17.

17. Wood KE. Major pulmonary embolism: review of a pathophysiologic approach to the golden hour of hemodynamically significant pulmonary embolism. Chest 2002;121:877–905.

18. Kasper W, Geibel A, Tiede N, et al. Patent foramen ovale in patients with haemodynamically significant pulmonary embolism. Lancet 1992;340:561–4.

19. Wells PS, Anderson DR, Rodger M, et al. Derivation of a simple clinical model to categorize patients probability of pulmonary embolism: increasing the models utility with the SimpliRED D-dimer. Thromb Haemost 2000;83(3):416–20.

20. Le Gal G, Righini M, Roy PM, et al. Prediction of pulmonary embolism in the emergency department: the revised Geneva score. Ann Intern Med 2006;144:165–71.

21. Aujesky D, Obrosky DS, Stone RA, et al. Derivation and validation of a prognostic model for pulmonary embolism. Am J Respir Crit Care Med 2005;172(8):1041–6.

22. van Belle A, Büller HR, Huisman MV, et al, Christopher Study Investigators. Effectiveness of managing suspected pulmonary embolism using an algorithm combining clinical probability, D-dimer testing, and computed tomography. JAMA 2006;295(2):172–9.

23. Worsley DF, Alavi A, Aronchick JM, et al. Chest radiographic findings in patients with acute PE: observations from the PIOPED study. Radiology 1993;189:133–6.

24. Elliott CG, Goldhaber SZ, Visani L, et al. Chest radiographs in acute pulmonary embolism. Results from the International Cooperative Pulmonary Embolism Registry. Chest 2000;118:33–8.

25. Stein PD, Beemath A, Matta F, et al. Clinical characteristics of patients with acute pulmonary embolism: data from PIOPED II. Am J Med 2007;120:871–9.

26. Stein PD, Fowler SE, Goodman LR, et al. Multidetector computed tomography for acute pulmonary embolism. N Engl J Med 2006;354:2317–27.

27. Miniati M, Pistolesi M, Marini C, et al. Value of perfusion lung scan in the diagnosis of pulmonary embolism: results of the Prospective Investigative Study of Acute Pulmonary Embolism Diagnosis (PISA-PED). Am J Respir Crit care Med 1996;154:1387–93.

28. Di Nisio M, Squizzato A, Rutjes AW, et al. Diagnostic accuracy of D-dimer test for exclusion of venous thromboembolism: a systematic review. J Thromb Haemost 2007;5:296–304.

29. Carrier M, Righini M, Djurabi RK, et al. VIDAS D-dimer in combination with clinical pre-test probability to rule out pulmonary embolism. A systematic review of management outcome studies. Thromb Haemost 2009;101:886–92.

30. Righini M, Le Gal G, De Lucia S, et al. Clinical usefulness of D-dimer testing in cancer patients with suspected pulmonary embolism. Thromb Haemost 2006;95:715–9.

31. Shimony A, Filion KB, Mottillo S, et al. Meta-analysis of usefulness of D-dimer to diagnose acute aortic dissection. Am J Cardiol 2011;107(8):1227–34.

32. Kreit JW. The impact of right ventricular dysfunction on the prognosis and therapy of normotensive patients with pulmonary embolism. Chest 2004;125:1539–45.

33. Kjaergaard J, Schaadt BK, Lund JO, et al. Quantitative measures of right ventricular dysfunction by echocardiography in the diagnosis of acute non-massive pulmonary embolism. J Am Soc Echocardiogr 2006;19:1264–71.

34. Fremont B, Pacouret G, Jacobi D, et al. Prognostic value of echocardiographic right/left ventricular end-diastolic diameter ratio in patients with acute pulmonary embolism: results from a monocenter registry of 1,416 patients. Chest 2008;133:358–62.

35. Pruszczyk P, Torbicki A, Kuch-Wocial A, et al. Diagnostic value of transoesophageal echocardiography in suspected haemodynamically significant pulmonary embolism. Heart 2001;85:628–34.

36. Binder L, Pieske B, Olschewski M, et al. N-terminal pro-brain natriuretic peptide or troponin testing followed by echocardiography for risk stratification of acute pulmonary embolism. Circulation 2005;112:1573–9.

37. Douketis JD, Crowther MA, Stanton EB, et al. Elevated cardiac troponin levels in patients with submassive pulmonary embolism. Arch Intern Med 2002;162:79–81.

38. Konstantinides S, Geibel A, Olschewski M, et al. Importance of cardiac troponins I and T in risk stratification of patients with acute pulmonary embolism. Circulation 2002;106:1263–8.

39. Kruger S, Merx MW, Graf J. Utility of brain natriuretic peptide to predict right ventricular dysfunction and clinical outcome in patients with acute pulmonary embolism. Circulation 2003;108:e94–5.

40. Becattini C, Vedovati MC, Agnelli G. Prognostic value of troponins in acute pulmonary embolism: a meta-analysis. Circulation 2007;116:427–33.

41. ten Wolde M, Tulevski II, Mulder JW, et al. Brain natriuretic peptide as a predictor of adverse

outcome in patients with pulmonary embolism. Circulation 2003;107:2082–4.

42. Stein PD, Terrin ML, Hales CA, et al. Clinical, laboratory, roentgenographic, and electrocardiographic findings in patients with acute pulmonary embolism and no pre-existing cardiac or pulmonary disease. Chest 1991;3:598–603.

43. Rodger M, Makropoulos D, Turek M, et al. Diagnostic value of the electrocardiogram in suspected pulmonary embolism. Am J Cardiol 2000;86:807–9 A10.

44. Geibel A, Zehender M, Kasper W, et al. Prognostic value of the ECG on admission in patients with acute major pulmonary embolism. Eur Respir J 2005;25:843–8.

45. Punukollu G, Gowda RM, Vasavada BC, et al. Role of electrocardiography in identifying right ventricular dysfunction in acute pulmonary embolism. Am J Cardiol 2005;96:450–2.

46. Bergqvist D, Lindblad B. A 30-year survey of pulmonary embolism verified at autopsy: an analysis of 1274 surgical patients. Br J Surg 1985;72:105–8.

47. Stulz P, Schlapfer R, Feer R, et al. Decision making in the surgical treatment of massive pulmonary embolism. Eur J Cardiothorac Surg 1994;8:188–93.

48. Quinlan DJ, McQuillan A, Eikelboom JW. Low-molecular-weight heparin compared with intravenous unfractionated heparin for treatment of pulmonary embolism: a meta-analysis of randomized, controlled trials. Ann Intern Med 2004;140:175–83.

49. Warkentin TE, Levine MN, Hirsh J, et al. Heparin-induced thrombocytopenia in patients treated with low-molecular-weight heparin or unfractionated heparin. N Engl J Med 1995;332:1330–5.

50. Buller HR, Davidson BL, Decousus H, et al. Subcutaneous fondapari nux versus intravenous unfractionated heparin in the initial treatment of pulmonary embolism. N Engl J Med 2003;349:1695–702.

51. Kearon C, Akl EA, Comerota AJ, et al, American College of Chest Physicians. Antithrombotic therapy for VTE disease: antithrombotic therapy and prevention of thrombosis, 9th ed: American College of Chest Physicians evidence-based clinical practice guidelines. Chest 2012;141(Suppl 2):e419S–94S.

52. Hull RD, Raskob GE, Rosenbloom D, et al. Heparin for 5 days as compared with 10 days in the initial treatment of proximal venous thrombosis. N Engl J Med 1990;322:1260–4.

53. Warkentin TE, Greinacher A, Koster A, et al, American College of Chest Physicians. Treatment and prevention of heparin-induced thrombocytopenia: American College of Chest Physicians evidence-based clinical practice guidelines (8th edition). Chest 2008;133(Suppl):340S–80S.

54. Bell WR. Present-day thrombolytic therapy: therapeutic agents: pharmacokinetics and pharmacodynamics. Rev Cardiovasc Med 2002; 3(Suppl 2):S34–44.

55. Dalla-Volta S, Palla A, Santolicandro A, et al. PAIMS 2: alteplase combined with heparin versus heparin in the treatment of acute pulmonary embolism. Plasminogen activator Italian multicenter study 2. J Am Coll Cardiol 1992;20:520–6.

56. Dong B, Jirong Y, Liu G, et al. Thrombolytic therapy for pulmonary embolism. Cochrane Database Syst Rev 2006;(8):CD004437.

57. Wan S, Quinlan DJ, Agnelli G, et al. Thrombolysis compared with heparin for the initial treatment of pulmonary embolism: a meta-analysis of the randomized controlled trials. Circulation 2004;110:744–9.

58. Ly B, Arnesen H, Eie H, et al. A controlled clinical trial of streptokinase and heparin in the treatment of major pulmonary embolism. Acta Med Scand 1978;203:465–70.

59. Daniels LB, Parker JA, Patel SR, et al. Relation of duration of symptoms with response to thrombolytic therapy in pulmonary embolism. Am J Cardiol 1997;80:184–8.

60. Konstantinides S, Geibel A, Heusel G, et al, Management Strategies and Prognosis of Pulmonary Embolism-3 Trial Investigators. Heparin plus alteplase compared with heparin alone in patients with submassive pulmonary embolism. N Engl J Med 2002;347:1143–50.

61. Ramakrishnan N. Thrombolysis is not warranted in submassive pulmonary embolism: a systematic review and meta-analysis. Crit Care Resusc 2007; 9(4):357–63.

62. Steering Committee. Single-bolus tenecteplase plus heparin compared with heparin alone for normotensive patients with acute pulmonary embolism who have evidence of right ventricular dysfunction and myocardial injury: rationale and design of the Pulmonary Embolism Thrombolysis (PEITHO) trial. Am Heart J 2012;163(1):33–8.

63. Jerjes-Sanchez C, Ramirez-Rivera A, de Lourdes García M, et al. Streptokinase and heparin versus heparin alone in massive pulmonary embolism: a randomized controlled trial. J Thromb Thrombolysis 1995;2:227–9.

64. Levine M, Hirsh J, Weitz J, et al. A randomized trial of a single bolus dosage regimen of recombinant tissue plasminogen activator in patients with acute pulmonary embolism. Chest 1990;98:1473–9.

65. Goldhaber SZ, Haire WD, Feldstein ML, et al. Alteplase versus heparin in acute pulmonary embolism: randomised trial assessing right-ventricular function and pulmonary perfusion. Lancet 1993; 341:507–11.

66. Fiumara K, Kucher N, Fanikos J, et al. Predictors of major hemorrhage following thrombolysis for acute pulmonary embolism. Am J Cardiol 2006;97:127–9.

67. Torbicki A, Galie N, Covezzoli A, et al. Right heart thrombi in pulmonary embolism: results from the International Cooperative Pulmonary Embolism Registry. J Am Coll Cardiol 2003;41:2245–51.

68. He C, Von Segesser LK, Kappetein PA, et al. Acute pulmonary embolectomy. Eur J Cardiothorac Surg 2013;43(6):1087–95.

69. Aklog L, Williams CS, Byrne JG, et al. Acute pulmonary embolectomy: a contemporary approach. Circulation 2002;105:1416–9.

70. Rosenberger P, Shernan SK, Mihaljevic T, et al. Transesophageal echocardiography for detecting extrapulmonary thrombi during pulmonary embolectomy. Ann Thorac Surg 2004;78(3):862–6.

71. Leacche M, Unic D, Goldhaber SZ, et al. Modern surgical treatment of massive pulmonary embolism: results in 47 consecutive patients after rapid diagnosis and aggressive surgical approach. J Thorac Cardiovasc Surg 2005;129(5):1018–23.

72. Gulba DC, Schmid C, Borst HG, et al. Medical compared with surgical treatment for massive pulmonary embolism. Lancet 1994;343(8897):576–7.

73. Sareyyupoglu B, Greason KL, Suri RM, et al. A more aggressive approach to emergency embolectomy for acute pulmonary embolism. Mayo Clin Proc 2010;85(9):785–90.

74. Clarke DB, Abrams LD. Pulmonary embolectomy: a 25 year experience. J Thorac Cardiovasc Surg 1986;92(3 Pt 1):442–5.

75. Aymard T, Kadner A, Widmer A, et al. Massive pulmonary embolism: surgical embolectomy versus thrombolytic therapy–should surgical indications be revisited? Eur J Cardiothorac Surg 2013;43(1):90–4.

76. Ullmann M, Hemmer W, Hannekum A. The urgent pulmonary embolectomy: mechanical resuscitation in the operating theatre determines the outcome. Thorac Cardiovasc Surg 1999;47:5–8.

77. Gray HH, Morgan JM, Paneth M, et al. Pulmonary embolectomy for acute massive pulmonary embolism. An analysis of 71 cases. Br Heart J 1988;60:196–200.

78. Girard P, Simonneau G. Catheter fragmentation of pulmonary emboli. Chest 1999;115:1759.

79. Kuo WT. Endovascular therapy for acute pulmonary embolism. J Vasc Interv Radiol 2012;23(2):167–79.

80. Chechi T, Vecchio S, Spaziani G, et al. Rheolytic thrombectomy in patients with massive and submassive acute pulmonary embolism. Catheter Cardiovasc Interv 2009;73:506–13.

81. Chamsuddin A, Nazzal L, Kang B, et al. Catheter-directed thrombolysis with the Endowave system in the treatment of acute massive pulmonary embolism: a retrospective multicenter case series. J Vasc Interv Radiol 2008;19:372–6.

82. Francis CW, Blinc A, Lee S, et al. Ultrasound accelerates transport of recombinant tissue plasminogen activator into clots. Ultrasound Med Biol 1995;21:419–24.

83. Schmitz-Rode T, Janssens U, Duda SH, et al. Massive pulmonary embolism: percutaneous emergency treatment by pigtail rotation catheter. J Am Coll Cardiol 2000;36:375–80.

84. Biederer J, Charalambous N, Paulsen F, et al. Treatment of acute pulmonary embolism: local effects of three hydrodynamic thrombectomy devices in an ex vivo porcine model. J Endovasc Ther 2006;13:549–60.

85. Schmitz-Rode T, Kilbinger M, Gunther RW. Simulated flow pattern in massive pulmonary embolism: significance for selective intrapulmonary thrombolysis. Cardiovasc Intervent Radiol 1998;21:199–204.

86. Kuo WT, Gould MK, Louie JD, et al. Catheter-directed therapy for the treatment of massive pulmonary embolism: systematic review and meta-analysis of modern techniques. J Vasc Interv Radiol 2009;20:1431–40.

87. Verstraete M, Miller GA, Bounameaux H, et al. Intravenous and intrapulmonary recombinant tissue-type plasminogen activator in the treatment of acute massive pulmonary embolism. Circulation 1988;77:353–60.

88. Voelkel NF, Quaife RA, Leinwand LA, et al. Right ventricular function and failure: report of a National Heart, Lung, and Blood Institute Working Group on Cellular and Molecular Mechanisms of Right Heart Failure. Circulation 2006;114:1883–91.

89. Lee FA. Hemodynamics of the right ventricle in normal and disease states. Cardiol Clin 1992;10:59–67.

90. Prewitt RM. Hemodynamic management in pulmonary embolism and acute hypoxemic respiratory failure. Crit Care Med 1990;18:S61–9.

91. Mercat A, Diehl JL, Meyer G, et al. Hemodynamic effects of fluid loading in acute massive pulmonary embolism. Crit Care Med 1999;27:540–4.

92. Piazza G, Goldhaber SZ. The acutely decompensated right ventricle. Pathways for diagnosis and management. Chest 2005;128:1836–52.

93. Molloy DW, Lee KY, Girling L, et al. Treatment of shock in a canine model of pulmonary embolism. Am Rev Respir Dis 1984;130:870–4.

94. Belenkie I, Dani R, Smith ER, et al. Effects of volume loading during experimental acute pulmonary embolism. Circulation 1989;80:178–88.

95. Ghignoue M, Girling L, Prewitt RM. Volume expansion vs. norepinephrine in treatment of low cardiac output complicating an acute increase in right ventricular afterload in dogs. Anesthesiology 1984;60:132–5.

96. Ducas J, Prewitt RM. Pathophysiology and therapy of right ventricular dysfunction due to pulmonary embolism. Cardiovasc Clin 1987;17:191–202.

97. Layish DT, Tapson VF. Pharmacologic hemodynamic support in massive pulmonary embolism. Chest 1997;111:218–24.

98. Jardin F, Genevray B, Brun-Ney D, et al. Dobutamine: a hemodynamic evaluation in pulmonary embolism shock. Crit Care Med 1985;13:1009–12.

99. Kucher N, Goldhaber SZ. Management of massive pulmonary embolism. Circulation 2005; 112(2):e28–32.

100. Kerbaul F, Gariboldi V, Giorgi R, et al. Effects of levosimendan on acute pulmonary embolism-induced right ventricular failure. Crit Care Med 2007;35: 1948–54.

101. Webb SA, Stott S, van Heerden PV. The use of inhaled aerosolized prostacyclin (IAP) in the treatment of pulmonary hypertension secondary to pulmonary embolism. Intensive Care Med 1996;22: 353–5.

102. Capelller G, Jacques I, Balvay P, et al. Inhaled nitric oxide in patients with pulmonary embolism. Intensive Care Med 1997;23:1089–92.

103. Moreno H Jr, Tanus-Santos JE. Nitric oxide inhalation during massive pulmonary embolism. Anesth Analg 1999;88:1188.

104. Szold O, Khoury W, Biderman P, et al. Inhaled nitric oxide improves pulmonary functions following massive pulmonary embolism: a report of four patients and review of the literature. Lung 2006;184: 1–5.

105. Summerfield DT, Desai H, Levitov A, et al. Inhaled nitric oxide as salvage therapy in massive pulmonary embolism: a case series. Respir Care 2012; 57(3):444–8.

106. Jardin F, Vieillard-Baron A. Is there a safe plateau pressure in ARDS? The right heart only knows. Intensive Care Med 2007;33(3):444–7.

107. Sevransky JE, Levy MM, Marini JJ. Mechanical ventilation in sepsis-induced acute lung injury/acute respiratory distress syndrome: an evidence-based review. Crit Care Med 2004; 32(Suppl 11):S548–53.

108. Price LC, Wort SJ, Finney SJ, et al. Pulmonary vascular and right ventricular dysfunction in adult critical care: current and emerging options for management: a systematic literature review. Crit Care 2010;14(5):R169.

109. Rich S, Seidlitz M, Dodin E, et al. The short-term effects of digoxin in patients with right ventricular dysfunction from pulmonary hypertension. Chest 1998;114:787–92.

110. Dubin AM, Feinstein JA, Reddy VM, et al. Electrical resynchronization: a novel therapy for the failing right ventricle. Circulation 2003;107:2287–9.

111. Malekan R, Saunders PC, Yu CJ, et al. Peripheral extracorporeal membrane oxygenation: comprehensive therapy for high-risk massive pulmonary embolism. Ann Thorac Surg 2012;94(1):104–8.

112. Belohlavek J, Rohn V, Jansa P, et al. Veno-arterial ECMO in severe acute right ventricular failure with pulmonary obstructive hemodynamic pattern. J Invasive Cardiol 2010;22(8):365–9.

113. Lango R, Kowalik MM, Klajbor K, et al. Circulatory support with right ventricular assist device and intra-aortic balloon counterpulsation in patient with right ventricle failure after pulmonary embolectomy. Interact CardioVasc Thorac Surg 2008;7:643–5.

114. ELSO Guidelines for Cardiopulmonary Extracorporeal Life Support. Extracorporeal Life Support Organization; 2009. Version 1:1.

115. Kaufman JA, Kinney TB, Streiff MB, et al. Guidelines for the use of retrievable and convertible vena cava filters: report from the Society of Interventional Radiology multidisciplinary consensus conference. J Vasc Interv Radiol 2006;17:449–59.

116. Sarosiek S, Crowther M, Sloan JM. Indications, complications, and management of inferior vena cava filters: the experience in 952 patients at an academic hospital with a level I trauma center. JAMA Intern Med 2013;173(7):513–7.

117. Decousus H, Leizorovicz A, Parent F, et al. A clinical trial of vena caval filters in the prevention of pulmonary embolism in patients with proximal deep-vein thrombosis: Prevention du Risque d'Embolie Pulmonaire par Interruption Cave Study Group. N Engl J Med 1998;338:409–15.

118. Hull R, Delmore T, Genton E, et al. Warfarin sodium versus low-dose heparin in the long-term treatment of venous thrombosis. N Engl J Med 1979;301:855–8.

119. Kearon C, Gent M, Hirsh J, et al. A comparison of three months of anticoagulation with extended anticoagulation for a first episode of idiopathic venous thromboembolism. N Engl J Med 1999;340:901–7.

120. Schulman S, Kearon C, Kakkar AK, et al, RECOVER Study Group. Dabigatran versus warfarin in the treatment of acute venous thromboembolism. N Engl J Med 2009;361:2342–52.

121. EINSTEIN–PE Investigators, Büller HR, Prins MH, Lensin AW, et al. Oral rivaroxaban for the treatment of symptomatic pulmonary embolism. N Engl J Med 2012;366(14):1287–97.

122. Casazza F, Becattini C, Bongarzoni A, et al. Clinical features and short term outcomes of patients with acute pulmonary embolism. The Italian Pulmonary Embolism Registry (IPER). Thromb Res 2012; 130(6):847–52.

123. Pepke-Zaba J, Delcroix M, Lang I, et al. Chronic thromboembolic pulmonary hypertension (CTEPH): results from an international prospective registry. Circulation 2011;124(18):1973–81.

Mechanical Complications of Acute Myocardial Infarction

Ramesh S. Kutty, MBBS, MRCS[a],
Nicola Jones, MA, BM BCh, MRCP, FRCA, FFICM[b],
Narain Moorjani, MB ChB, MRCS, MD, FRCS (C-Th)[a],*

KEYWORDS

- Acute myocardial infarction • Ventricular septal rupture • Papillary muscle rupture
- Left ventricular free wall rupture • Infarct exclusion technique

KEY POINTS

- The major mechanical complications after acute myocardial infarction (AMI) include rupture of the left ventricular free wall, papillary muscle rupture, and ventricular septal rupture.
- Primary percutaneous coronary intervention has significantly reduced major mechanical complications since its introduction as a treatment strategy in AMI.
- Echocardiography with color-flow Doppler is the investigation of choice in the diagnosis and differentiation of the conditions.
- Preoperative optimization, with an intra-aortic balloon pump and vasodilators, may help to reduce the afterload on the compromised ventricle following AMI and may improve cardiac output in the short term, but should not delay expedient surgical intervention.
- Surgical intervention remains the mainstay of treatment in patients with mechanical complications of AMI, with dismal outcomes for patients treated medically.

INTRODUCTION

Acute myocardial infarction (AMI) can result in ischemic, mechanical, arrhythmic, embolic, or inflammatory complications. The development of mechanical complications following AMI is associated with a significantly reduced short-term and long-term survival (**Fig. 1**).[1] Since the introduction of primary percutaneous coronary intervention (PCI) as the principal reperfusion strategy following acute ST-elevation myocardial infarction (STEMI), the incidence of mechanical complications has reduced significantly to less than 1%, including rupture of the left ventricular free wall (0.52%), papillary muscle (0.26%), and ventricular septum (0.17%).[1]

VENTRICULAR SEPTAL RUPTURE
Introduction

Ventricular septal rupture (VSR) represents a defect in the interventricular septum caused by ischaemic necrosis following AMI. Before the introduction of thrombolysis and primary PCI, VSR occurred in 1% to 2% of patients following AMI and usually presented between 3 and 5 days after AMI.[2,3] Since the introduction of early reperfusion therapy, however, the incidence

The authors have nothing to disclose.
[a] Department of Cardiothoracic Surgery, Papworth Hospital, University of Cambridge, Cambridge CB23 3RE, UK; [b] Department of Cardiothoracic Intensive Care, Papworth Hospital, University of Cambridge, Cambridge CB23 3RE, UK
* Corresponding author.
E-mail address: narain.moorjani@papworth.nhs.uk

Cardiol Clin 31 (2013) 519–531
http://dx.doi.org/10.1016/j.ccl.2013.07.004
0733-8651/13/$ – see front matter © 2013 Elsevier Inc. All rights reserved.

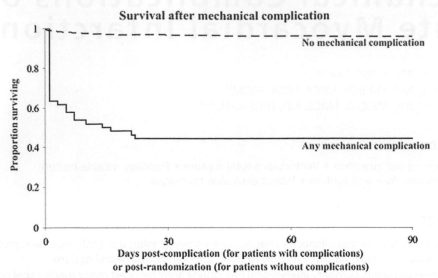

Fig. 1. Ninety-day survival following acute myocardial infarction, comparing patients with and without mechanical complications. (*From* French JK, Hellkamp AS, Armstrong PW, et al. Mechanical complications after percutaneous coronary intervention in ST elevation myocardial infarction (from APEX-AMI). Am J Cardiol 2010;105:62; with permission.)

of VSR has decreased to 0.17% and is usually diagnosed within the first 24 hours following presentation of AMI.[4]

Pathophysiology

VSR occurs following a transmural infarct, and may be subclassified into simple and complex VSR.[5] A simple VSR represents a single defect with openings in both ventricles at approximately the same level, whereas a complex VSR represents a meshwork of serpiginous channels with hemorrhage and disruption of myocardial tissue, which are more commonly found following posteroinferior AMI.

Before the introduction of early reperfusion, risk factors for VSR included hypertension, age, female sex, and the absence of previous history of ischemic heart disease (angina or myocardial infarction [MI]).[6–8] The presence of angina or MI may have led to development of collateral coronary vessels as well as myocardial preconditioning, both of which reduce the risk of a transmural infarct and subsequent VSR development.[8] In patients undergoing thrombolysis, advanced age, female sex, and the absence of smoking have been described as risk factors for the development of VSR, whereas the absence of prior angina or infarction has not been associated with an increased risk.[5,9]

AMI complicated with VSR can progress into left ventricular (LV) or right ventricular (RV) failure, cardiogenic shock, and potentially irreversible

end-organ malperfusion.[10] The immediate effect of VSR is shunting of blood from the left to the right ventricle. The magnitude of this shunt is determined by the left- and right-sided pressures, as well as the size of the defect, which in turn determines the extent of hemodynamic compromise. Whereas LV dysfunction is related to the extent of the AMI, RV dysfunction is related to the volume overload produced by the intraventricular shunt as well as the initial infarct.

Diagnosis

Patients characteristically present for the first time following AMI, with no previous history of angina and with increasing dyspnea, often deteriorating rapidly into cardiogenic shock.[11] A harsh pansystolic murmur, which is heard loudest at the left sternal edge, is present in 90% of patients, with a parasternal thrill palpable in 50% of patients.[12] Mitral regurgitation (MR) secondary to papillary muscle rupture is an important differential diagnosis but has a murmur loudest at the apex.

Electrocardiography confirms primarily an anterior or inferior STEMI, with an associated atrioventricular conduction block noted in approximately 40% of patients.[13] Chest radiography is generally nonspecific and may demonstrate cardiomegaly, pulmonary congestion, or pleural effusions.

Echocardiography with color-flow Doppler is the gold standard for diagnosis, monitoring, and planning treatment, distinguishing between papillary muscle rupture and VSR, as well as assessing

LV and RV function. The sensitivity and specificity of color Doppler echocardiography has been reported in the literature to be as high as 100%.[14,15] Echocardiography can identify the rupture, characterize the site and size of the defect, and the estimate the degree of left-to-right shunt by assessing flow across the pulmonary and aortic valves.

Although right heart catheterization has now been superseded by echocardiography as a diagnostic tool, it can help to provide a diagnosis if the echocardiographic data are unclear. A demonstrated "step-up" between samples taken from the right atrium and pulmonary artery confirms the presence of a ventricular shunt.[16] The ratio of flows between the pulmonary and systemic circulations provides an estimate of the size of the shunt. The excess pulmonary blood flow represents the amount of blood passing through the defect. Oxygen saturation samples are taken simultaneously to estimate the pulmonary to systemic flow ratio from the right atrium (Svo_2), pulmonary artery ($Spao_2$), and systemic artery (Sao_2), which represents aortic saturations. Oxygen saturations from the pulmonary veins ($Spvo_2$) are not usually measured, but are assumed in a patient with healthy lungs to be fully oxygenated at 100%. The shunt ratio can then be calculated by the following formula:

$$Q_p/Q_s = (Sao_2 - Svo_2)/(Spvo_2 - Spao_2)$$

where Q_p is pulmonary blood flow and Q_s is systemic blood flow.

A Q_p/Q_s ratio of greater than 2 suggests a large shunt, which is usually poorly tolerated by patients. Standard pulmonary artery catheter reference values need to be interpreted with caution in patients with a shunt, and other continuous real-time hemodynamic monitoring tools, such as the LiDCO (London, UK) or PiCCO (Pulsion AG, Munich, Germany) systems, may be more useful.[17]

Preoperative Resuscitation and Optimization

Patients presenting with VSR are often in extremis, secondary to acute pulmonary congestion. Management of these patients may require intubation for a definitive airway or noninvasive ventilatory support. The mainstay of medical treatment is to achieve afterload reduction, using pharmacologic and nonpharmacologic methods.[18]

Pharmacologic agents include angiotensin-converting enzyme inhibitors, intravenous nitrates, or hydralazine.[19,20] Phosphodiesterase-3 inhibitors, such as milrinone and enoximone, are also used as inodilators, as they increase myocardial contractility as well as producing vasodilation.[21,22]

The calcium sensitizer, levosimendan, has also been used to beneficial effect to counteract the ventricular stunning associated with reperfusion injury following AMI.[23] Levosimendan improves ventricular function as it acts as a positive inotrope by increasing the sensitivity of myofilaments to calcium by binding to troponin C, thereby increasing contractility without increasing myocardial oxygen consumption. It also has vasodilatory effects, thereby reducing preload and afterload as well as increasing coronary blood flow. Patients with significant RV dysfunction may also benefit from pulmonary vasodilators, such as inhaled nitric oxide.[24]

Nonpharmacologic measures include the use of an intra-aortic balloon pump (IABP),[25] the Impella Recover device (Abiomed, Aachen, Germany),[26] extracorporeal membrane oxygenation (ECMO),[27] a ventricular assist device (VAD),[28] a total artificial heart[29] to unload the failing myocardium, and hemofiltration to treat the volume overload and manage fluid status.[30] Insertion of an IABP decreases LV afterload, thereby reducing the volume of the shunt, and improves coronary blood flow. The resultant increased cardiac output produces improved systemic pressures and end-organ perfusion. The quest for optimization, however, should not delay definitive surgical treatment.

Operative Technique

Standard surgical repair of a postinfarction VSR involves using the infarct exclusion technique (Fig. 2).[31] This procedure comprises a left ventriculotomy through the infarcted anterior or inferior wall, 2 to 3 cm parallel to the left anterior descending artery or posterior descending artery, respectively. A glutaraldehyde-fixed bovine pericardial patch is then sutured to healthy endocardium deep in the left ventricle, to exclude the infarct and VSR from the high-pressure area of the left ventricle. This patch is then brought out through the ventriculotomy and incorporated in the closure. The ventriculotomy is closed in 2 layers, buttressed by Teflon strips. Using this technique, LV geometry and volume can be restored. Surgical repair of a posterior VSR is technically more difficult because of access to the inferobasal LV wall, especially involving necrotic and friable myocardium immediately after an AMI. Involvement of the posteromedial papillary muscle, either in the ischemic area of the infarct or by the suture line of the repair, increases the risk of papillary muscle dysfunction with resultant compromise of the mitral valve apparatus. In these patients, concomitant mitral valve repair or replacement might be required. Once surgical repair of the

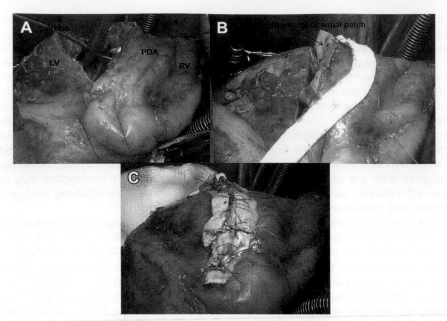

Fig. 2. Operative images demonstrating (*A*) posterior ventricular septal rupture, illustrated following ventriculotomy with the probe passing from the left ventricle through the defect in the ventricular septum into the right ventricle; (*B*) exclusion of the infarct and septal rupture, by suturing a bovine pericardial patch to noninfarcted muscle deep in the left ventricle; and (*C*) 2-layered closure of the ventriculotomy, buttressed by Teflon felt strips and BioGlue. LV, left ventricle; PDA, posterior descending artery; RV, right ventricle.

VSR is complete, coronary artery bypass grafting (CABG) is completed.

Percutaneous closure

The role of percutaneous devices to primarily close defects following VSR is limited at present to selected patients with simple defects that are less than 15 mm in diameter and after approximately 3 weeks following AMI.[32] Percutaneous closure has also been used in the acute setting, with variable results.[33] VSR without a suitable rim or a basal VSR in the vicinity of the mitral apparatus or the aortic valve represent a contraindication to percutaneous closure. In the majority of cases, rapid hemodynamic stabilization occurs by reducing the left-to-right shunt, and may provide a bridge to definitive surgery.[34] Percutaneous closure devices are also used for patients with residual defects after surgical repair.

Postoperative management

The principal goal of postoperative care in these patients is optimizing cardiac output and reversing any end-organ dysfunction that may have occurred following the AMI or in the perioperative period.[35] This care involves continuation of preoperative cardiac support, including the use of an IABP, positive inotropic agents, antiarrhythmic agents, and vasodilatory agents, to reduce the preload and afterload on the impaired myocardium. In

particular, optimization of RV function may be required with phosphodiesterase-3 inhibitors, nitric oxide, or an RV assist device. In addition, renal replacement therapy with hemodialysis, nasogastric feeding, and prolonged ventilator support is often required in these patients.

Controversial Issues

Should surgery be performed on all patients with a VSR?

Although current guidelines recommend immediate surgical treatment for patients with VSR following AMI to avoid end-organ failure and improve survival, certain patients are likely to have a poor outcome despite optimal medical or surgical management.[36] Risk factors predisposing patients to increased operative mortality include cardiogenic shock, age, RV failure, and renal impairment.[37] Some patients with multiple comorbid risk factors may be best suited to a trial of maximal nonoperative management, and undergo operative intervention if they can be hemodynamically stabilized.[38]

Concomitant coronary revascularization or not?

There has previously been controversy in the surgical literature over the benefits of concomitant CABG at the time of surgical VSR repair. Initial studies demonstrated that concomitant CABG did not confer a long-term survival advantage and that performing a left heart catheterization is time consuming, which may contribute to perioperative morbidity and mortality in these already hemodynamically compromised patients.[39] In most series, however, more than 60% of patients with septal rupture have significant involvement of at least 1 vessel in the noninfarcted area.[40] More recently, incomplete myocardial revascularization has been demonstrated to be a significant predictor of late mortality following surgical repair of postinfarction VSR.[41] In view of this, concomitant CABG to all stenotic coronary arteries, including those supplying the noninfarcted area, is recommended for patients undergoing surgical repair of VSR.[42] The improvement of the collateral flow to the myocardium is thought to contribute to enhanced ventricular recovery.

Is there a role for delayed surgery?

The strategy of operating following stabilization for around 6 weeks, often with IABP counterpulsation, is an attractive option, as it allows an infarcted septum to "mature" with fibrotic healing.[43] The sickest patients fail to survive this trial of delayed surgery, through a process of "unnatural selection."[44] As outcomes of immediate and delayed surgery have been shown to be similar, more patients who otherwise may not survive to 6 weeks could potentially be saved by early surgery.[38] The use of nonpharmacologic cardiac support in acute VSR management is predominantly limited to IABP support. However, in some patients who are at high risk of perioperative death but in whom surgery cannot be safely deferred, the use of mechanical circulatory support, such as using an ECMO circuit or Impella Recover device, may provide hemodynamic stability and the potential to correct multiorgan dysfunction, until a definitive procedure is performed.[26–28]

Outcomes

Patients treated medically have a universally dismal prognosis, with 24% mortality at 24 hours, 46% mortality at 1 week, and 82% mortality within 2 months.[45] In a review of 64 patients presenting with VSR, medically treated patients had a 30-day mortality of 100% (**Fig. 3**).[10]

Recent data from the Society of Thoracic Surgeons registry of 2876 patients presenting with postinfarction VSR demonstrated an overall operative mortality of 42.9%.[46] Patients who underwent surgical repair within 7 days from MI (54.1%) had a higher operative morality compared with those in whom the surgical repair was performed more than 7 days following the MI (18.4%). Multivariable analysis identified several factors associated with increased risk of operative death, including preoperative dialysis, age, female sex, cardiogenic shock, preoperative IABP, mitral insufficiency, and redo cardiac operation.[45] The Swedish national registry data of 189 patients undergoing surgical repair of postinfarction VSR reported a 30-day mortality rate of 41% and 5 year survival of 38% (**Fig. 4**).[47] For patients that survived the first 30 days (n = 112), the 5-year cumulative survival was 67%. The investigators observed that posterior septal rupture was independently associated with an increased risk of operative death.

Summary of Ventricular Septal Rupture

VSR requires the expeditious stabilization of a hemodynamically compromised patient followed by

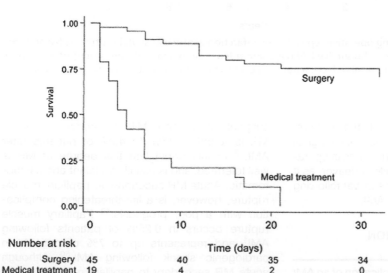

Fig. 3. Short-term cumulative survival in medically and surgically treated patients. (*From* Poulsen SH, Praestholm M, Munk K, et al. Ventricular septal rupture complicating acute myocardial infarction: clinical characteristics and contemporary outcome. Ann Thorac Surg 2008;85(5):1593; with permission.)

Number at risk				
Surgery	45	40	35	34
Medical treatment	19	4	2	0

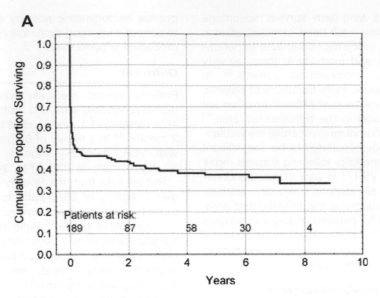

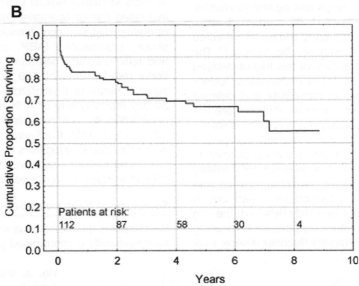

Fig. 4. Cumulative survival following operative repair of postinfarction ventricular septal rupture in (*A*) all surgical patients and (*B*) surgical patients who survived 30 days. (*From* Jeppsson A, Liden H, Johnsson P, et al. Surgical repair of post infarction ventricular septal defects: a national experience. Eur J Cardiothorac Surg 2005;27:217–8; with permission.)

prompt surgical management of the rupture. Despite the high mortality associated with surgical repair of VSR, good long-term outcomes in operative survivors make it a worthwhile endeavor, as it is potentially the only option for survival following this mechanical complication of AMI.

ACUTE MITRAL REGURGITATION
Introduction

Acute MR is a catastrophic complication of an AMI that, if recognized, is amenable to emergent

surgical intervention. Mild to moderate chronic MR is found in 15% to 45% of patients after AMI.[48] In this population this degree of MR is well tolerated, and is usually transient and asymptomatic. Acute MR secondary to papillary muscle rupture, however, is a life-threatening complication with a poor prognosis.[49] Papillary muscle rupture occurs in 0.25% of patients following AMI[1] and represents up to 7% of patients in cardiogenic shock following AMI.[50] Although acute MR secondary to papillary muscle rupture is usually diagnosed between 2 to 7 days after

AMI, the median time to papillary muscle rupture is approximately 13 hours.[36] Papillary muscle rupture following AMI may be partial (occurring at either one of the muscle heads) or complete.

Pathophysiology

Following AMI, papillary muscle dysfunction or rupture, in combination with changes in LV shape and regional wall function, results in acute MR.[49,51] Even slight modifications of LV geometry caused by regional wall-motion abnormality may contribute to the increased frequency of MR after AMI.[52] In the acute setting, pulmonary edema and cardiogenic shock may ensue, as there is not enough time for the left ventricle to dilate or compensate. Acute MR secondary to papillary muscle dysfunction or rupture occurs most commonly following an inferior MI, owing to the single blood supply to the posteromedial papillary muscle from the posterior descending coronary artery.[53,54] The anterolateral papillary muscle, however, has a dual blood supply (left anterior descending and circumflex coronary arteries) and, therefore, is more likely to be protected following an AMI in a single-vessel territory.

Diagnosis

When acute MR accompanies complete papillary muscle rupture, patients may present with immediate pulmonary edema, hypotension, and, in some cases, cardiogenic shock. A new pansystolic murmur is heard loudest at the cardiac apex, with a diastolic component, and radiates to the axilla. VSR secondary to AMI is an important differential diagnosis, and can be distinguished by a harsh pansystolic murmur heard loudest at the left sternal edge.

Electrocardiography usually confirms an inferior or posterior MI. Chest radiography demonstrates pulmonary edema, which occasionally is localized to the right upper lobe, if the flow is directed at the right superior pulmonary vein.[55]

Echocardiography with color-flow Doppler is the standard for diagnosis, monitoring, and planning of surgical treatment, distinguishing between papillary muscle rupture and VSR, as well as assessing LV and RV function. It usually identifies either a flail chord or papillary muscle, with resultant leaflet prolapse and MR.[56] Echocardiography usually overestimates the LV function, as the ventricle is hyperdynamic in the presence of MR. Transesophageal echocardiography is particularly useful in identifying the anatomy of the mitral valve and demonstrating the pathology of the MR (**Fig. 5**).

Right heart catheterization has limited use in the diagnosis of acute MR, but can be useful in differentiating it from VSR (see earlier discussion). The pulmonary capillary wedge pressure (PCWP) trace may show giant V waves but these are generally

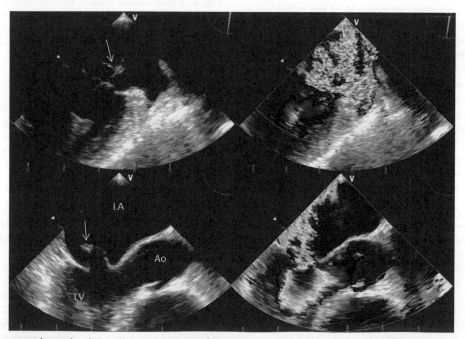

Fig. 5. Transesophageal echocardiogram images demonstrating prolapse of the anterior mitral valve leaflet, secondary to flail papillary muscle (*arrow*), and corresponding color-flow Doppler images illustrating a resultant posteriorly directed jet of severe mitral regurgitation. Ao, aorta; LA, left atrium; LV, left ventricle.

nonspecific, as they may also be seen in VSR or severe LV failure.[57]

Treatment

Prompt diagnosis with immediate initiation of aggressive medical therapy is vital until emergent surgical intervention can be performed. Urgent cardiac catheterization needs to be performed to identify coronary anatomy, as concomitant revascularization during mitral valve surgery is associated with improved short-term and long-term outcomes (**Fig. 6**).[58,59]

Medical therapy aims to reduce the afterload, with a resultant decreased regurgitant fraction and increased forward stroke volume and cardiac output.[60] This goal can be achieved pharmacologically with vasodilators and inodilators, such as nitrites, sodium nitroprusside, diuretics, and phosphodiesterase-3 inhibitors.[61,62] Intra-aortic balloon counterpulsation during acute MR decreases afterload, resulting in less MR and more forward flow from the left ventricle into the aorta.[25] Similarly to patients with VSR, these patients may also benefit from mechanical cardiac support, such as an Impella Recover device,[26] ECMO circuit,[27] or VAD.[28] In addition, positive-pressure ventilation is used with great effect in such patients with acute pulmonary edema and pulmonary congestion.[63] As medical therapy is associated with a very poor survival, emergent surgery remains the cornerstone of treatment.[58] During the operation, careful assessment of the mitral valve and the subvalvular apparatus will allow for decision making regarding repair or replacement. If there is evidence of papillary muscle necrosis or there are concerns about subtle, ongoing progression of ischemic injury, mitral valve replacement provides a definitive treatment of the failing mitral valve apparatus.[64] Intra-aortic balloon counterpulsation should continue for at least 24 hours following surgery, in addition to the supportive postoperative care that will be required for these patients with multiorgan dysfunction (see the section on postoperative management of VSR).[65]

Outcomes

Acute postinfarction MR is associated with an in-hospital mortality of between 70% and 80% with medical treatment.[49] In the largest series of patients (N = 126) who underwent surgical intervention for papillary muscle rupture, operative mortality was 26.9% with a 15-year survival of 39%.[58] Although there was no difference in early mortality between patients undergoing concomitant CABG and those who were not revascularized at the time of emergent mitral surgery (CABG

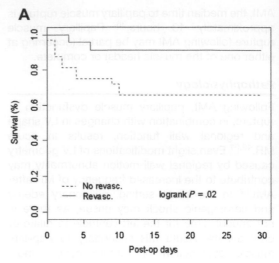

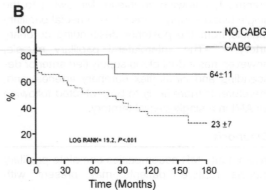

Fig. 6. Kaplan-Meier graphs demonstrating (*A*) perioperative and (*B*) 15-year actuarial survival benefit in patients undergoing concomitant coronary revascularization following acute postinfarction mitral regurgitation. ([A] *From* Chevalier P, Burri H, Fahrat F, et al. Perioperative outcome and long-term survival of surgery for acute post-infarction mitral regurgitation. Eur J Cardiothorac Surg 2004;26(2): 332, with permission; and [B] *Adapted from* Lorusso R, Gelsomino S, De Cicco G, et al. Mitral valve surgery in emergency for severe acute regurgitation: analysis of postoperative results from a multicentre study. Eur J Cardiothorac Surg 2008;33(4):577, with permission.)

27.3% vs no CABG 26.4%; *P*>.9), long-term survival was significantly improved in patients undergoing concomitant revascularization at 15 years (CABG 64% vs no CABG 23%; *P*<.001). In a more recent study, concomitant CABG has also been shown to improve operative mortality (odds ratio 0.18; 95% confidence interval 0.04–0.83; *P* = .011).[66] However, no significant difference in 5-year survival has been demonstrated between mitral valve repair or mitral valve replacement in this patient cohort (62.1% vs 66.7%; *P* = .48).[66]

Of note, the 5-year survival rate of the operative survivors following surgical repair of postinfarction papillary muscle rupture (79.4%) is similar to that of matched controls with an uncomplicated MI.[66]

Summary of Acute Mitral Regurgitation

Patients presenting with the catastrophic mechanical complication of acute MR secondary to papillary muscle rupture following MI benefit from combined mitral valve surgery and myocardial revascularization, with satisfactory early and late outcomes despite the increased operative mortality. Mitral valve replacement rather than repair may be indicated in patients following acute papillary muscle rupture, or in cases with severe restriction of the mitral valve caused by papillary muscle dysfunction after AMI.

RUPTURE OF LEFT VENTRICULAR FREE WALL
Introduction

Rupture of the LV free wall occurs in 0.5% of patients following AMI and is associated with 20% mortality.[1] A high index of suspicion and early diagnosis are vital to the survival of these high-risk patients. Approximately 50% of patients with free-wall rupture are diagnosed within 5 days of the AMI, with 90% diagnosed within 2 weeks.[5] Risk factors for the development of free-wall rupture following AMI include age, female gender, hypertension, first MI, and poor coronary artery collateralization.[6]

Pathophysiology

Early free-wall rupture, seen within the first 24 hours, represents a small-tear, full-thickness rupture, which is temporarily sealed by clot and fibrinous pericardial adhesions. The use of thrombolysis may result in the necrotic tissue developing into a hemorrhagic infarct, with a sudden "blow-out" rupture, which is associated with 35% to 60% mortality.[67] Late free-wall rupture develops 1 to 3 days following the AMI and is due to erosion at the border zone between infarction and normal myocardium.[68] Since the advent of thrombolytic agents and primary PCI, there has been a reduction in the incidence of late rupture.[69] Cardiac rupture has been also been classified according to pathology, with type I representing an abrupt myocardial tear in the absence of myocardial thinning; type II representing erosion of the infarcted myocardium followed by dehiscence and subsequent covering by thrombus; and type III representing myocardial thinning and perforation at the center of the ventricular aneurysm.[70] Pseudoaneurysm of the left ventricle represents free-wall rupture that is contained by pericardial adhesions. The culprit coronary lesion associated with LV rupture has been reported as the left anterior descending artery in 42% of patients, the circumflex coronary artery in 40% of patients, and the right coronary artery in 18% of patients.[71]

Diagnosis

Sudden onset of pain following coughing or straining may be suggestive of myocardial rupture following AMI. A proportion of patients who develop free-wall rupture will present with a subacute course of pain in keeping with pericarditis, nausea, and hypotension.[72] Acute rupture, however, often presents as electromechanical dissociation and sudden death (type I) or hemorrhage, tamponade, hypotension, and state of low cardiac output (types II and III).[73] The nature of acute rupture does not always lend itself to diagnostic investigation. If time allows, echocardiography is the modality of choice, with a sensitivity and specificity of 93% to 98%.[74] Echocardiography will demonstrate a pericardial collection with signs of cardiac tamponade, including collapse of the right atrium and ventricle in diastole, a dilated inferior vena cava, and marked respiratory variation in mitral and tricuspid valve inflow. Similarly, if a pulmonary artery catheter is in situ, it will demonstrate the hemodynamic abnormality of cardiac tamponade with equalization of right atrial, RV diastolic, and pulmonary capillary wedge pressures.[75] Computed tomography or magnetic resonance imaging may also be useful in determining the extent of the free-wall rupture or pseudoaneurysm (**Fig. 7**).

Management

LV wall rupture requires emergent salvage surgery. The use of emergency pericardiocentesis is controversial.[76] Although emergency pericardiocentesis may provide hemodynamic short-term improvement by relieving the tamponade, it can cause a dangerous increase in blood pressure with increased tension on damaged myocardium, with the potential for extension of a small tear to a rupture. Traditionally surgical repair is performed by direct suture of the myocardium over the infarct zone with reinforcement by Teflon felt strip,[77] or repair using the infarct exclusion technique.[31] More recently, a bovine pericardial patch has been used over the repair, reinforced with surgical glue beneath the patch, with or without epicardial suture on the patch borders (patch and glue technique).[78] Angiographically guided complete revascularization should be attempted following repair of the rupture. If angiography is not performed,

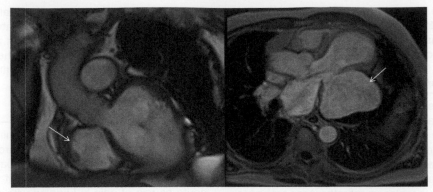

Fig. 7. Cardiac magnetic resonance images demonstrating a large (9 cm) pseudoaneurysm (*arrow*) in the basal and mid inferior and inferolateral aspects of the left ventricle, with a rim of mural thrombus.

complete revascularization to the noninfarcted areas is recommended.[79,80]

Outcomes

Successful surgical management of patients with LV rupture has been reported in small series (N = 25), with an operative mortality of 12% to 30%.[78,81] The long-term outcomes of these patients is primarily related to cardiac function following the AMI rather than recurrent rupture, with a 7-year survival of 68%.[78]

Summary of Rupture of LV Free Wall

Rupture of the LV free wall represents a significant mechanical complication of AMI, associated with a high mortality. Patients with contained rupture of the left ventricle benefit from expeditious diagnosis and emergent surgical intervention. If possible, avoiding the use of cardiopulmonary bypass by using a minimally invasive operative approach to repair the free-wall rupture (patch and glue technique) may be beneficial in patients with an already hemodynamically compromised myocardium.

SUMMARY

Mechanical complications after AMI, including VSR, papillary muscle rupture, and rupture of the LV free wall, are surgical emergencies that require urgent diagnosis and rapid intervention for optimal outcomes. Diagnosis in the emergent setting can be difficult in patients with dyspnea and shock. A high index of suspicion and appropriate investigation with echocardiography is vital for rapid diagnosis followed by emergent surgical treatment, if possible. Preoperative optimization with IABP and vasodilators may help to reduce the afterload on the compromised ventricle following AMI and improve cardiac output in the short term, but

should not delay expedient surgical intervention. Despite high operative mortality, the lack of an effective medical alternative makes surgical repair the mainstay of current management for these patients.

REFERENCES

1. French JK, Hellkamp AS, Armstrong PW, et al. Mechanical complications after percutaneous coronary intervention in ST-elevation myocardial infarction (from APEX-AMI). Am J Cardiol 2010;105:59–63.
2. Pohjola-Sintonen S, Muller JE, Stone PH, et al. Ventricular septal and free wall rupture complicating acute myocardial infarction: experience in the Multicenter Investigation of Limitation of Infarct Size. Am Heart J 1989;117(4):809–18.
3. Radford MJ, Johnson RA, Daggett WM Jr, et al. Ventricular septal rupture: a review of clinical and physiologic features and an analysis of survival. Circulation 1981;64(3):545–53.
4. Holmes DR Jr, Bates ER, Kleiman NS, et al. Contemporary reperfusion therapy for cardiogenic shock: the GUSTO-I trial experience. The GUSTO-I Investigators. Global Utilization of Streptokinase and Tissue Plasminogen Activator for Occluded Coronary Arteries. J Am Coll Cardiol 1995;26(3):668–74.
5. Crenshaw BS, Granger CB, Birnbaum Y, et al. Risk factors, angiographic patterns, and outcomes in patients with ventricular septal defect complicating acute myocardial infarction. Circulation 2000;101:27–32.
6. Shapira I, Isakov A, Burke M, et al. Cardiac rupture in patients with acute myocardial infarction. Chest 1987;92:219–23.
7. Oskoui R, Van Voorhees LB, DiBianco R, et al. Timing of ventricular septal rupture after acute myocardial infarction and its relation to thrombolytic therapy. Am J Cardiol 1996;78:953–5.

8. Prêtre R, Rickli H, Ye Q, et al. Frequency of collateral blood flow in the infarct-related coronary artery in rupture of the ventricular septum after acute myocardial infarction. Am J Cardiol 2000;85:497–9.

9. Skehan JD, Carey C, Norrell MS, et al. Patterns of coronary artery disease in post-infarction ventricular septal rupture. Br Heart J 1989;62:268–72.

10. Poulsen SH, Praestholm M, Munk K, et al. Ventricular septal rupture complicating acute myocardial infarction: clinical characteristics and contemporary outcome. Ann Thorac Surg 2008;85:1591–6.

11. Figueras J, Cortadellas J, Soler-Soler J. Comparison of ventricular septal and left ventricular free wall rupture in acute myocardial infarction. Am J Cardiol 1998;81:495–7.

12. Lemery R, Smith HC, Giuliani ER, et al. Prognosis in rupture of the ventricular septum after acute myocardial infarction and role of early surgical intervention. Am J Cardiol 1992;70:147–51.

13. Vlodaver Z, Edwards JE. Rupture of ventricular septum or papillary muscle complicating myocardial infarction. Circulation 1977;55:815–22.

14. Smyllie JH, Sutherland GR, Geuskens R, et al. Doppler color flow mapping in the diagnosis of ventricular septal rupture and acute mitral regurgitation after myocardial infarction. J Am Coll Cardiol 1990;15:1449–55.

15. Fortin DF, Sheikh KH, Kisslo J. The utility of echocardiography in the diagnostic strategy of postinfarction ventricular septal rupture: a comparison of two-dimensional echocardiography versus Doppler color flow imaging. Am Heart J 1991;121:25–32.

16. Selzer A, Gerbode F, Kerth WJ. Clinical, hemodynamic, and surgical considerations of rupture of the intraventricular septum after myocardial infarction. Am Heart J 1969;78:598.

17. Schwarzkopf K, Simon S, Preussler NP, et al. Measurement of cardiac output in ventricular rupture following acute myocardial infarction–pulmonary artery catheter vs transpulmonary thermodilution–a case report. Middle East J Anesthesiol 2009;20(1):105–6.

18. Khan MM, Patterson GC, O'Kane HO, et al. Management of ventricular septal rupture in acute myocardial infarction. Br Heart J 1980;44(5):570–6.

19. Tecklenberg PL, Fitzgerald J, Allaire BI, et al. Afterload reduction in the management of postinfarction ventricular septal defect. Am J Cardiol 1976;38:956–8.

20. DiSegni E, Kaplinsky E, Klein HO, et al. Treatment of ruptured interventricular septum with afterload reduction. Arch Intern Med 1978;138:1427–9.

21. Hentschel T, Yin N, Riad A, et al. Inhalation of the phosphodiesterase-3 inhibitor milrinone attenuates pulmonary hypertension in a rat model of congestive heart failure. Anesthesiology 2007;106:124–31.

22. Lahm T, McCaslin CA, Wozniak TC, et al. Medical and surgical treatment of acute right heart failure. J Am Coll Cardiol 2010;56:1435–46.

23. Husebye T, Eritsland J, Müller C, et al. Levosimendan in acute heart failure following primary percutaneous coronary intervention-treated acute ST-elevation myocardial infarction. Results from the LEAF trial: a randomized, placebo-controlled study. Eur J Heart Fail 2013;15(5):565–72.

24. George I, Xydas S, Topkara VK, et al. Clinical indication for use and outcomes after inhaled nitric oxide therapy. Ann Thorac Surg 2006;82:2161–9.

25. Ryan TJ, Antman EM, Brooks NH, et al. 1999 update: ACC/AHA guidelines for the management of patients with acute myocardial infarction. A report of the American College of Cardiology/American Heart Association Task Force on Practice Guidelines (Committee on Management of Acute Myocardial Infarction). J Am Coll Cardiol 1999;34:890–911.

26. Dixon SR, Henriques JP, Mauri L, et al. A prospective feasibility trial investigating the use of the Impella 2.5 system in patients undergoing high-risk percutaneous coronary intervention (the PROTECT 1 trial): initial US experience. JACC Cardiovasc Interv 2009;2:91–6.

27. Sheu JT, Tsai TH, Lee FY, et al. Early extracorporeal membrane oxygenator-assisted primary percutaneous coronary intervention improved 30-day clinical outcomes in patients with ST-segment elevation myocardial infarction complicated with profound cardiogenic shock. Crit Care Med 2010;38:1810–7.

28. Leshnower BG, Gleason TG, O'Hara ML, et al. Safety and efficacy of left ventricular assist device support in postmyocardial infarction cardiogenic shock. Ann Thorac Surg 2006;81:1365–70.

29. Slepian MJ, Copeland JG. The total artificial heart in refractory cardiogenic shock: saving the patient versus saving the heart. Nat Clin Pract Cardiovasc Med 2008;5:64–5.

30. Vidal S, Richebé P, Barandon L, et al. Evaluation of continuous veno-venous hemofiltration for the treatment of cardiogenic shock in conjunction with acute renal failure after cardiac surgery. Eur J Cardiothorac Surg 2009;36(3):572–9. http://dx.doi.org/10.1016/j.ejcts.2009.04.018.

31. David TE, Dale L, Sun Z. Postinfarction ventricular septal rupture: repair by endocardial patch with infarct exclusion. Thorac Cardiovasc Surg 1995;110(5):1315–22.

32. Attia R, Blauth C. Which patients might be suitable for a septal occluder device closure of postinfarction ventricular septal rupture rather than immediate surgery? Interact Cardiovasc Thorac Surg 2010;11(5):626–9. http://dx.doi.org/10.1510/icvts.2010.233981.

33. Maltais S, Ibrahim R, Basmadjian AJ, et al. Postinfarction ventricular septal defects: towards a new treatment algorithm? Ann Thorac Surg 2009;87: 687–92.

34. Costache VS, Chavanon O, Bouvaist H, et al. Early Amplatzer occluder closure of a postinfarct ventricular septal defect as a bridge to surgical procedure. Interact Cardiovasc Thorac Surg 2007;6(4): 503–4.

35. Menon V, Hochman JS. Management of cardiogenic shock complicating acute myocardial infarction. Heart 2002;88:531–7.

36. Menon V, Webb JG, Hillis LD, et al. Outcome and profile of ventricular septal rupture with cardiogenic shock after myocardial infarction: a report from the SHOCK Trial Registry. J Am Coll Cardiol 2000;36(Suppl A):1110–6.

37. Birnbaum Y, Fishbein MC, Blanche C, et al. Ventricular septal rupture after acute myocardial infarction. N Engl J Med 2002;347(18):1426–32.

38. Norell MS, Gershlick AH, Pillai R, et al. Ventricular septal rupture complicating myocardial infarction: is earlier surgery justified? Eur Heart J 1987;8: 1281–6.

39. Dalrymple-Hay MJ, Langley SM, Sami SA, et al. Should coronary artery bypass grafting be performed at the same time as repair of a post-infarct ventricular septal defect? Eur J Cardiothorac Surg 1998;13(3):286–92.

40. Cox F, Morshius W, Thijs Plokker H, et al. Importance of coronary revascularization for late survival after postinfarction ventricular septal rupture. A reason to perform coronary angiography prior to surgery. Eur Heart J 1996;17:1841–5.

41. Barker TA, Ramnarine IR, Woo EB, et al. Repair of post-infarct ventricular septal defect with or without coronary artery bypass grafting in the northwest of England: a 5-year multi-institutional experience. Eur J Cardiothorac Surg 2003;24(6):940–6.

42. Perrotta S, Lentini S. In patients undergoing surgical repair of post-infarction ventricular septal defect, does concomitant revascularization improve prognosis? Interact Cardiovasc Thorac Surg 2009;9(5):879–87.

43. Giuliani ER, Danielson GK, Pluth JR, et al. Postinfarction ventricular septal rupture: surgical considerations and results. Circulation 1974;49:455–9.

44. Honey M, Belcher JR, Hasan M, et al. Successful early repair of acquired ventricular septal defect after myocardial infarction. Br Heart J 1967;29:453.

45. Westaby S, Kharbanda R, Banning AP. Cardiogenic shock in ACS. Part 1: prediction, presentation and medical therapy. Nat Rev Cardiol 2011; 9(3):158–71.

46. Arnaoutakis GJ, Zhao Y, George TJ, et al. Surgical repair of ventricular septal defect after myocardial infarction: outcomes from the Society of Thoracic Surgeons National Database. Ann Thorac Surg 2012;94(2):436–43.

47. Jeppsson A, Liden H, Johnsson P, et al. Surgical repair of post infarction ventricular septal defects: a national experience. Eur J Cardiothorac Surg 2005;27:216–21.

48. Aronson D, Goldsher N, Zukermann R, et al. Ischemic mitral regurgitation and risk of heart failure after myocardial infarction. Arch Intern Med 2006;166(21):2362–8.

49. Kishon Y, Oh JK, Schaff HV, et al. Mitral valve operation in postinfarction rupture of a papillary muscle: immediate results and long-term followup of 22 patients. Mayo Clin Proc 1992;67:1023–30.

50. Thompson CR, Buller CE, Sleeper LA, et al. Cardiogenic shock due to acute severe mitral regurgitation complicating acute myocardial infarction: a report from the SHOCK Trial Registry. SHould we use emergently revascularize Occluded Coronaries in cardiogenic shocK? J Am Coll Cardiol 2000;36(3 Suppl A):1104–9.

51. Glasson JR, Komeda M, Daughters GT, et al. Early systolic mitral leaflet "loitering" during acute ischemic mitral regurgitation. J Thorac Cardiovasc Surg 1998;116:193–205.

52. Lamas GA, Mitchell GF, Flaker GC, et al. Survival and Ventricular Enlargement Investigators. Clinical significance of mitral regurgitation after acute myocardial infarction. Circulation 1997;96:827–33.

53. Barbour DJ, Roberts WC. Rupture of a left ventricular papillary muscle during acute myocardial infarction: analysis of 22 necropsy patients. J Am Coll Cardiol 1986;8:558–65.

54. Voci P, Bilotta F, Caretta Q, et al. Papillary muscle perfusion pattern: a hypothesis for ischemic papillary muscle dysfunction. Circulation 1995;91: 1714–8.

55. Raman S, Pipavath S. Images in clinical medicine. Asymmetric edema of the upper lung due to mitral valvular dysfunction. N Engl J Med 2009;361(5):e6.

56. Gueret P, Khalife K, Jobic Y, et al, Study Investigators. Echocardiographic assessment of the incidence of mechanical complications during the early phase of myocardial infarction in the reperfusion era: a French multicentre prospective registry. Arch Cardiovasc Dis 2008;101(1):41–7.

57. Kageji Y, Oki T, Iuchi A, et al. Relationship between pulmonary capillary wedge V wave and transmitral and pulmonary venous flow velocity patterns in various heart diseases. J Card Fail 1996;2:215–22.

58. Chevalier P, Burri H, Fahrat F, et al. Perioperative outcome and long-term survival of surgery for acute post-infarction mitral regurgitation. Eur J Cardiothorac Surg 2004;26(2):330–5.

59. Lorusso R, Gelsomino S, De Cicco G, et al. Mitral valve surgery in emergency for severe acute regurgitation: analysis of postoperative results from a

multicentre study. Eur J Cardiothorac Surg 2008; 33(4):573–82.

60. Stout KK, Verrier ED. Acute valvular regurgitation. Circulation 2009;119:3232–41.

61. Berkowitz C, McKeever L, Gunnar TM. Comparative response to dobutamine and nitroprusside in patients with low output cardiac failure. Circulation 1977;56:918.

62. Chen EP, Bittner HB, Davis RD Jr, et al. Milrinone improves pulmonary hemodynamics and right ventricular function in chronic pulmonary hypertension. Ann Thorac Surg 1997;63:814–21.

63. Bellone A, Barbieri A, Ricci C, et al. Acute effects of non-invasive ventilatory support on functional mitral regurgitation in patients with exacerbation of congestive heart failure. Intensive Care Med 2002;28(9):1348–50.

64. Tavakoli R, Weber A, Brunner-La Rocca H, et al. Results of surgery for irreversible moderate to severe mitral valve regurgitation secondary to myocardial infarction. Eur J Cardiothorac Surg 2002;21(5):818–24.

65. Hasdai D, Topol EJ, Califf RM, et al. Cardiogenic shock complicating acute coronary syndromes. Lancet 2000;356:749–56.

66. Russo A, Suri RM, Grigioni F, et al. Clinical outcome after surgical correction of mitral regurgitation due to papillary muscle rupture. Circulation 2008;118: 1528–34.

67. Coletti G, Torracca L, Zogno M, et al. Surgical management of left ventricular free wall rupture after acute myocardial infarction. Cardiovasc Surg 1995;3(2):181–6.

68. Purcaro A, Costantini C, Ciampani N, et al. Diagnostic criteria and management of subacute ventricular free wall rupture complicating acute myocardial infarction. Am J Cardiol 1997;80(4): 397–405.

69. Moreno R, López-Sendón J, García E, et al. Primary angioplasty reduces the risk of left ventricular free wall rupture compared with thrombolysis in patients with acute myocardial infarction. J Am Coll Cardiol 2002;39(4):598–603.

70. Becker AE, van Mantgem JP. Cardiac tamponade. A study of 50 hearts. Eur J Cardiol 1975;3:349–58.

71. Markowicz-Pawlus E, Nożyński J, Duszańska A, et al. The impact of a previous history of ischaemic episodes on the occurrence of left ventricular free wall rupture in the setting of myocardial infarction. Kardiol Pol 2012;70(7):713–7.

72. Oliva PB, Hammill SC, Edwards WD. Cardiac rupture, a clinically predictable complication of acute myocardial infarction: report of 70 cases with clinicopathologic correlations. J Am Coll Cardiol 1993;22(3):720–6.

73. Figueras J, Curos A, Cortadellas J, et al. Reliability of electromechanical dissociation in the diagnosis of left ventricular free wall rupture in acute myocardial infarction. Am Heart J 1996;131:861–4.

74. Pollak H, Diez W, Spiel R, et al. Early diagnosis of subacute free wall rupture complicating acute myocardial infarction. Eur Heart J 1993;14(5):640–8.

75. Fillmore SF, Scheidt S, Killip T. Objective assessment of pericardial tamponade; right heart catheterization at the bedside. Chest 1971;59(3):312–5.

76. Fitch MT, Nicks BA, Pariyadath M, et al. Videos in clinical medicine. Emergency pericardiocentesis. N Engl J Med 2012;366(12):e17.

77. Pretre R, Benedikt P, Turina MI. Experience with postinfarction left ventricular free wall rupture. Ann Thorac Surg 2000;69(5):1342–5.

78. Zoffoli G, Battaglia F, Venturini A, et al. A novel approach to ventricular rupture: clinical needs and surgical technique. Ann Thorac Surg 2012; 93(3):1002–3.

79. Mantovani V, Vanoli D, Chelazzi P, et al. Post-infarction cardiac rupture: surgical treatment. Eur J Cardiothorac Surg 2002;22(5):777–80.

80. Sutherland FW, Guell FJ, Pathi VL, et al. Postinfarction ventricular free wall rupture: strategies for diagnosis and treatment. Ann Thorac Surg 1996; 61(4):1281–5.

81. Flajsig I, Castells y Cuch E, Mayosky AA, et al. Surgical treatment of left ventricular free wall rupture after myocardial infarction: case series. Croat Med J 2002;43(6):643–8.

Novel Antiplatelet and Anticoagulant Agents in the Cardiac Care Unit

Vaani Panse Garg, MD, Jonathan L. Halperin, MD*

KEYWORDS

- Acute coronary syndrome • Anticoagulants • Antiplatelet drugs • Atrial fibrillation
- Percutaneous coronary intervention • Stroke • Venous thromboembolism

KEY POINTS

- Prasugrel and ticagrelor are more effective than clopidogrel for preventing ischemic events in patients with acute coronary syndromes (ACS) at the cost of a slightly higher risk of bleeding.
- Prasugrel is approved by the U.S. Food and Drug Association (FDA) for use in patients with ACS undergoing percutaneous coronary intervention (PCI), whereas ticagrelor is approved for use with or without PCI.
- Dabigatran, rivaroxaban, and apixaban proved noninferior to warfarin for preventing stroke and systemic embolism in patients with nonvalvular atrial fibrillation.
- These novel anticoagulants were associated with much lower rates of intracerebral bleeding than warfarin.
- Rivaroxaban is the first novel anticoagulant to gain FDA approval for preventing and treating venous thromboembolism.
- The absence of validated reversal strategies to use in the event of major bleeding during treatment with a new antithrombotic agent is a potential limitation.

Atherothrombotic vascular disease causes most cases of acute coronary syndrome (ACS) and ischemic stroke, contributing substantially to cardiovascular morbidity and mortality worldwide.[1] Patients with ACS often require urgent treatment in the intensive care unit (ICU) for symptom relief, hemodynamic stabilization, and prevention and control of complications. Secondary thromboembolic events, including deep vein thrombosis and pulmonary embolism, and atrial fibrillation occur frequently in critically ill patients in the ICU. Comprehensive knowledge of conventional and novel antithrombotic drugs is therefore essential.

Platelets play a central role in thrombosis, leading to acute ischemic events in coronary, cerebral, and other vascular beds.[2] Dual antiplatelet therapy (DAPT) with aspirin plus a thienopyridine or $P2Y_{12}$ adenosine diphosphate (ADP) receptor inhibitor has become standard of care for patients with ACS, with clopidogrel the conventional agent.[3–5] Although this regimen is widespread, limitations inspired the development of alternative drugs.

Although the newer agents also target the ADP pathway, they cause more complete inhibition of platelet aggregation than clopidogrel. When given in combination with aspirin in clinical trials of ACS, prasugrel and ticagrelor displayed greater efficacy than clopidogrel at the cost of increased bleeding.[6,7] Novel oral anticoagulants approved as alternatives to warfarin for preventing stroke and systemic embolism in patients with nonvalvular atrial fibrillation and prevention and treatment

Disclosures: Dr Garg has no financial conflicts of interests to disclose. Dr Halperin - see statement.
Department of Medicine, The Cardiovascular Institute, Mount Sinai Medical Center, Icahn School of Medicine at Mount Sinai, Fifth Avenue at 100th Street, New York, NY 10029-6574, USA
* Corresponding author.
E-mail address: jonathan.halperin@mssm.edu

Cardiol Clin 31 (2013) 533–544
http://dx.doi.org/10.1016/j.ccl.2013.07.001

of venous thromboembolism (VTE) showed comparable or greater antithrombotic efficacy, with an overall decrease in intracerebral bleeding, translating into net clinical benefit for appropriately selected patients.[8–11]

This article reviews the landmark studies of the novel antiplatelet and anticoagulant agents and discusses the clinical use of these drugs in the cardiac care unit (CCU).

ANTIPLATELET AND ANTICOAGULANT THERAPY
Conventional Antiplatelet Agents

Aspirin irreversibly inhibits cyclooxygenase-1 in the arachidonic acid pathway, reducing the formation of key activators, such as prostacyclin and thromboxane A_2, on platelet receptors (**Fig. 1, Table 1**). The benefits of aspirin in the prevention and treatment of ischemic events have been well established.[12–15] The United States Veterans Administration Cooperative study found a 51% reduction in the incidence of death or acute myocardial infarction in patients with ACS randomized to aspirin compared with placebo ($P = .0005$),[12] and investigations of aspirin for long-term secondary coronary prevention after myocardial infarction demonstrated its value well beyond the acute phase.

Clopidogrel irreversibly inhibits the platelet $P2Y_{12}$ ADP receptor, a mechanism distinct from that of aspirin, although both impede platelet activation and aggregation. Clopidogrel has fewer side effects than the thienopyridine ticlopidine, which more often caused bone marrow suppression. Clopidogrel has applications across a wide spectrum of acute and chronic cardiovascular disease states.[16–19] Dual antiplatelet therapy with aspirin and clopidogrel is recommended for patients with unstable angina (UA) and/or non–ST elevation myocardial infarction (NSTEMI).[3]

Limitations of Conventional Platelet Inhibitor Drugs

Among the limitations of aspirin are a dose-dependent risk of gastrointestinal intolerance and allergy.[2,3] Clopidogrel is generally well tolerated but may cause allergic reactions, diarrhea, and, rarely, thrombocytopenia; like all antithrombotic agents, aspirin and clopidogrel can cause or exacerbate bleeding. Both agents also have variable platelet inhibition among individuals. Proposed mechanisms for clopidogrel involve genetic polymorphisms in the CYP450 enzyme, specifically CYP2C19, which decrease the amount of active metabolite available for platelet inhibition[2,20,21] in up to one-third of patients.[22,23]

Newer Antiplatelet Agents

Prasugrel, a prodrug, requires one-step hepatic activation by CYP450 isoenzymes to irreversibly inhibit the $P2Y_{12}$ ADP receptor.[2] As a result, platelet inhibition is more rapid after administration of prasugrel (within 30 minutes) than after clopidogrel (6 hours).[24] Platelet inhibition is also more complete after a loading dose of prasugrel (60 mg) compared with high-dose clopidogrel (600 mg),[25] and the platelet inhibitory effects of a maintenance dose of prasugrel were greater than those with clopidogrel, even at a higher than conventional daily dosage (150 vs 75 mg, respectively).[26]

Ticagrelor, neither a thienopyridine nor a prodrug, is a cyclopentyl-triazolo-pyrimidine that also inhibits the $P2Y_{12}$ ADP receptor. Unlike thienopyridines that inhibit the receptor site for the life of the platelet, ticagrelor reversibly changes the conformation of the receptor, allowing ADP

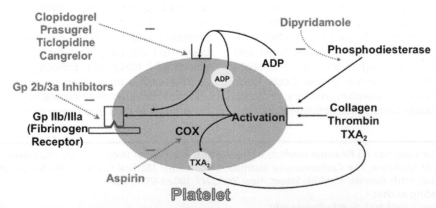

Fig. 1. Targets for antiplatelet therapy. COX, cyclooxygenase; Gp, glycoprotein; TXA$_2$, thromboxane A$_2$. (*Adapted from* Schafer AI. Antiplatelet therapy. Am J Med 1996;101:199–209; with permission.)

Table 1
Comparison of oral antiplatelet agents

Antiplatelet Agents	Aspirin	Clopidogrel	Prasugrel	Ticagrelor
Target	Cyclooxygenase-1	$P2Y_{12}$ ADP receptor	$P2Y_{12}$ ADP receptor	$P2Y_{12}$ ADP receptor
Chemical structure	Acetylsalicylic acid (NSAID)	Thienopyridine	Thienopyridine	Cyclopentyl-triazolo-pyrimidine
Receptor binding	Irreversible	Irreversible	Irreversible	Reversible
Prodrug	No	Yes	Yes	No
Bioavailability (%)	50–75	>50 (active metabolite)	70–80 (active metabolite)	30–40
Time to peak	1–3 h	6 h*	30 min–4 h*	30 min–2 h*
Half-life (h)	2.0–30.0 (dose-dependent)	0.5	7.0–12.0	6.0–9.0
Renal excretion (%)	75	50	60–70	1–5
FDA-approved	Primary and secondary prevention of stroke and MI; ACS +/− PCI; peripheral vascular disease	ACS +/− PCI; secondary prevention	ACS + PCI	ACS +/− PCI
Contraindications or warnings	Gastrointestinal bleeding; allergy; children/adolescents (Reye syndrome)	Allergy; known resistance	History of stroke/TIA or age >75 y; use lower dose (5 mg) for weight <60 kg	May have higher risk of stent thrombosis if missed doses
Hold before surgery (d)	7	7	5	7

Abbreviations: MI, myocardial infarction; NSAID, nonsteroidal anti-inflammatory drug; PCI, percutaneous coronary intervention; TIA, transient ischemic attack.
    * After loading dose.

to bind without inducing signaling.[2] This function, plus diminished inhibition after 12 hours, allows for more rapid reversal of the antiplatelet effect that, although potentially advantageous if an invasive procedure is required, might increase the risk of thrombotic complications after missed doses. Ticagrelor does not require hepatic activation and, like prasugrel, produces peak platelet inhibition 30 minutes after a loading dose.[27]

Anticoagulants

Anticoagulation has been a mainstay for the management of patients with ACS, prevention of stroke and systemic embolism in patients with atrial fibrillation, and prevention and treatment of VTE. Several studies compared unfractionated heparin (UFH), low-molecular-weight heparins (LMWHs; eg, enoxaparin, dalteparin), the parenteral antithrombin agent bivalirudin, and the factor Xa inhibitor fondaparinux, in patients with ACS.[15,26,28,29] Unfractionated heparin, enoxaparin, or fondaparinux is recommended for

patients managed without initial revascularization.[4] For those undergoing percutaneous coronary intervention (PCI), bivalirudin is another option. For patients with nonvalvular atrial fibrillation, aspirin or an anticoagulant is prescribed based on the individual's risk profile.[30] For those with acute VTE, LMWHs and fondaparinux are alternatives to therapy with UFH followed by a vitamin K antagonist.[31]

Limitations of Conventional Anticoagulants

Among the parenteral anticoagulants used in the ICU, UFH requires monitoring of the activated partial thromboplastin time (aPTT) to assure therapeutic dosing, whereas, except in cases of heparin-induced thrombocytopenia, bivalirudin, fondaparinux, and enoxaparin do not. Anticoagulation initiated with these agents is usually followed by a transition to oral warfarin for extended therapy. Among the limitations of warfarin are numerous interactions with foods and other drugs, requiring routine monitoring of anticoagulation intensity.[32] These limitations stimulated development of newer anticoagulants.

Newer Anticoagulant Agents

The novel oral anticoagulants directly inhibit thrombin (coagulation factor IIa) or factor Xa (**Fig. 2, Table 2**). They have a wide therapeutic window, and minimal food interaction or interpatient variability, allowing administration in fixed doses without routine coagulation monitoring. Dabigatran etexilate, a prodrug, inhibits thrombin, reaches peak plasma concentrations 30 minutes to 2 hours after ingestion, has a half-life of 12 to 17 hours,[33,34] and is approximately 80% cleared by the kidneys.[35] Potent P-glycoprotein (P-gp) inhibitors, such as quinidine, increase plasma concentrations of dabigatran and should be avoided.[36]

Rivaroxaban and apixaban, oral direct factor Xa inhibitors, block free and clot-bound factor Xa activity. Both reach peak plasma concentrations within 1 to 3 hours but, unlike dabigatran, are highly protein-bound in the active form and are only 25% to 33% cleared renally.[37] Concurrent therapy with CYP3A4 or P-gp inhibitors, such as ketoconazole or ritonavir, increases serum drug concentrations and should be avoided.

ANTITHROMBOTIC THERAPY IN THE CCU: ACS

Plaque rupture and platelet activation and aggregation are involved in most cases of ACS. Initial management involves DAPT with parenteral anticoagulation, regardless of whether an invasive or conservative treatment strategy is planned. Although clopidogrel is conventional, prasugrel and ticagrelor (each combined with aspirin) are increasingly chosen, and the LMWHs or fondaparinux are reasonable alternatives to UFH and bivalirudin.[12]

The TRITON-TIMI 38 trial compared prasugrel with clopidogrel in 13,608 patients with moderate-to-high risk ACS on aspirin scheduled for PCI, stratified based on UA/NSTEMI (10,074 patients) or ST elevation myocardial infarction (STEMI) (3534 patients).[6] Patients were randomized to prasugrel (60 mg load, 10 mg/d) or clopidogrel (300 mg load, 75 mg/d). Drug-eluting and bare metal stents were balanced; approximately 50% of patients were treated with platelet glycoprotein IIb/IIIa inhibitors during index hospitalization. The primary end point (cardiovascular death, nonfatal myocardial infarction, or nonfatal stroke) occurred in 12.1% of patients in the clopidogrel group versus 9.9% in the prasugrel group (hazard ratio [HR], 0.81; 95% confidence interval [CI], 0.73–0.90; P<.001). Patients with UA/NSTEMI on prasugrel showed a reduction in the primary end point (HR, 0.82; 95% CI, 0.73–0.93; P = .002); the advantage was similar for patients with STEMI (HR, 0.79; 95% CI, 0.65–0.97; P = .02). A 52% reduction in stent thrombosis and a reduction in the secondary end point of cardiovascular death, nonfatal myocardial infarction, or urgent target vessel revascularization were seen with prasugrel.

Prasugrel was associated with a higher risk of fatal (0.4% vs 0.1%; P = .002) and nonfatal (1.1% vs 09%; P = .23) life-threatening bleeding and greater requirement for blood transfusion (4% vs 3%; P<.001). Several post hoc analyses suggested a net harm of prasugrel in patients who had a previous stroke or transient ischemic attack (TIA; HR, 1.54; 95% CI, 1.02–2.32; P = .04) and no benefit among patients older than 75 years or weighing

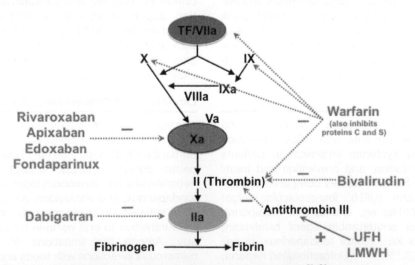

Fig. 2. Targets for anticoagulant therapy. TF, tissue factor. (*Data from* Refs.[62–64])

Table 2
Comparison of oral anticoagulant agents

Oral Anticoagulant Agent	Warfarin	Dabigatran	Rivaroxaban	Apixaban
Target	Vitamin K	IIa	Xa	Xa
Prodrug	No	Yes	No	No
Bioavailability (%)	95	6–8	60–80	50
Time to peak (h)	24	2	3–4	1–3
Half-life (h)	36–38	12–17	8–9	7–8
Renal excretion (%)	90	80	35	25
FDA-approved indications	Standard of care anticoagulation for various conditions (eg, AF, DVT, PE, mechanical heart valves, LV thrombus)	Nonvalvular AF	Nonvalvular AF; acute VTE (DVT, PE); prophylaxis of VTE after elective knee or hip replacement	Nonvalvular AF
Contraindications or warnings	Pregnancy, especially first trimester (fetal warfarin syndrome); several food and drug interactions	Black box warning for use with mechanical heart valves; avoid concurrent use with P-gp inhibitors (quinidine)	Avoid concurrent use with CYP3A4 or P-gp inhibitors (ketoconazole, ritonavir)	

Abbreviations: AF, atrial fibrillation; DVT, deep vein thrombosis; LV, left ventricle; PE, pulmonary embolism; P-gp, P-glycoprotein.

less than 60 kg. The U.S. Food and Drug Administration (FDA) approval for prasugrel warns against use in patients with previous stroke, TIA, or bleeding risk and in patients older than 75 years because of an increased risk of fatal intracranial hemorrhage. For those weighing less than 60 kg, the increased bleeding risk is attributed to an increased exposure to active metabolites. A lower dosage (5 mg/d) has been cautiously recommended but not investigated in prospective trials.[4]

The PLATO trial compared ticagrelor and clopidogrel in patients with ACS with and without ST-segment elevation.[7] A total of 18,624 patients were randomized to ticagrelor (180 mg load, 90 mg twice daily) or clopidogrel (300 or 600 mg load, 75 mg/d) plus aspirin (75–100 mg/d; for those not previously receiving aspirin, the preferred loading dosage of 325 mg/d was permitted for up to 6 months). PCI was performed in 64.3% of patients. After 1 year, the primary end point of death from vascular causes, myocardial infarction, or stroke occurred in 9.8% of patients randomized to ticagrelor versus 11.7% with clopidogrel. The difference in efficacy appeared 30 days after randomization and continued to the end of the study. Ticagrelor was associated with a reduction in all-cause mortality (4.5% vs 5.9% per year; *P*<.001). Bleeding unrelated to coronary artery bypass graft (CABG) surgery, specifically fatal intracranial hemorrhage, was higher with ticagrelor. Other adverse effects included dyspnea (13.8% vs 7.8%; *P*<.001) and increased serum uric acid and creatinine levels. Outcomes for those with prior stroke or TIA were not reported. Subgroup analyses found that the benefit of ticagrelor was attenuated in patients weighing less than average, those not taking lipid-lowering medication, and those from study centers in North America (*P* = .045), where the dose of aspirin was often higher than in other regions.[38]

Of the novel antiplatelet therapies, only ticagrelor is FDA-approved for patients with ACS managed without revascularization. Among 5216 patients in PLATO (28% of the study population) who did not undergo PCI, ticagrelor was associated with a reduction in primary events (12% vs 14.3% per year; HR, 0.85; 95% CI, 0.73–1.00; *P* = .04) and mortality.[39] For the management of ACS without PCI, antiplatelet therapy with clopidogrel or ticagrelor is recommended for 12 months.

Prasugrel was investigated in 9326 patients with UA or NSTEMI managed without revascularization in the Targeted Platelet Inhibition to Clarify Optimal Strategy to Medically Manage Acute Coronary Syndromes (TRILOGY ACS) study.[40] The results were inconclusive, because divergence in rates of primary events (cardiovascular death, myocardial infarction, or stroke) after 12 months did not reach significance ($P = .07$).

The CHAMPION-PCI and CHAMPION-PLATFORM trials compared cangrelor, an intravenous $P2Y_{12}$ ADP receptor inhibitor, with clopidogrel in patients with ACS undergoing PCI. Both studies were terminated early based on futility assessments regarding the primary end point (death, myocardial infarction, revascularization, or stent thrombosis 48 hours after randomization).[41] The CHAMPION-PHOENIX trial involving 11,145 patients, using a more restricted definition of myocardial infarction, found a primary end point rate of 4.7% with cangrelor versus 5.9% with clopidogrel ($P = .005$).[42] Adverse events were low in both arms, but stent thrombosis was less frequent in the cangrelor group.

Timing of Antiplatelet Drug Therapy

Either clopidogrel or ticagrelor can be administered in patients with ACS before an invasive or conservative strategy is determined, but prasugrel is not recommended this early. Before PCI, timing of loading is crucial: clopidogrel (600 mg) or ticagrelor (180 mg) should be given as early as possible before PCI is performed, and prasugrel (60 mg) should be given after coronary anatomy is defined when PCI is planned. After deployment of bare metal stents, antiplatelet therapy should continue for up to 1 year (clopidogrel, 75 mg/d; prasugrel, 10 mg/d; or ticagrelor, 90 mg twice daily). With drug-eluting stents for ACS, DAPT should generally continue for at least 12 months, although earlier interruption may be safe with later-generation (eg, everolimus-eluting) stents.

Concurrent Anticoagulation

Patients with ACS should be treated with parenteral anticoagulation (UFH, LMWH, or fondaparinux). Bivalirudin is generally restricted to the catheterization laboratory. In the ATLAS ACS-2-TIMI-51 trial, rivaroxaban, 2.5 mg twice daily, plus DAPT reduced cardiovascular death, myocardial infarction, and stroke compared with DAPT alone in patients with ACS. Increased bleeding in patients receiving rivaroxaban was comparable to that with prasugrel or ticagrelor in the TRITON and PLATO trials.[6,7,43] Rivaroxaban was approved in Europe in March 2013 for use in conjunction with

antiplatelet therapy in patients with ACS; however, a few weeks earlier, the FDA deferred approval pending further review.

ATRIAL FIBRILLATION

Atrial fibrillation is associated with, on average, a 5-fold increased risk of ischemic stroke. When atrial fibrillation develops after coronary intervention, after cardiac or noncardiac surgery, or during critical illness, the initial focus is on controlling the ventricular rate, unless hemodynamic instability or an accessory bypass tract requires cardioversion. Anticoagulation is not an immediate concern. In patients at high risk of thromboembolism, however, UFH is most often used in the ICU to prevent thromboembolism, although the safety and efficacy of this approach are not validated. In patients with ongoing or recurrent atrial fibrillation for whom long-term antithrombotic prophylaxis is necessary, warfarin is the conventional anticoagulant, but several novel agents (dabigatran, rivaroxaban, and apixaban) have been approved for patients with nonvalvular atrial fibrillation.[8,9,11,44] A fourth agent, edoxaban, is under investigation.[45]

The oral direct thrombin inhibitor dabigatran (110 or 150 mg twice daily) was compared with warfarin (goal international normalized ratio [INR], 2–3) in 18,113 patients (mean age, 71 years; mean $CHADS_2$ score, 2.1) with nonvalvular atrial fibrillation in the Randomized Evaluation of Long-Term Anticoagulation Therapy (RE-LY) trial.[8] The primary end point (all stroke, ischemic or hemorrhagic) or systemic embolism occurred at a rate of 1.69% per year with warfarin versus 1.53% per year with dabigatran, 110 mg twice daily (relative risk [RR], 0.91; 95% CI, 0.74–1.11; noninferiority $P<.001$), and 1.11% per year with dabigatran, 150 mg twice daily (RR, 0.66; 95% CI, 0.53–0.82; superiority $P<.001$). Annual rates of major bleeding were 3.36% with warfarin, 2.71% with dabigatran 110 mg twice daily ($P = .003$), and 3.11% with dabigatran 150 mg twice daily ($P = .31$). Hemorrhagic stroke rates were lower in both dabigatran groups than the warfarin group. Dabigatran, 150 mg twice daily, was FDA-approved in 2010 for patients with nonvalvular atrial fibrillation, stroke risk factors, and creatinine clearance of 30 mL/min or greater. A dosage of 75 mg twice daily was approved for patients with creatinine clearance of 15 to 30 mL/min, but the agent should not be used in patients with creatinine clearance less than 15 mL/min or who are undergoing dialysis. Dabigatran at a dosage of 110 mg twice daily was not approved for use in the United States.[46]

The Rivaroxaban Once Daily Oral Direct Factor Xa Inhibition Compared with Vitamin K Antagonism for Prevention of Stroke and Embolism Trial in Atrial Fibrillation (ROCKET-AF) randomized 14,264 patients (median age, 73 years; mean CHADS$_2$ score, 3.5) with nonvalvular atrial fibrillation to rivaroxaban (20 mg/d; 15 mg/d for those with creatinine clearance of 30–49 mL/min) or warfarin (goal INR, 2–3).[9] Rivaroxaban was noninferior for preventing ischemic or hemorrhagic stroke and systemic embolism (1.7 vs 2.2 events per 100 patient-years; HR, 0.79; 95% CI, 0.66–0.96; P<.001). No difference was seen in major and nonmajor clinically relevant bleeding rates. Patients taking rivaroxaban developed intracranial hemorrhage (0.5% vs 0.7%; P = .02) and fatal bleeding (0.2% vs 0.5%; P = .003) less often than those on warfarin. Rivaroxaban was FDA-approved in 2011 for this indication.

The Apixaban Versus Acetylsalicylic Acid to Prevent Stroke in Atrial Fibrillation Patients Who Have Failed or Are Unsuitable for Vitamin K Antagonist Treatment (AVERROES) trial, randomized 5599 patients to apixaban (5 mg twice daily) or aspirin (81–324 mg/d) over a mean of 1.1 years.[44] The study was terminated when it became apparent that the rate of stroke or systemic embolism was significantly lower with apixaban (1.6% vs 3.7% per year), bleeding risk was similar in the 2 groups, and mortality was lower with apixaban.

In the Apixaban for Reduction in Stroke and Other Thromboembolic Events in Atrial Fibrillation (ARISTOTLE) study, 18,201 patients were randomized to apixaban (5 mg twice daily, reduced to 2.5 mg twice daily in patients with 2 of the following factors: age ≥80 years, weight <60 kg, or serum creatinine >1.5 mg/dL) or warfarin (goal INR, 2–3). The median age was 70 years and the mean CHADS$_2$ score 2.2. The primary event rate was lower (1.27% vs 1.6% per year; HR, 0.79; 95% CI, 0.66–0.95; superiority P = .01), major bleeding was 2.1% versus 3.1% per year (P<.001), and all-cause mortality was 3.52% versus 3.94% per year (P = .047) with apixaban, which was approved for this indication in December 2012.

Anticoagulation for Cardioversion

Anticoagulation is recommended for 3 or more weeks before and after cardioversion, unless transesophageal echocardiography is used to exclude thrombus in the left atrium or left atrial appendage. With either approach, anticoagulation must be maintained during and after cardioversion for a period based on the intrinsic thromboembolic risk.

A subgroup analysis evaluated dabigatran in 1270 patients undergoing 1983 cardioversion procedures (647 on warfarin, 672 on dabigatran at

110 mg twice daily, and 664 on dabigatran at 150 mg twice daily) performed during the RE-LY trial, with most taking the assigned drug for 3 or more weeks.[45] In those undergoing transesophageal echocardiography, the incidence of spontaneous echo contrast or intracardiac thrombus was similar in all groups. By 30 days, stroke or systemic embolism occurred in 0.60% of patients cardioverted on warfarin, compared with 0.77% treated with dabigatran at 110 mg twice daily (P = .71) and 0.30% treated with dabigatran at 150 mg twice daily (P = .40). The rate of major bleeding was low in all groups (0.6%, 0.6%, and 1.7%, respectively).

ACUTE VTE

Approximately 500,000 patients are hospitalized with acute VTE annually in the United States.[47] In the CCU, acute VTE typically presents secondary to immobilization during critical illness or intrinsic coagulopathy.[48–50] Conventional management begins with parenteral followed by oral anticoagulation for periods varying based on severity and likelihood of recurrence. Rivaroxaban is approved in the United States for treating patients with acute symptomatic deep vein thrombosis or pulmonary embolism, to improve outcomes and reduce risk of recurrence. In the RE-MEDY and RE-SONATE trials, extended dabigatran therapy after initial warfarin management showed lower rates of VTE but more bleeding and drug discontinuation in patients treated with dabigatran.[51]

Acute Deep Vein Thrombosis

The EINSTEIN-DVT study involved 3449 patients randomized to oral rivaroxaban (15 mg twice daily for 3 weeks, then 20 mg/d) versus subcutaneous enoxaparin followed by warfarin or acenocoumarol for 3, 6, or 12 months. The Continued Treatment Study evaluated rivaroxaban (20 mg/d) versus placebo for 6 or 12 additional months in 1196 patients after completing 6 to 12 months treatment. Recurrent VTE occurred in 2.1% in the rivaroxaban group versus 3% with enoxaparin and vitamin K antagonist (HR, 0.68; 95% CI, 0.44–1.04; P<.001). Rates of major bleeding were similar. Compared with placebo for extended treatment, fewer recurrences occurred with rivaroxaban (1.3% vs 7.1%; HR, 0.18; 95% CI, 0.09–0.39; P<.001).[10]

Acute Pulmonary Embolism

In EINSTEIN-PE, 4832 patients with acute symptomatic pulmonary embolism were randomized to rivaroxaban (15 mg twice daily for 3 weeks, then

20 mg/d) or enoxaparin followed by vitamin K antagonist for 3, 6, or 12 months to prevent recurrence.[52] Rivaroxaban (2.1% per year) was noninferior to standard therapy (1.8% per year; HR, 1.12; 95% CI, 0.75–1.68; noninferiority $P = .003$) was associated with less frequent instances of major bleeding (superiority $P = .003$). The FDA approved rivaroxaban for VTE treatment in 2012.

Thromboprophylaxis During Acute Medical Illness

Rivaroxaban (10 mg/d) was compared with subcutaneous enoxaparin (40 mg/d) in preventing asymptomatic or symptomatic VTE for up to 10 (for noninferiority) or 35 days (for superiority) in 8101 patients hospitalized with acute medical illnesses.[53] The median hospital stay was 11 days. The primary efficacy outcome occurred in 2.7% of patients in each arm (RR, 0.97; 95% CI, 0.71–1.31; noninferiority $P = .003$ at day 10). After 35 days, a reduction was seen in VTE (RR, 0.77; 95% CI, 0.62–0.96; superiority $P = .02$), but more bleeding occurred in the rivaroxaban group. Although rivaroxaban is approved for thromboprophylaxis in adults undergoing elective hip or knee replacement surgery, it is not approved for preventing VTE in medically ill patients.[54]

SPECIAL CONSIDERATIONS
Mechanical Heart Valve Prostheses

The dabigatran package insert carries a black-box warning against use in patients with mechanical heart valves based on the phase II RE-ALIGN study, which was terminated because of excess thromboembolism and bleeding with dabigatran compared with vitamin K antagonist therapy.[30] Research is ongoing to establish a safer and more effective dabigatran regimen for this indication.

Triple Therapy

The combined use of clopidogrel, aspirin, and an oral anticoagulant (so-called triple therapy) in patients undergoing PCI is associated with significantly higher rates of bleeding than antithrombotic monotherapy. The combination of clopidogrel and an oral anticoagulant (without aspirin) as an alternative to triple therapy was evaluated in the open-label, multicenter WOEST trial that randomized 573 patients on an oral anticoagulant undergoing PCI to either clopidogrel alone or clopidogrel plus aspirin.[55] The primary outcome was the rate of major, minor, and minimal bleeding over a year, based on the Thrombolysis in Myocardial Infarction score. Significantly less bleeding was seen in the

clopidogrel plus oral anticoagulant group than in the triple therapy group (HR, 0.36; 95% CI, 0.26–0.50; $P<.001$). The combination of death, myocardial infarction, stroke, target vessel revascularization, and stent thrombosis (safety end point) was also significantly lower in the dual-therapy group than the triple therapy group (11.3% and 17.7%, respectively; $P = .025$). All-cause mortality was 2.5% per year with dual therapy versus 6.4% with triple therapy ($P<.03$). Although underpowered for efficacy end points, and the primary end point included minimal, minor, and major bleeding (some of which is subjectively assessed), the results suggest a potential role for therapy with clopidogrel rather than triple therapy in patients on oral anticoagulants undergoing PCI.

Rivaroxaban is currently under investigation in patients with atrial fibrillation undergoing PCI in the 3-arm PIONEER AF-PCI trial which will randomize an anticipated 2100 patients to (1) rivaroxaban, 15 mg/d plus clopidogrel, 75 mg/d; (2) rivaroxaban, 2.5 mg twice daily plus DAPT; or (3) vitamin K antagonist (goal INR, 2–3) plus DAPT for a treatment duration of 12 months. The primary end point is major and minor bleeding events.

Control of Bleeding

Compared with no antithrombotic therapy, aspirin is associated with a 60% greater risk of major bleeding, clopidogrel with a 38% greater risk, and prasugrel with a 32% greater risk.[6,16] In the PLATO trial of patients receiving aspirin concurrently, major bleeding unrelated to CABG surgery, including intracranial hemorrhage, was 25% higher with ticagrelor than with clopidogrel.[7] If excessive bleeding develops during treatment with prasugrel or ticagrelor, the drug should be stopped and platelets transfused as necessary. Off prasugrel, platelet inhibition resolves within 7 to 10 days.[55] Ticagrelor is more reversible, but metabolites may interfere with transfused platelets. Interruption of antiplatelet therapy during the first several months after coronary intervention increases the risk of stent thrombosis.

Among the advantages of the novel oral anticoagulants are their pharmacokinetic profiles, with half-lives of 12 to 17 hours for dabigatran, 8 to 9 hours for rivaroxaban, and 7 to 8 hours for apixaban, compared with 36 to 38 hours for warfarin.[35] Withholding the drugs may be sufficient in cases of minor or non–life-threatening bleeding, and activated charcoal may reduce drug absorption within 2 to 3 hours of ingestion. For more severe bleeding, treatment includes transfusion of fresh frozen plasma or packed erythrocytes, although the efficacy of plasma is unconfirmed. No specific antidotes are available to reverse the anticoagulation effects of the new agents. Activated 4-factor prothrombin complex concentrate (not available in the United States) corrected the aPTT in normal subjects taking rivaroxaban ($P<.001$) but did not reverse the dabigatran effect on aPTT.[56] Dialysis may reduce plasma concentrations of dabigatran but will not reverse rivaroxaban or apixaban. To manage bleeding during treatment with a novel anticoagulant, intravenous fluid should be given. Factor VIII inhibitor–binding activator or recombinant factor VII may be useful, but these have not been investigated clinically and carry a risk of thrombosis.

On an investigational level, a humanized monoclonal antibody fragment against dabigatran is in preclinical development as a specific reversal agent. The compound proved effective in vitro and in vivo in monkeys, and reduced dabigatran-related blood loss in a rat tail bleeding model.[34,57,58] Specific factor Xa antidotes currently under development include factor Xa derivatives lacking binding activity. These agents reversed laboratory markers of anticoagulation induced by rivaroxaban and apixaban in vitro and in animal models,[59,60] and reduced rivaroxaban-induced blood loss in a rabbit liver laceration model.[61] Human studies are in formative stages, made complex because of the importance of showing a reduction of clinical bleeding rather than simply a correction of laboratory coagulation measurements.

Perioperative Use

Elective surgery should be deferred for at least 4 to 6 weeks after PCI with bare metal stents and at least 6 months after drug-eluting stents.[5] Prasugrel should be discontinued at least 7 days and ticagrelor or clopidogrel 5 days before surgery. For urgent CABG surgery, the risk of bleeding must be weighed against the benefit of continuing $P2Y_{12}$ therapy. The use of intravenous cangrelor after cessation of oral antiplatelet therapy before CABG surgery is associated with a greater degree of platelet inhibition but no excess in major bleeding compared with placebo.[58] Cangrelor is not currently available for clinical use. In patients undergoing urgent noncardiac surgery, antiplatelet therapy should generally be continued unless the risk of stent thrombosis and myocardial infarction is lower than the risk of bleeding. Vitamin K antagonists should be stopped 5 days preoperatively, and in patients with mechanical heart valves, bridging therapy with UFH or LMWH is recommended. Less evidence exists for bridging in anticoagulated patients with atrial fibrillation or VTE.

SUMMARY

The development of novel antiplatelet and anticoagulant agents has broadened therapeutic options with favorable benefit to risk ratios compared to conventional agents. When combined with aspirin in patients with ACS, prasugrel and ticagrelor are more effective than clopidogrel in preventing ischemic events but carry a slightly high risk of bleeding, particularly intracranial hemorrhage. Dabigatran, rivaroxaban, and apixaban are all noninferior to warfarin in preventing stroke and systemic embolism in patients with nonvalvular atrial fibrillation, apixaban caused less major bleeding, and all agents caused less intracranial hemorrhage than warfarin. Although statistical significance varied, the new anticoagulants reduced all-cause mortality by approximately 10% compared with warfarin, an indicator of net clinical benefit. Only rivaroxaban is approved in the United States for preventing and treating VTE, but evidence with the others is accumulating. Although fixed oral dosing without routine coagulation monitoring, relatively few drug and food interactions, and the potential to reduce hospital length of stay make these agents appealing, the lack of reversal strategies and high cost are limitations.

Future investigation should focus on gaps in clinical applications and alternative pathways for inhibition of platelet function or coagulation.[2] Among the uncertainties is how to manage patients with recurrent ischemic events during treatment, with an aim to better understand the mechanisms of events, such as a ceiling effect limiting $P2Y_{12}$ inhibition, genetic polymorphisms affecting platelet reactivity, or thrombophilia. An urgent need exists for specific reversal agents to terminate the antithrombotic effects and for accurate ways to assess effects when patients require surgery or other invasive procedures. On balance, however, the new antiplatelet and anticoagulant agents have significant therapeutic advantages, offering substantial value in the management of patients with a variety of acute and chronic cardiovascular disease states before, during, and after their care in the CCU.

REFERENCES

1. Writing Group Members, Lloyd-Jones D, Adams RJ, Brown TM, et al. Heart disease and stroke statistics—2010 update: a report from the American Heart Association. Circulation 2010;121(7):e46–215.
2. Gurbel PA, Tantry US. Combination antithrombotic therapies. Circulation 2010;121(4):569–83.
3. Anderson JL, Adams CD, Antman EM, et al. 2011 ACCF/AHA focused update incorporated into the ACC/AHA 2007 guidelines for the management of

patients with unstable angina/non-ST-elevation myocardial infarction: a report of the American College of Cardiology Foundation/American Heart Association task force on practice guidelines. Circulation 2011;123(18):e426–579.

4. Jneid H, Anderson JL, Wright RS, et al. 2012 ACCF/AHA focused update of the guideline for the management of patients with unstable angina/non-ST-elevation myocardial infarction (updating the 2007 guideline and replacing the 2011 focused update): a report of the American College of Cardiology Foundation/American Heart Association task force on practice guidelines. J Am Coll Cardiol 2012;60(7):645–81.

5. Guyatt GH, Norris SL, Schulman S, et al. Methodology for the development of antithrombotic therapy and prevention of thrombosis guidelines: antithrombotic therapy and prevention of thrombosis, 9th ed: American College of Chest Physicians evidence-based clinical practice guidelines. Chest 2012;141(Suppl 2):53S–70S.

6. Wiviott SD, Braunwald E, McCabe CH, et al. Prasugrel versus clopidogrel in patients with acute coronary syndromes. N Engl J Med 2007;357(20): 2001–15.

7. Wallentin L, Becker RC, Budaj A, et al. Ticagrelor versus clopidogrel in patients with acute coronary syndromes. N Engl J Med 2009;361(11):1045–57.

8. Connolly SJ, Ezekowitz MD, Yusuf S, et al. Dabigatran versus warfarin in patients with atrial fibrillation. N Engl J Med 2009;361(12):1139–51.

9. Patel MR, Mahaffey KW, Garg J, et al. Rivaroxaban versus warfarin in nonvalvular atrial fibrillation. N Engl J Med 2011;365(10):883–91.

10. EINSTEIN Investigators, Bauersachs R, Berkowitz SD, Brenner B, et al. Oral rivaroxaban for symptomatic venous thromboembolism. N Engl J Med 2010;363(26):2499–510.

11. Granger CB, Alexander JH, McMurray JJ, et al. Apixaban versus warfarin in patients with atrial fibrillation. N Engl J Med 2011;365(11):981–92.

12. Lewis HD Jr, Davis JW, Archibald DG, et al. Protective effects of aspirin against acute myocardial infarction and death in men with unstable angina. Results of a Veterans Administration Cooperative study. N Engl J Med 1983;309(7):396–403.

13. Popma JJ, Ohman EM, Weitz J, et al. Antithrombotic therapy in patients undergoing percutaneous coronary intervention. Chest 2001;119(Suppl 1): 321S–36S.

14. Barnathan ES, Schwartz JS, Taylor L, et al. Aspirin and dipyridamole in the prevention of acute coronary thrombosis complicating coronary angioplasty. Circulation 1987;76(1):125–34.

15. Theroux P, Ouimet H, McCans J, et al. Aspirin, heparin, or both to treat acute unstable angina. N Engl J Med 1988;319(17):1105–11.

16. Yusuf S, Zhao F, Mehta SR, et al. Effects of clopidogrel in addition to aspirin in patients with acute coronary syndromes without ST-segment elevation. N Engl J Med 2001;345(7):494–502.

17. Steinhubl SR, Berger PB, Mann JT 3rd, et al. Early and sustained dual oral antiplatelet therapy following percutaneous coronary intervention: a randomized controlled trial. J Am Med Assoc 2002;288(19):2411–20.

18. Sabatine MS, Cannon CP, Gibson CM, et al. Addition of clopidogrel to aspirin and fibrinolytic therapy for myocardial infarction with ST-segment elevation. N Engl J Med 2005;352(12):1179–89.

19. Chen ZM, Jiang LX, Chen YP, et al. Addition of clopidogrel to aspirin in 45,852 patients with acute myocardial infarction: randomised placebo-controlled trial. Lancet 2005;366(9497):1607–21.

20. Fintel DJ. Oral antiplatelet therapy for atherothrombotic disease: overview of current and emerging treatment options. Vasc Health Risk Manag 2012; 8:77–89.

21. Kim L, Charitakis K, Swaminathan RV, et al. Novel antiplatelet therapies. Curr Atheroscler Rep 2012; 14(1):78–84.

22. Gurbel PA, Bliden KP, Hiatt BL, et al. Clopidogrel for coronary stenting: response variability, drug resistance, and the effect of pretreatment platelet reactivity. Circulation 2003;107(23): 2908–13.

23. Serebruany VL, Steinhubl SR, Berger PB, et al. Variability in platelet responsiveness to clopidogrel among 544 individuals. J Am Coll Cardiol 2005; 45(2):246–51.

24. Jernberg T, Payne CD, Winters KJ, et al. Prasugrel achieves greater inhibition of platelet aggregation and a lower rate of non-responders compared with clopidogrel in aspirin-treated patients with stable coronary artery disease. Eur Heart J 2006; 27(10):1166–73.

25. Wiviott SD, Trenk D, Frelinger AL, et al. Prasugrel compared with high loading- and maintenance-dose clopidogrel in patients with planned percutaneous coronary intervention: the prasugrel in comparison to clopidogrel for inhibition of platelet activation and aggregation-thrombolysis in myocardial infarction 44 trial. Circulation 2007; 116(25):2923–32.

26. Stone GW, McLaurin BT, Cox DA, et al. Bivalirudin for patients with acute coronary syndromes. N Engl J Med 2006;355(21):2203–16.

27. Cannon CP, Husted S, Harrington RA, et al. Safety, tolerability, and initial efficacy of AZD6140, the first reversible oral adenosine diphosphate receptor antagonist, compared with clopidogrel, in patients with non-ST-segment elevation acute coronary syndrome: primary results of the DISPERSE-2 trial. J Am Coll Cardiol 2007;50(19):1844–51.

28. Cohen M, Demers C, Gurfinkel EP, et al. A comparison of low-molecular-weight heparin with unfractionated heparin for unstable coronary artery disease. Efficacy and safety of subcutaneous enoxaparin in non-Q-wave coronary events study group. N Engl J Med 1997;337(7):447–52.

29. Fifth Organization to Assess Strategies in Acute Ischemic Syndromes Investigators, Yusuf S, Mehta SR, Chrolavicius S, et al. Comparison of fondaparinux and enoxaparin in acute coronary syndromes. N Engl J Med 2006;354(14):1464–76.

30. Mohr JP, Thompson JL, Lazar RM, et al. A comparison of warfarin and aspirin for the prevention of recurrent ischemic stroke. N Engl J Med 2001;345(20):1444–51.

31. Ridker PM, Goldhaber SZ, Danielson E, et al. Long-term, low-intensity warfarin therapy for the prevention of recurrent venous thromboembolism. N Engl J Med 2003;348(15):1425–34.

32. Rose AJ, Hylek EM, Ozonoff A, et al. Risk-adjusted percent time in therapeutic range as a quality indicator for outpatient oral anticoagulation: results of the Veterans Affairs study to improve anticoagulation (VARIA). Circ Cardiovasc Qual Outcomes 2011;4(1):22–9.

33. Stangier J, Eriksson BI, Dahl OE, et al. Pharmacokinetic profile of the oral direct thrombin inhibitor dabigatran etexilate in healthy volunteers and patients undergoing total hip replacement. J Clin Pharmacol 2005;45(5):555–63.

34. Van de Werf F, Brueckmann M, Connolly SJ, et al. A comparison of dabigatran etexilate with warfarin in patients with mechanical heart valves: the randomized, phase II study to evaluate the safety and pharmacokinetics of oral dabigatran etexilate in patients after heart valve replacement (RE-ALIGN). Am Heart J 2012;163(6):931–7.e1.

35. Donadini MP, Ageno W, Douketis JD. Management of bleeding in patients receiving conventional or new anticoagulants: a practical and case-based approach. Drugs 2012;72(15):1965–75.

36. Schulman S, Kearon C, Kakkar AK, et al. Dabigatran versus warfarin in the treatment of acute venous thromboembolism. N Engl J Med 2009;361(24):2342–52.

37. Scaglione F. New oral anticoagulants: comparative pharmacology with vitamin K antagonists. Clin Pharm 2013;52(2):69–82.

38. Mahaffey KW, Wojdyla DM, Carroll K, et al. Ticagrelor compared with clopidogrel by geographic region in the platelet inhibition and patient outcomes (PLATO) trial. Circulation 2011;124(5):544–54.

39. James SK, Roe MT, Cannon CP, et al. Ticagrelor versus clopidogrel in patients with acute coronary syndromes intended for non-invasive management: substudy from prospective randomised platelet inhibition and patient outcomes (PLATO) trial. BMJ 2011;342:d3527.

40. Roe MT, Armstrong PW, Fox KA, et al. Prasugrel versus clopidogrel for acute coronary syndromes without revascularization. N Engl J Med 2012;367(14):1297–309.

41. Bhatt DL, Lincoff AM, Gibson CM, et al. Intravenous platelet blockade with cangrelor during PCI. N Engl J Med 2009;361(24):2330–41.

42. Bhatt DL, Stone GW, Mahaffey KW, et al. Effect of platelet inhibition with cangrelor during PCI on ischemic events. N Engl J Med 2013;368(14):1303–13.

43. Mega JL, Braunwald E, Mohanavelu S, et al. Rivaroxaban versus placebo in patients with acute coronary syndromes (ATLAS ACS-TIMI 46): a randomised, double-blind, phase II trial. Lancet 2009;374(9683):29–38.

44. Connolly SJ, Eikelboom J, Joyner C, et al. Apixaban in patients with atrial fibrillation. N Engl J Med 2011;364(9):806–17.

45. Ruff CT, Giugliano RP, Antman EM, et al. Evaluation of the novel factor Xa inhibitor edoxaban compared with warfarin in patients with atrial fibrillation: design and rationale for the effective anticoagulation with factor Xa next generation in atrial fibrillation-thrombolysis in myocardial infarction study 48 (ENGAGE AF-TIMI 48). Am Heart J 2010;160(4):635–41.

46. Wann LS, Curtis AB, Ellenbogen KA, et al. 2011 ACCF/AHA/HRS focused update on the management of patients with atrial fibrillation (update on dabigatran): a report of the American College of Cardiology Foundation/American Heart Association task force on practice guidelines. Circulation 2011;123(10):1144–50.

47. Centers for Disease Control and Prevention (CDC). Venous thromboembolism in adult hospitalizations - United States, 2007-2009. MMWR Morb Mortal Wkly Rep 2012;61(22):401–4.

48. Marks PW. Coagulation disorders in the ICU. Clin Chest Med 2009;30(1):123–9, ix.

49. Pastores SM. Management of venous thromboembolism in the intensive care unit. J Crit Care 2009;24(2):185–91.

50. Rajasekhar A, Beyth R, Crowther MA. Newer anticoagulants in critically ill patients. Crit Care Clin 2012;28(3):427–51, vii.

51. Schulman S, Kearon C, Kakkar AK, et al. Extended use of dabigatran, warfarin, or placebo in venous thromboembolism. N Engl J Med 2013;368(8):709–18.

52. EINSTEIN-PE Investigators, Buller HR, Prins MH, Lensin AW, et al. Oral rivaroxaban for the treatment of symptomatic pulmonary embolism. N Engl J Med 2012;366(14):1287–97.

53. Cohen AT, Spiro TE, Buller HR, et al. Rivaroxaban for thromboprophylaxis in acutely ill medical patients. N Engl J Med 2013;368(6):513–23.

54. Eriksson BI, Kakkar AK, Turpie AG, et al. Oral rivar-oxaban for the prevention of symptomatic venous thromboembolism after elective hip and knee replacement. J Bone Joint Surg Br 2009;91(5): 636–44.

55. Hirsh J, Guyatt G, Albers GW, et al. Antithrombotic and thrombolytic therapy: American College of Chest Physicians evidence-based clinical practice guidelines (8th edition). Chest 2008;133(Suppl 6): 110S–2S.

56. Levy JH, Faraoni D, Spring JL, et al. Managing new oral anticoagulants in the perioperative and intensive care unit setting. Anesthesiology 2013; 118(6):1466–74.

57. van Ryn J, Litzenberger T, Gan G, et al. In vitro characterization, pharmacokinetics and reversal of supratherapeutic doses of dabigatran-induced bleeding in rats by a specific antibody fragment antidote to dabigatran [abstract]. Presented at the 54th ASH Annual Meeting and Exposition. Atlanta, December 8–10, 2012. Abstract 3418.

58. Toth J, van Ryn J, Dursema H, et al. Reversal of dabigatran's anticoagulant activity in the monkey by a specific antidote and pharmacokinetic and pharmacodynamic modeling [abstract]. Presented at the 54th ASH Annual Meeting and Exposition. Atlanta, December 8–10, 2012. Abstract 22.

59. Lu G, DeGuzman FR, Lakhotia S, et al. Recombinant antidote for reversal of anticoagulation by factor Xa inhibitors [abstract]. Presented at the 50th ASH Annual Meeting and Exposition. San Francisco, December 6–9, 2008. Abstract 983.

60. Lu GP, Peng L, Hollenbach SJ, et al. Reconstructed recombinant factor Xa as an antidote to reverse anticoagulation by factor Xa inhibitors. J Thromb Haemost 2009;7:309.

61. Hollenbach SJ, Lu G, Tan S, et al. PRT064445 but not recombinant FVIIa reverses rivaroxaban induced anticoagulation as measured by reduction in blood loss in a rabbit liver laceration model [abstract]. Presented at the 54th ASH Annual Meeting and Exposition. Atlanta, December 8–10, 2012. Abstract 3414.

62. Weitz JI, Bates SM. New anticoagulants. J Thromb Haemost 2005;3:1843.

63. Turpie AG. New oral anticoagulants in atrial fibrillation. Eur Heart J 2007;29:155.

64. Geurtin KR, Choi YM. The discovery of the Factor Xa inhibitor otamixaban: from lead identification to clinical development. Curr Med Chem 2007;14: 2471.

The Pulmonary Artery Catheter
A Critical Reappraisal

Umesh K. Gidwani, MD[a,b,*], Bibhu Mohanty, MD[c],
Kanu Chatterjee, MB, FRCP (Lond), FRCP (Edin), MACP[d,e]

KEYWORDS

- Swan-Ganz catheter • Pulmonary artery catheter • Cardiac critical care

KEY POINTS

- The pulmonary artery catheter (PAC) is a simple diagnostic intervention, done at the bedside and widely used in cardiac critical care; however, over time evidence has developed that harm could result if is not used judiciously.
- Many technologies seek to supplant the PAC, but none has been subjected to as much clinical use and scrutiny.
- It is paramount that the user be intimately familiar with the pitfalls and complications, the dangers of misinterpretation, and the potential complications of this device.
- Thoughtful patient selection and judicious use of this device can mitigate any possible harm and maximize utility.

Beware of false knowledge; it is more dangerous than ignorance.
—George Bernard Shaw

INTRODUCTION

Balloon floatation pulmonary artery catheters (PACs) have been used for hemodynamic monitoring in cardiac, medical, and surgical intensive care units (ICUs) since the 1970s. In cardiac catheterization laboratories, balloon floatation catheters are routinely used for right heart catheterization. It was estimated in 2000 that approximately 1.5 million balloon floatation catheters were sold annually in the United States.[1] Approximately 30% of these catheters were used in cardiac surgery, 30% in coronary care units and cardiac catheterization laboratories, 25% in high-risk surgical and trauma patients, and 15% in medical ICUs. Right heart catheterization is performed primarily to determine hemodynamics and measure cardiac output, typically for the purpose of establishing a diagnosis of underlying pathology and also to guide therapy. With the availability of noninvasive diagnostic modalities, particularly echocardiography, the frequency of diagnostic pulmonary artery (PA) catheterization has declined.

In this review, the evolution of PACs, the results of nonrandomized and randomized studies in various clinical scenarios, the uses and abuses of bedside hemodynamic monitoring, and current indications of PA catheterization in critical care units are discussed.

EVOLUTION OF PA CATHETERS

The history of cardiac catheterization dates back to the early nineteenth century.[2] In 1844, Claude

Disclosures: None.
[a] Cardiac Critical Care, Zena and Michael A. Weiner Cardiovascular Institute, Mount Sinai Hospital, One Gustave Levy Place, New York, NY 10029, USA; [b] Cardiology, Pulmonary, Critical Care and Sleep Medicine, Icahn School of Medicine at Mount Sinai, One Gustave Levy Place, New York, NY 10029, USA; [c] Zena and Michael A. Weiner Cardiovascular Institute, Mount Sinai Hospital, One Gustave Levy Place, New York, NY 10029, USA; [d] The Carver College of Medicine, University of Iowa, 375 Newton Rd, Iowa City, IA 52242, USA; [e] University of California San Francisco, 500 Parnassus Avenue, San Francisco, CA 94143, USA
* Corresponding author. One Gustave L. Levy Place, Box 1030, New York, NY 10029.
E-mail address: umesh.gidwani@mountsinai.org

Cardiol Clin 31 (2013) 545–565
http://dx.doi.org/10.1016/j.ccl.2013.07.008
0733-8651/13/$ – see front matter © 2013 Elsevier Inc. All rights reserved.

Bernard performed right ventricular (RV) and left ventricular (LV) catheterization in horses by inserting glass tubes into the jugular veins and carotid arteries.[3,4] In the 1800s, the performance of cardiac catheterization in horses to measure intracardiac pressures became a common practice among other notable physiologists as well, including Jean-Baptiste Chauveau and Etienne Marey.[3,5] In the early 1900s, Fritz Bleichroder, Ernest Unger, and W. Loeb performed cardiac catheterization in dogs, testing the effect of drugs injected into the central circulation.[2,3]

Dr Werner Forssmann is credited with performing the first human right heart catheterization.[6] In 1929, he introduced a urethral catheter into his left antecubital vein and advanced the catheter to his right atrium (RA), documenting this self-catheterization by x-ray. Unfortunately, following publication of this landmark effort, Dr Forssmann lost his clinical practice privileges because of unfavorable press.[2,7–9]

In the 1940s, Drs Andre Cournand, Hilmert Ranges, and Dickinson Richards developed catheters that could be advanced into the pulmonary artery and used these catheters in the cardiac catheterization laboratory to study hemodynamics in patients with congenital and acquired heart diseases.[10–12] Working at Bellevue Hospital in New York, Andre Cournand and Dickinson Richards used PACs not only to measure intracardiac pressures, but also to obtain true mixed venous blood samples from the PA. This permitted measurement of cardiac output by the direct Fick principle for the first time.[13,14] Cournand and Richards also used PA catheterization for analysis of blood gases, pH, respiratory gas exchange, and blood volume in healthy individuals as well as in patients with cardiopulmonary disease.[3,11,15,16] In 1956, Drs Andre Cournand, Dickinson Richards, and Werner Forssmann were awarded the Nobel Prize in Physiology or Medicine for their pioneering contributions in cardiac catheterization.[8,17]

In 1949, the concept and technique of measuring pulmonary capillary wedge pressure (PCWP) was developed in the cardiac catheterization laboratory of Dr Lewis Dexter at the Brigham and Women's Hospital, Harvard Medical School.[18] PCWP was measured by advancing the PAC to the distal branches of the PA. It was assumed that PCWP reflected LV diastolic pressure. In 1953, Lategola and Rahn developed a self-guiding balloon-tipped catheter that could be advanced into the PA and thence into the wedge position.[19]

The development of PACs for a variety of clinical scenarios continued. Dr H.J.C. 'Jeremy' Swan, an Irishman and cardiovascular researcher in London moved to the US for a fellowship at the Mayo Clinic in 1951. There he worked with Earl Wood and furthered his interest in cardiac and pulmonary vascular physiology. In 1964, R. D. Bradley, a British intensivist whom Swan had mentored whilst in the UK, developed miniature catheters that could be guided into the PA.[20] In 1965, Drs Fife and Lees constructed self-guiding PACs and used these catheters for a variety of physiologic studies.[21] In 1969, Dr Melvin Scheinman and his colleagues at San Francisco General Hospital, used flow directed catheters to measure right heart pressures.[22]

Meanwhile, Dr Swan at Cedars-Sinai, where he had moved in 1965, was having little success with Bradley's catheters and wrestled with a design to make it easier to 'float' the PAC into the right heart and beyond. In his words: "In the fall of 1969, I was on the beach in Santa Monica, California, with my young children and noted a sailboat with a large spinnaker making good progress in a calm sea. I wondered whether a sail or parachute at the tip of a flexible catheter would solve the problem. I had been a consultant to Edwards Laboratories for several years and brought this proposal for discussion. David Chonette, new product manager, did not favor the solutions suggested, but proposed a small inflatable balloon that would be relatively easy to fabricate. The balloon worked superbly, and sail and parachute were abandoned."[23] In 1970, Drs Jeremy Swan, William Ganz, and Forrester published details of the first 'balloon tipped flow directed' catheters (**Fig. 1**) which could be used in patients in the intensive care unit without the use of fluoroscopy.[24] These catheters had two lumens – one to inflate the balloon and the other to record pressure.

The "Swan-Ganz" catheter was further developed by Ganz to measure cardiac output by the thermodilution method.[25] Chatterjee and colleagues[26] subsequently introduced balloon floatation catheters with pacing electrodes, which could be used for atrial, ventricular, and atrioventricular sequential pacing. Following this, further modifications included adding additional ports for hemodynamic monitoring and medication infusion, cardiac pacing, and even placing an oximeter at the tip, which allowed for continuous SvO_2 monitoring. **Fig. 2** shows the most common device in use today. It is a 7.5-Fr catheter inserted through an 8.5-Fr introducer sheath and has 3 ports for pressure monitoring and infusions, a thermistor probe 3 cm proximal to the tip, and a balloon at the tip inflated via a valve at the hub.[27]

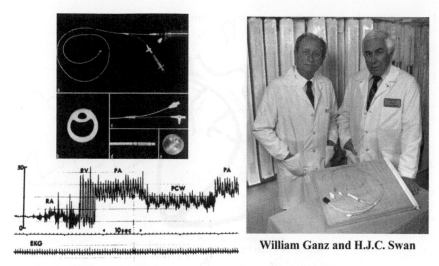

Fig. 1. The original "Swan-Ganz" catheter. (*Courtesy of* Dr Peter Ganz, MD, San Francisco, CA.)

PLACEMENT OF BALLOON FLOATATION CATHETERS AND HEMODYNAMIC MEASUREMENTS

The PAC is typically placed at the bedside without fluoroscopy. Access is established in a central vein as usual and a 10-cm 8.5-Fr introducer inserted. The PAC is then ensheathed in a sterile sleeve (that allows for future sterile manipulation) and passed through the valve in the introducer hub. Between 11 cm and 15 cm, the balloon is inflated and the catheter advanced. The balloon should always be fully inflated during catheter advancement, and fully deflated during catheter withdrawal.

As the catheter is advanced, its position can be identified by characteristic pressure wave forms. When the catheter is in the RA, the RA pressure wave form is noted. The RA pressure wave forms are characterized by two positive waves: an "a," which occurs during RA systole and a "v," which occurs during the end of right ventricular (RV) systole. It should be appreciated that in atrial fibrillation, "a" waves are absent. There are also two

negative waves: the "x" descent caused by atrial relaxation and the "y" descent, which occurs during RV rapid filling. In atrial fibrillation, the "a" upstroke and the "x" descent are absent. A positive wave called the "c" wave is frequently recognized during the "x" descent. The "c" wave results from doming of the tricuspid valve into RA during RV isovolumic systole.

With further advancement of the catheter, the balloon tip crosses the tricuspid valve and an RV pressure wave form is seen (**Fig. 3**). The RV pressure waveform is characterized by a sharp upstroke during the isovolumic phase of systole. During the ejection phase, there is much slower rise in pressure. During the isovolumic relaxation phase, there is a sharp down stroke in the RV pressure wave form. Because of the tricuspid valve, the RV systolic pressure is always higher than the RA pressure. During diastole, a rapid filling wave, diastasis, and atrial filling waves are recognized. During the rapid filling phase, RV diastolic pressure rises with inflow of blood from the RA. During the phase of diastasis, there is no further rise in RV pressure, as inflow from the

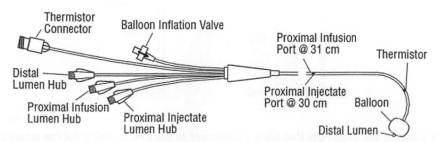

Fig. 2. A standard PAC. (*From* McGee WT, Headley JM, Frazier JA, et al. Quick guide to cardiopulmonary care. 2nd edition. Irwin, CA: Edwards Critical Care Education; 2009; with permission.)

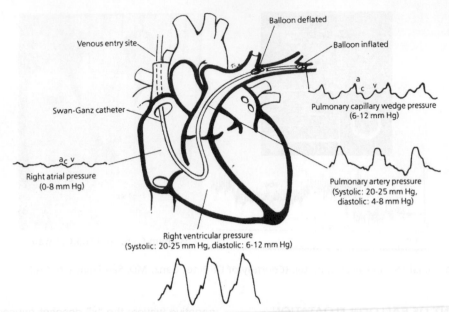

Fig. 3. Hemodynamic waveforms in the RA, RV, PA, and wedge (PCWP) positions of the PAC. (*From* Disease-a-month. The Swan-Ganz Catheter. Dis Mon 1991;37(8):509–43; with permission.)

RA ceases due to the lack of a pressure gradient between the 2 chambers. The atrial filling wave is related to RA contraction at the end of diastole. In atrial fibrillation, the atrial filling wave is absent.

When the catheter with the balloon inflated is advanced from the RV, it crosses the pulmonic valve and floats into the PA (**Fig. 3**), ultimately arriving at the wedge position recognized by a characteristic pressure wave form (**Fig. 3**). When the balloon is deflated, the PA pressure waveform is restored (**Fig. 3**). The PA pressure waveform is characterized by a sharp upstroke and a down stroke interrupted by the dicrotic notch and dicrotic wave. The PCWP wave form is similar to the RA pressure wave form, but at a higher pressure and later in the cardiac cycle (when timed against the QRS complex).

The PCWP is commonly used to assess pulmonary venous and left atrial pressures, which also reflects LV diastolic pressure in the absence of mitral valve obstruction. It should be appreciated that for determination of left atrial pressure by measuring the PCWP, presence of a continuous fluid column between the distal tip of the catheter and the left atrium is necessary (**Fig. 4**). The continuous fluid column is absent when the alveolar pressure is considerably higher than pulmonary capillary pressure. In these circumstances, the small pulmonary veins and capillaries collapse. This zone of the lung is called West zone 1, and typically correlates anatomically with the upper air fields above the level of the left atrium.[28] The continuous fluid column between the distal tip of the catheter and left atrium can be maintained

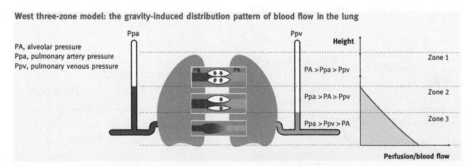

Fig. 4. West's zones of the lung; note that Zone 3 placement of the PAC is critical for the accurate estimation of the left ventricle end diastolic pressure from the PCWP. (*From* de Beer JM, Gould T. Principles of artificial ventilation. Anaesth Intensive Care Med 2013;14(3):83–93; with permission.)

only when the catheter is placed in an area of the lung where the PCWP is considerably higher than the alveolar pressure. This area is termed West zone 3, located in the most dependent part of the lung below the level of the left atrium.

The wedge position can be verified by withdrawing blood with the balloon inflated for determination of oxygen saturation. If the catheter is in proper wedge position, withdrawn blood will be "arterialized" with an oxygen saturation of 95% or higher. There may be considerable inaccuracy in proper measurement of PCWP by the waveform analysis alone and considerable interobserver variability as well.[29]

At the time of catheter placement, the difference between PA end-diastolic and mean PCWP should be determined. If the difference does not exceed 5 mm Hg, PA end-diastolic pressure can be used in place of PCWP.[30–32] The normal range of RA pressure is 0 to 7 mm Hg. The RA "a" wave pressure is higher than the "v" wave pressure. The normal range of RV systolic pressure is 15 to 25 mm Hg and the normal range of RV end-diastolic pressure is between 0 and 8 mm Hg. The PA systolic pressure is similar to that of RV systolic pressure in the absence of RV outflow obstruction. The normal mean PA pressure (MPAP) is less than 18 mm Hg and the normal mean PCWP is 15 mm Hg or less. The "a" wave pressure is lower than the "v" wave pressure in PCWP.

When the RA and RV are markedly dilated or in patients with severe pulmonary arterial hypertension (not uncommon in the cardiac ICU), it may become necessary to use fluoroscopy for PAC placement because coiling and knotting in the RA or RV can occur.

During hemodynamic monitoring in critical care units, RA, PA, and PCW pressures are typically monitored, in addition to arterial pressure and cardiac output. Arterial and mixed venous oxygen saturations can be used to assess changes in cardiac output.

The RA pressure reflects RV diastolic pressure in the absence of tricuspid valve obstruction. Jugular venous pressure is similar to RA pressure in the absence of superior vena cava or innominate vein obstruction. Thus, bedside measurement of jugular venous pressure provides a reasonable estimate of RA and RV diastolic pressure, meaning that RV filling pressure can be assessed without the use of a PAC. PCWP reflects LV diastolic pressure in the absence of non–Zone III placement and pulmonary venous, left atrial, and mitral valve obstruction. PCWP, however, cannot be estimated without right heart catheterization, even with the use of sophisticated Doppler

echocardiography. In the absence of cardiopulmonary disease, RA pressure has only a modest correlation to PCWP.[33] In the presence of valvular, myocardial, or pericardial disease, this correlation is even worse.[34,35]

The RA and PCW pressures are, at best, surrogates for RV and LV filling pressures respectively, which in turn are used to assess RV and LV function. Although it is commonly assumed that right atrial pressure (RAP) and PCWP represent RV and LV preloads, it should be appreciated that true preload refers to ventricular end-diastolic volume. As ventricular volumes are difficult to determine at the bedside in critical care units, RAP and PCWP are used as surrogates for ventricular filling pressures. Ventricular function curves are constructed by relating stroke volume or cardiac output to the ventricular filling pressure (Frank-Starling relation). Stroke volume is calculated by dividing cardiac output by heart rate. Cardiac output is usually determined by the thermodilution method when a PAC is used. Cardiac output can also be determined by dividing total body oxygen consumption by the arterial and mixed venous oxygen content difference (Fick principle).

To construct a ventricular function curve, stroke volume is plotted on the vertical axis and ventricular filling pressure on the horizontal axis (**Fig. 5**). Obviously, in the absence of mitral or tricuspid valve regurgitation or intracardiac shunts, RV and LV stroke volumes are the same.

Both RV and LV function curves have an initial steep portion and a relatively flat terminal portion. On the steep portion of the function curve, for a given increase in filling pressure, there is a substantial increase in stroke volume. This may occur, for example, during volume expansion by administration of fluids. On the flat portion of the function curve, a similar increase in filling pressure is associated with a smaller increase in stroke volume. In the failing ventricle, the ventricular function curve moves downward and to the right. The steep portion of the depressed ventricular function curve is relatively shorter and the flat portion longer (see **Fig. 5**). Thus, in failing hearts, for a given increase in filling pressure, the degree of rise in stroke volume is much smaller.

The RV and LV are structurally different: the RV free wall is thinner than that of the LV. The determinants of RV and LV stroke volume are also different. For example, systemic arterial pressure, a component of LV afterload, is higher than PA pressure, a component of RV afterload. The RV is also more compliant than the LV. Thus, RV filling pressure is much lower than that of the LV for a similar end-diastolic volume. As such, the RV function curve sits to the left of the LV function curve

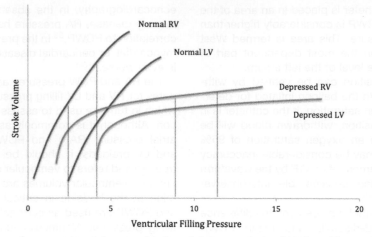

Fig. 5. Starling curves for normal and decreased left and right ventricular function. (Illustration: N. Jethmalani.)

(**Fig. 5**). An understanding of the difference between the RV and LV function curves is clinically important. During volume expansion therapy, for a given increase in stroke volume, RV filling pressure increases much less than LV filling pressure. When stroke volume increases from 15 mL to 40 mL, RA pressure (RV filling pressure) increases from 5 to 10 mm Hg. However, PCWP (LV filling pressure) increases from 15 to 30 mm Hg, and can result in pulmonary edema.

Although in clinical practice, RA and PCW pressures are used as RV and LV filling pressures, true ventricular filling pressures are transmural. The transmural pressure is the difference between the ventricular distending pressure and the pressure-resisting ventricular distention. Pericardial and mediastinal pressures comprise resisting pressure. Normally, the intrapericardial pressure is 0 and the mediastinal pressure is between −1 mm Hg and −3 mm Hg. Thus, in normal conditions, RAP and PCWP are assumed to accurately reflect RV and LV filling pressures. However, when intrapericardial and mediastinal pressures change, transmural pressure changes. For example, in pericardial effusion, the intrapericardial pressure is increased. To estimate RV and LV filling (transmural) pressures, pericardial pressure should be subtracted from the RA and PCW pressures.

The cardiac pressure waveforms can vary with the respiratory phase. Typically, the respiratory influence on the waveform is most neutral at end-expiration, where end-expiration depends on whether the patient is breathing spontaneously or is on positive-pressure (assisted) ventilation (**Fig. 6**).

In various arrhythmias, both PCWP and RAP are altered. In atrial fibrillation, "a" waves are absent and in atrial flutter, flutter waves can be visualized. In the presence of PVCs, cannon waves distort the RAP and PCWP wave forms. Cannon waves are produced when atrial systole occurs while the atrioventricular valves are closed during ventricular systole, such as with complete heart block.

CARDIAC OUTPUT

Cardiac output can be determined by the thermo-dilution technique with a PAC by using the Stewart-Hamilton equation. A fixed volume of

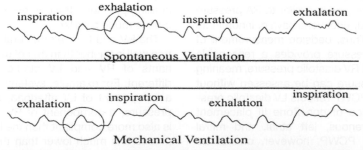

Fig. 6. The effect of respiration on the "wedge" waveform. The wedge should be measured at end-expiration. (*From* Daily EK. Hemodynamic waveform analysis. J Cardiovasc Nursing 2001;15(2):6–22, 87–8; with permission.)

cold fluid (typically 10 mL of normal saline at room temperature) is injected as a bolus into the proximal lumen of the PAC, and the resulting change in the PA blood temperature is recorded by the thermistor at the catheter tip. As the cooler mixed blood flows by the thermistor, the rate of change of temperature and a return back to body temperature is reflected in a temperature concentration curve (**Fig. 7**). The quicker the rate of change in blood temperature, the greater the flow rate, and, thus, the higher the cardiac output. Conversely, a slower rate of change in blood temperature indicates lower cardiac output.

In certain circumstances, cardiac output cannot be determined accurately by the thermodilution technique. In patients with severe tricuspid regurgitation and intracardiac shunts, prolonged indicator transit time and recycling of the indicator can cause overestimation or underestimation of cardiac output.[27] Lower limb compression devices, ubiquitous in the ICU, have even been shown to confound thermodilution cardiac output measurement.[36] Low basal blood temperature, for example during therapeutic hypothermia, may also introduce error in measured cardiac output by the thermodilution technique.

The analysis of arterial pulse pressure wave forms (APWA) method has also been used for measurement of cardiac output. This method estimates intravascular volume status through the use of stroke volume variation (SVV) and, thus, estimates cardiac output.[37] This technique can be used only in patients on a ventilator. The variables that can be determined by the APWA method are cardiac index (CI) and SVV. A CI of at least 2.8 L/min/m² measured by this technique has been reported to indicate a favorable prognosis.[37] It has been also reported that SVV can be used to assess volume responsiveness. It should be noted that a poor correlation between the APWA method and thermodilution has been reported.[38]

A transpulmonary thermodilution technique also can be used to measure cardiac output (CO). In this method, a thermal injectate is delivered into the RA by a central venous catheter and the change in temperature of the blood circulating through the pulmonary and arterial circulation is sensed by a thermistor mounted at the tip of the radial artery. A high correlation exists between CO determined by this technique and CO determined by thermodilution with a PAC.[39] The transpulmonary thermodilution technique can be used with global and diastolic volume and lung water.

Transthoracic and transesophageal echocardiography (TTE and TEE, respectively) are being used increasingly in ICUs to assess LV and RV function and filling pressures. Transesophageal echocardiography can be used to assess RV and LV volumes and ejection fraction even in patients

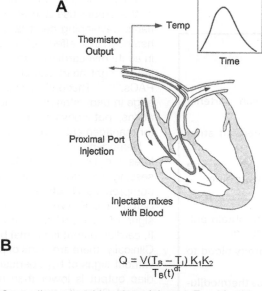

$$Q = \frac{V(T_B - T_I) K_1 K_2}{T_B(t)^{dt}}$$

Q= cardiac output, V= volume injected, T_B = blood temperature, T_I = injectate temperature, K_1 and K_2 = computational constants, and $T_B(t)^{dt}$ = change in blood temperature as a function of time.

Fig. 7. The temperature change versus time graph (*A*) applied to the Stewart Hamilton equation. (*B*) Notice that the rate of change of temperature is inversely proportional to the cardiac output. (*From* Marino PL. The ICU book. 2nd edition. Philadelphia: Lippincott Williams and Wilkins; 1997; with permission.)

on ventilators. RV systolic pressure can also be determined from the tricuspid regurgitation jet.[40,41] The measurement of inferior vena cava diameter has been used to assess central venous pressure.[42] Studies on the correlation between Doppler and thermodilution methods of cardiac output determination have varied, some suggesting poor correlation and others reporting reasonable correlation.[43,44]

PULMONARY ARTERY DATA

A plethora of data can be obtained from the PAC (**Box 1**, **Table 1**). Once the monitoring system is properly calibrated, zeroed to atmospheric pressure, and the transducer leveled to the phlebostatic axis, the central venous pressure (CVP) and pulmonary artery pressure (PAP) are displayed on the monitor. Typically the blood pressure and heart rate are also displayed. The next step is to aspirate a blood sample from the PA port to obtain the SvO_2, Inflate the balloon with 1.5 mL of air and measure the wedge pressure at end expiration, and inject 10 mL of normal saline in the RA port of the PAC to obtain cardiac output by thermodilution. With these primary measurements at hand, one can populate various equations as shown in **Table 1** and obtain derived data. **Fig. 8** illustrates the determinants of SvO_2 and the utility of monitoring SvO_2, which is a less operator-dependent variable and quite useful when waveform analysis or thermodilution are in question.

Box 1
Organization of PAC data

1. Observe

   a. MAP: Blood pressure/mean arterial pressure

   b. RAP: Central venous pressure/right atrial pressure

   c. PAP/MPAP: Pulmonary artery pressure and mean pulmonary artery pressure

2. Do

   a. PCWP: Inflate the balloon to obtain pulmonary capillary wedge pressure

   b. SvO_2: Aspirate pulmonary artery blood to obtain SvO_2

   c. CO: Obtain cardiac output by thermodilution via PAC

3. Derive

   a. Cardiovascular dynamics

   b. Oxygen dynamics

CLINICAL APPLICATIONS
Cardiac Catheterization Laboratory

Balloon floatation catheters are routinely used in cardiac catheterization laboratories for right heart catheterization to record intracardiac pressures and cardiac output. Cardiac output is usually determined by thermodilution, as described earlier. Cardiac output also should be determined by measuring oxygen consumption and arteriovenous oxygen difference (Fick equation), especially in patients with severe tricuspid regurgitation and intracardiac shunts.

In the presence of a large left-to-right shunt, pulmonary blood flow is higher than systemic flow and cardiac output determined by thermodilution will overestimate the true cardiac output. In the presence of a right-to-left shunt, pulmonary blood flow is lower than systemic flow and cardiac output determined by thermodilution will underestimate the true systemic cardiac output.

Acute Coronary Syndromes

When the PAC was first introduced, hemodynamic monitoring by right heart catheterization was routinely performed in patients with acute coronary syndromes (ACS) in myocardial infarction research units, and in coronary care units. Numerous studies were performed seeking to identify such features as the optimal left heart filling pressure,[45] the best medical therapy for ACS by application of hemodynamic subsets,[46,47] or the proper use and effects of diuretics in patients developing heart failure during ACS.[48] The hemodynamic effects of various vasoactive agents in acute myocardial infarction (MI) were also studied by right heart catheterization with the use of PACs.[49–51] These studies provided useful knowledge in understanding of the hemodynamic alterations, pathophysiologic changes, and rationale for management of patients with acute MI.

Hemodynamic subsets and their clinical correlates in patients with acute MI were useful for assessing severity of cardiac and hemodynamic compromise (**Table 2**).[46,47] In subset I, cardiac output and PCWP are normal and there are no signs of hypoperfusion or congestion. In subset II, cardiac output is normal but PCWP is elevated. Clinically, there are signs of pulmonary congestion without signs of hypoperfusion. In subset III, cardiac output is lower than normal and PCWP is normal. Clinically, there are signs of hypoperfusion without signs of pulmonary congestion. In subset IV, cardiac output is reduced and PCWP is elevated. Clinically, there are signs of hypoperfusion and of pulmonary congestion. Patients in cardiogenic shock fall under subset IV and are

Table 1
Derived parameters for cardiovascular and oxygen dynamics

Cardiovascular Dynamics	
Cardiac index (L/min/m^2) = $\dfrac{CO\left(\frac{L}{min}\right)}{BSA\ (m^2)}$	2.5–4 L/min/m^2
Stroke volume (L/beat) = $\dfrac{CO\left(\frac{L}{min}\right)}{HR\left(\frac{beats}{min}\right)}$	0.06–0.1 L/beat
Stroke volume index (L/beat/m^2) = $\dfrac{SV\left(\frac{L}{beat}\right)}{BSA\ (m^2)}$	0.033–0.047 L/beat/m^2
MAP (mm Hg) = $\dfrac{2\text{Diastolic} + \text{Systolic}}{3}$	70–110 mm Hg
SVR (dyne-sec-cm^{-5}) = $\dfrac{MAP\ (mm\ Hg) - MRAP\ (mm\ Hg)}{CO\left(\frac{L}{min}\right)} \times 80$	800–1200 dyne-sec-cm^{-5}
SVRI ([dyne-sec-cm^{-5}]/m^2) = $\dfrac{MAP\ (mm\ Hg) - MRAP\ (mm\ Hg)}{CI\left(\frac{L}{min}\right)} \times 80$	1970–2390 [dyne-sec-cm^{-5}]/m^2
PVR (dyne-sec-cm^{-5}) = $\dfrac{mPAP\ (mm\ Hg) - PCWP\ (mm\ Hg)}{CO\left(\frac{L}{min}\right)} \times 80$	<250 dyne-sec-cm^{-5}
PVRI ([dyne/sec/cm^{-5}]/m^2) = $\dfrac{mPAP\ (mm\ Hg) - PCWP}{CI} \times 80$	255–285 [dyne-sec-cm^{-5}]/m^2
LVSWI (g-m/m^2/beat) = 0.0136[SVI × (MAP − PCWP)]	50–62 g-m/m^2/beat
RVSWI (g-m/m^2/beat) = 0.0136[SVI × (mPAP − RAP)]	5–10 g-m/m^2/beat
Oxygen Dynamics	
DO$_2$ (ml /min/m^2) = CO $\left(\frac{mL}{min}\right)$ × CaO$_2$ = CO [(Hb × SaO$_2$ × 1.34) + (PaO$_2$ × 0.0031)]	500–600 mL/min
VO$_2$ (mL/min) = 13.4[CO × Hb × (SaO$_2$ − SvO$_2$)]	200–250 mL/min
O$_2$ER (%) = O$_2$ ER = 100$\left(\frac{VO_2}{DO_2}\right)$	25%–30%

Abbreviations: BSA, body surface area; CaO$_2$, arterial O$_2$ content; CI, cardiac index; CO, cardiac output; DO$_2$, oxygen delivery; Hb, hemoglobin; HR, heart rate; LVSWI, left ventricular stroke work index; MAP, mean arterial pressure; O$_2$ ER, oxygen extraction ratio; mPAP, mean pulmonary artery pressure; PCWP, pulmonary capillary wedge pressure; PVR, pulmonary vascular resistance; PVRI, pulmonary vascular resistance index; RAP, right atrial pressure; RVSWI, right ventricular stroke work index; SV, stroke volume; SVI, stroke volume index; SvO$_2$, mixed venous saturation; SVR, systemic vascular resistance; SVRI, systemic vascular resistance index; VO$_2$, oxygen consumption.

additionally hypotensive, with an arterial pressure of 90 mm Hg or less.

It should be noted that these hemodynamic studies were performed before the era of echocardiography and immediate revascularization. With the advent of echocardiography, the need for invasive hemodynamic monitoring has declined markedly. For practical purposes, RV and LV filling pressures and cardiac output can be only approximated by echo-Doppler studies.[41,42,52] An analysis of data from the multinational Global Registry of Acute Coronary Events (GRACE) revealed that the rate of PA catheterization was 3.0% in 2007 compared with 5.4% in 2000.[53] In the United States, this number dropped from 10.4% in 2000 to 1.5% in 2007. Furthermore, it was observed that PA catheterization is associated with increased mortality and longer length of hospital stay.[54] Mortality at 30 days was substantially higher among patients with PAC for both unadjusted (odds ratio [OR] 8.7; 95% confidence interval [CI] 7.3–10.2) and adjusted analyses (OR 6.4; 95% CI 5.4–7.6) in all groups except in patients with cardiogenic shock (OR 0.99; 95% CI 0.80–1.23).

Gore and colleagues,[55] showed that in patients with heart failure secondary to acute MI, in-hospital mortality was 44.8% in those receiving PA catheterization versus 25.3% in those who did not. In patients with hypotension, the mortality was 48.3% in patients who received PA catheterization versus 32.2% in patients who did not. In patients with cardiogenic shock complicating ACS, however, there was no difference in mortality between patients who received PA catheterization (74.4%) and those who did not (79.1%). In the

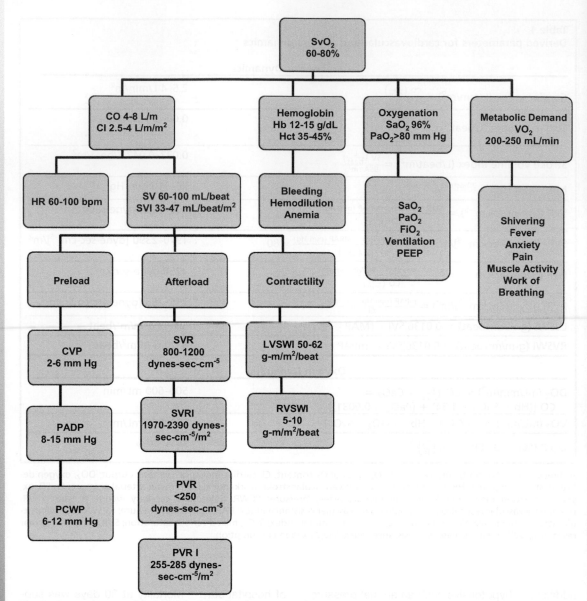

Fig. 8. Determinants of SvO₂ with normal values. Note that when Hb, SaO₂, and VO₂ are constant, changes in SaO₂ reflect changes in cardiac output.

GUSTO trial,[54] the hazard ratio of 30-day mortality in patients without cardiogenic shock who received PA catheterization was 4.80 (95% CI 3.56–6.47) compared with those who did not. Yet, in patients with cardiogenic shock, there was no difference in the risk of mortality; the hazard ratio was 0.99 (95% CI 0.80–1.23). In a broad retrospective registry analysis of 5841 hospitalized patients with ACS, mortality was higher in patients who received PA catheterization.[56] The results of these studies suggest that there is no indication for routine PA catheterization in patients with

ACS, unless there is concomitant cardiogenic shock or other complications. In this setting, hemodynamic monitoring with PACs may be necessary to guide appropriate therapy, particularly when vasoactive drugs are being used.

RV-MI

Diagnosis of Right Ventricular Myocardial Infarction (RV-MI) can be established by characteristic hemodynamic findings.[57] RA pressure is elevated and is frequently equal to or higher than PCWP.

Table 2
Hemodynamic Subsets in pump failure due to acute myocardial infarction

Subset	Clinical Signs: PC (Wet/Dry) HYP (Cold/Warm)		Cardiac Index (L/min/m²)	PAWP (mm Hg)	Hospital Mortality (%)
I	PC HYP	No (dry) No (warm)	>2.2	<18	3
II	PC HYP	Yes (wet) No (warm)	>2.2	>18	9
III	PC HYP	No (dry) Yes (cold)	<2.2	<18	23
IV	PC HYP	Yes (wet) Yes (cold)	<2.2	>18	51

Abbreviations: HYP, peripheral hypoperfusion; PAWP, pulmonary artery wedge pressure; PC, pulmonary congestion.
   Data from Forrester JS, Diamond G. Chatterjee K, et al. Medical therapy of acute myocardial infarction by application of hemodynamic subsets. N Engl J Med 1976;295:1356.

In patients with severe RV dysfunction, RV systolic pressure is not as elevated as in patients with pre-capillary pulmonary hypertension due to the RV's inability to generate high pressure. However, the most distinctive feature of acute RV infarction is a distorted PA pressure waveform (**Fig. 9**). Although a PAC is not needed for diagnosis of acute RV infarct, hemodynamic monitoring may be helpful in patients with cardiogenic shock complicating RV infarction.

Mechanical Complications of ACS

Acute mitral regurgitation and septal rupture are the 2 most striking mechanical complications of ACS. Acute mitral regurgitation due to papillary muscle infarction or rupture is associated with a giant "V" wave in the PCWP tracing or a reflected "V" wave in the PAP tracing (**Fig. 10**). Giant "V" waves are not diagnostic of acute severe mitral regurgitation as they can be observed in ventricular septal rupture and even in aortic and mitral

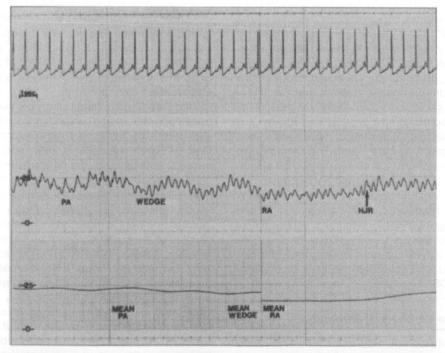

Fig. 9. Acute right ventricular infarct. Note that the PA waveform has a narrow pulse pressure due to decreased RV SV. The RA, PA and PCWP are difficult to differentiate. (*From* Sharkey SW. Beyond the wedge: clinical physiology and the Swan-Ganz catheter. Am J Med 1987;83(1):111–22.)

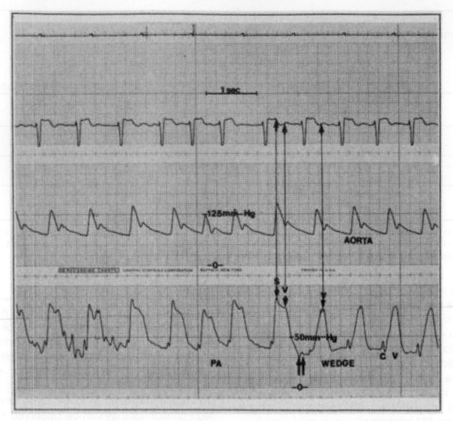

Fig. 10. Giant 'v' waves from acute MR reflected on the PA as well as the Wedge waveforms. (*From* Sharkey SW. Beyond the wedge: clinical physiology and the Swan-Ganz catheter. Am J Med 1987;83(1):111–22.)

stenosis. In these conditions, the magnitude of a normal "V" wave is accentuated if there is increased volume return to the left atrium. However, the reflected "V" wave in the PAP tracing is diagnostic of acute or subacute severe mitral regurgitation. Of course, papillary muscle infarction or rupture can be easily diagnosed by echocardiography.

Ventricular septal rupture is usually associated with a large left-to-right shunt. The characteristic hemodynamic feature is a large step up in O_2 saturation in pulmonary arterial and RV blood samples compared with that obtained from the RA (**Fig. 11**). Echocardiography, however, can be used not only for the diagnosis of the ventricular septal rupture but also to assess the magnitude of shunt. As such, PA catheterization is not required, nor recommended for diagnosis of mechanical complications of ACS.

Non Acute Coronary Syndromes

Hemodynamic monitoring with PACs is frequently used in intensive coronary units for management of patients with hypotension and shock not due to ACS or valvular heart disease. Determination

of PCWP can distinguish between hemodynamic (cardiogenic) and permeability (noncardiogenic) pulmonary edema. Hemodynamic pulmonary edema is characterized by a PCWP of 25 mm Hg or greater. In patients with permeability pulmonary edema, the PCWP is normal.

Septic and hypovolemic shock are two common conditions for which hemodynamic monitoring was frequently used in ICUs. Determination of RAP, PCWP, cardiac output, and systemic vascular resistance allows differentiation between cardiogenic, hypovolemic, and septic shock.

In cardiogenic shock, RAP and PCWP are usually elevated, but PCWP is higher than RAP. Cardiac output is reduced, systemic vascular resistance is usually elevated, and systemic systolic blood pressure is low. In hypovolemic shock, both RAP and PCWP are lower than normal, cardiac output and arterial pressure are reduced, and systemic vascular resistance is normal or elevated depending on the magnitude of hypotension and reduction of cardiac output. In septic shock, RAP and PCWP are normal before fluid therapy, cardiac output is normal or higher than normal, and systemic vascular resistance is abnormally low.

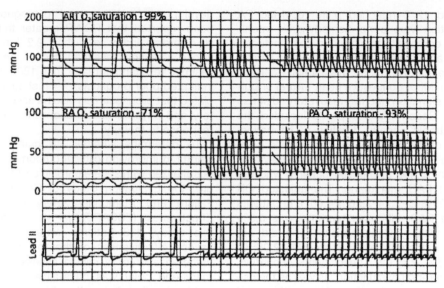

Fig. 11. Acute ventricular septal defect. Note the step up in O_2 saturation in PA and RV blood samples compared to that obtained from the RA. (*From* Disease-a-month. The Swan-Ganz Catheter. Dis Mon 1991;37(8):509–43; with permission.)

However, in critically ill patients with septic or hypovolemic shock, PA catheterization has been associated with an increased risk of mortality (OR of death was 1.24, 95% CI 1.03–1.049).[58]

In a randomized clinical trial performed in the United Kingdom, there was no difference in mortality, organ dysfunction, or length of hospital stay between patients receiving PA catheterization and patients who were not catheterized.[59] In a multicenter study, 676 patients with noncardiogenic shock or acute lung injury or both were randomized to receive PA catheterization or no catheterization. There was no difference in 30-day mortality between the 2 groups.[60]

In a randomized trial sponsored by National Heart, Lung, and Blood Institute, 1001 patients were randomized to receive PA catheterization or central venous catheter placement to assess the relative efficacy of PACs in decreasing mortality and morbidity of patients with acute respiratory distress syndrome.[61] In the PAC group, a slightly higher percentage of patients were in shock and received vasopressors. However, there was no difference in hospital mortality, ICU length of stay, or total hospital days. There was a higher incidence of arrhythmias in the PAC group. Also, although hospital costs were similar in both groups, the long-term cost was higher in the PAC group and there was a mean loss of 0.3 quality-adjusted life years in the PAC group.[62] Thus, PA catheterization did not provide any advantage over the use of central venous catheters in the management of patients with acute respiratory syndrome and routine use in this setting is not recommended.

PA catheterization has also been used for the management of high-risk surgical patients. In the perioperative setting, optimizing oxygen delivery by volume expansion therapy or hemodynamic manipulation with vasoactive drugs guided by PAC monitoring was associated with reduced mortality and morbidity and improved prognosis in high-risk surgical patients.[63,64] However, a randomized clinical trial of 1994 patients (after screening 3803) reported that there was no advantage of PA catheterization compared with standard care for the management of high-risk surgical patients in the perioperative period.[65] In-hospital mortality between the 2 groups was 7.7% and 7.8% in the standard care and catheterized groups, respectively. One-year survival was also similar in both groups. Although morbidity, including complications such as MI, heart failure, and arrhythmias, was similar in the 2 groups, the incidence of pulmonary embolism was higher in patients who received PA catheterization.

The need for perioperative and intraoperative hemodynamic monitoring with PACs in cardiac surgical patients remains controversial. In a prospective observational multicenter study, the effects of PA catheterization were assessed in 5065 patients undergoing coronary artery bypass surgery.[66] Some patients were monitored by transesophageal echocardiography only, whereas other patients were monitored by PA catheterization only. A third group received both TEE and PA catheterization and a fourth group received neither. Propensity score matched-pair analysis was used to statistically generate comparisons and yielded 1273 matched pairs receiving PA catheterization versus no hemodynamic monitoring. The composite primary end point included death from any cause, cerebral dysfunction (stroke or encephalopathy), renal dysfunction, cardiac dysfunction (MI or congestive heart failure) or pulmonary dysfunction (acute respiratory distress syndrome). Secondary end points included the use of inotropic agents, duration of intubation, and length of stay in ICUs. The primary end point occurred in 21.3% of the 271 patients receiving a PAC and in 15.4% of the 196 patients who did not receive PAC monitoring. The adjusted OR was 1.68 (95% CI 1.24–2.26; P<.001). In patients receiving a PAC, all-cause mortality was 3.5% compared with 1.7% in patients who did not receive PA catheterization (adjusted OR 2.08; CI 1.11%–3.88%, P = .02). The incidence of cardiac, renal, and cerebral dysfunction, as well as the use of inotropic drugs, duration of intubation, and length of stay in the ICU, was also higher in patients receiving PA catheterization. The results of this study thus suggest that PA catheterization can produce deleterious effects in patients undergoing coronary artery bypass surgery.

In another randomized trial, hemodynamic monitoring with PACs was compared with transpulmonary thermodilution (TTD) in patients undergoing combined valve repair surgery.[67] Patients were randomized in two equal groups of 40. In the PAC group, cardiac index, mean arterial pressure, and PCWP were monitored during goal-directed therapy. In the TTD group, global end-diastolic volume index, extravascular lung water index, and oxygen delivery index were additionally monitored. Hemodynamic improvement was greater in the TTD group and duration of mechanical ventilation was longer in the PAC group. The results of this study suggest that TTD is better than PAC during goal-directed therapy in patients undergoing combined valve repair surgery.

It should be recognized that in these studies, PA catheterization was performed not for the diagnosis of hemodynamic abnormality but for therapeutic guidance. This required prolonged catheterization, which may be associated with undesirable complications.

Chronic Systolic Heart Failure

In patients with severe chronic heart failure, PA catheterization has been performed to determine the severity of hemodynamic abnormalities to guide therapy and assess prognosis. In this context, clinical subsets based on hemodynamic abnormalities have been established and therapies specific to these subsets have also been developed.[68,69] With regard to prognosis, it has been reported that PCWP greater than 25 mm Hg, cardiac index less than 2.2 L/min/m^2, LV stroke work index less than 45 g/m^2, and systemic vascular resistance greater than 1800 dyn.s.cm^{-5} indicated poor prognosis.[70,71] It should be appreciated that prognosis can also be assessed by history and physical examination and evaluation of response to therapy.

To determine whether PA catheterization is helpful in improving clinical outcomes in patients hospitalized with severe chronic systolic heart failure, the Evaluation Study of Congestive Heart Failure and Pulmonary Artery Catheterization Effectiveness (ESCAPE) trial was performed.[72] In this study, 433 patients were randomized to assess effectiveness of therapy guided by PA catheterization or by clinical assessment. The primary end point was days-alive out of hospital within the first 6 months. The secondary end points were changes in quality of life, exercise tolerance, and biochemical and echocardiographic parameters. PAC use did not improve the primary outcome. The number of days-alive out of hospital in first 6 months was 133 days in the PAC group and 135 days in the clinical assessment group (hazard ratio 1.00, 95% CI 0.82–1.21; P = .99). Mortality in the PAC group was 10% and 9% in the clinical assessment group. In-hospital complications were 21.9% in the PAC group and 11.5% in the clinical assessment group (P = .04). These data suggest that routine use of PACs does not improve prognosis of patients with severe chronic heart failure and may be associated with a higher complication rate.

Pulmonary Hypertension

The etiology of pulmonary hypertension (PH) can be suspected by physical examination, heralded by the presence of a loud pulmonic component of the second heart sound. The presence or absence of mitral and aortic valve diseases and LV myocardial disease provides clues regarding whether PH is postcapillary, precapillary, or mixed. PH resulting from intracardiac shunts can also be suspected by bedside physical examination. Echo-Doppler studies should be routinely performed in all patients suspected of PH. However, right heart catheterization is necessary not only for diagnostic confirmation, but also to establish the etiology and guide therapeutic approach.[73,74]

A mean PA pressure at rest of greater than 25 mm Hg establishes the diagnosis of PH. Postcapillary pulmonary hypertension is defined when elevated PCWP is the principal mechanism for PH. In patients with postcapillary pulmonary hypertension, pulmonary vascular resistance is normal or only slightly elevated and the difference between PA end diastolic pressure and mean PCWP is 5 mm Hg or less.

In patients with precapillary pulmonary hypertension, PCWP is normal, pulmonary vascular resistance is markedly elevated, and the difference between the PA end diastolic pressure and mean PCWP is significantly greater than 5 mm Hg.

In patients with mixed-type pulmonary hypertension, PCWP is elevated and there is also increased pulmonary vascular resistance. The difference between PA end diastolic pressure and mean PCWP is greater than 5 mm Hg.

During hemodynamic evaluation of patients with pulmonary hypertension, oxygen saturations in the intracardiac chambers should be determined to exclude significant intracardiac shunts as well. The need and importance of PA catheterization in the diagnosis and management of patients with PH is apparent.

Transplantation

PA catheterization is routinely performed for evaluation of potential heart transplant recipients. In addition to determining PA pressure, pulmonary vascular resistance and the severity of right and left heart failure, the reversibility of pulmonary vascular resistance in response to pulmonary vasodilators is tested to determine whether heart, or combined heart and lung transplantation is indicated. Patients on continuous infusion of a single high-dose intravenous inotrope or multiple intravenous inotropes, in addition to continuous hemodynamic monitoring of LV filling pressures, are classified as Status 1A priority for purposes of heart transplantation.

Following transplantation, hemodynamics are monitored by PAC placement as well. Transient RV failure following cardiac or pulmonary transplantation therapy is common and therapies are frequently guided by hemodynamic abnormalities determined by PA catheterization.

COMPLICATIONS

Although the incidence of serious complications during hemodynamic monitoring with PACs is low, complications related to the placement and prolonged use do occur and can be significant.[75,76] Complications during insertion of PACs include inadvertent puncture of the arteries, production of large hematomas, formation of pseudoaneurysms, and hemothorax or pneumothorax. The incidence of inadvertent arterial puncture is approximately 3% to 9% and bleeding from the arterial puncture site can usually be

stopped by compression of the artery. Injury of the thoracic duct may occur during attempts to cannulate the left internal jugular or left subclavian vein and can lead to formation of chylothorax. The risk of catheter-related venous thrombosis is approximately 2% when subclavian veins are used, 8% when internal jugular veins are used, and 22% when femoral veins are used. These complications, however, are not unique to the use of PACs. The use of any central venous catheter can be associated with these complications. Air embolism, a potentially fatal complication in the presence of intracardiac shunts, occurs rarely.

Although cardiac arrhythmias occur frequently during placement of PACs, these arrhythmias are usually transient. Atrial and ventricular premature beats, nonsustained atrial and ventricular tachycardia, and conduction anomalies can occur during placement.[77,78] The incidence of arrhythmias ranges from 12.5% to 70.0% during placement of PACs. The incidence of ventricular premature beats is between 52% and 68% and that of nonsustained ventricular tachycardia is 1% to 53%. Sustained ventricular tachycardia or ventricular fibrillation requiring direct current shocks occurs in fewer than 1% of patients. In patients with preexisting left bundle branch block, complete heart block may be precipitated during insertion of PACs and pacing may be required.[79] The incidence of transient right bundle branch block is less than 5% and is benign.

Traumatic injury of the tricuspid valve apparatus can also occur.[80] Catheters can become entangled within the tricuspid valve chordate and severe tricuspid valve regurgitation can occur during removal of the entangled catheter.

As with any other central venous catheter, bacteremia, sepsis, and catheter site infection are potential complications as well. The reported incidence of sepsis and bacteremia is between 1.3% and 2.3%. Because the tricuspid valve can be traumatized during PAC placement, tricuspid valve endocarditis is potentially a serious complication. The reported incidence of right-sided endocarditis is between 2.2% and 7.1%.

Pulmonary artery rupture presents as sudden profuse hemoptysis and is almost always a fatal complication, but is rare, with a reported incidence between 0.03% and 0.20%.[81,82] The reported mortality is 70% and the risk factors are PA hypertension and older age. The forceful overinflation of the balloon and keeping the balloon inflated for prolonged periods of time are the most common causes of PA rupture. Rarely, PA dissection can be caused by the tip of the catheter, and can progress to complete rupture.

Knotting of pulmonary catheters is an uncommon complication, and the estimated incidence is 0.03%.[83] When the PA pressure wave form cannot be obtained despite advancing the PAC beyond 60 to 70 cm, use of fluoroscopy can reduce the risk of knotting. Catheter techniques for unknotting exist, although occasionally, extraction by venotomy is required.[76]

CONTROVERSY SURROUNDING THE PA CATHETER

There was tremendous enthusiasm following the introduction of the PAC, a technology that seemed to make it easy to estimate right and left heart-filling pressures and rapidly measure response to therapeutic interventions. Suddenly, it seemed, cardiopulmonary physiology could be studied without cumbersome technology and many physician scientists spent the good part of a decade exploring their favorite ideas. Cohn, an early surgical intensivist, for instance used the PAC to develop an "automated physiologic profile" to monitor hemodynamic, oxygen consumption and tissue utilization data in perioperative patients. Louis Del Guercio, a surgeon and one of the founders of the Society for Critical Care Medicine (SCCM) and its sixth president, used the "automated physiologic profile" to reduce operative mortality in elderly patients, using a variety of interventions.[84] Shoemaker, the third president of the SCCM, and others investigated whether "supranormal" oxygen delivery improved outcomes in high-risk surgical patients.[63,64] As discussed in the previous section, Forrester and colleagues[46,47] used the PAC in acute MI for prognostic and therapeutic purposes. The ability to easily generate reams of seemingly meaningful physiologic data was all too alluring for many intensivists to resist. Before long, the use of the PAC had become "routine" in all kinds of ICUs: cardiac, surgical, and medical. The rapidity of adoption of this technology was like few seen before. Indeed, Paul Marino remarked "The PAC is not just important for the specialty of critical care, it is *responsible* for the specialty of critical care".[85] Soon, there was an explosion of anecdotal data reporting improved outcomes, no difference at all, as well as worse outcomes in a variety of patient populations in uncontrolled settings. In 1996, Connors and colleagues[58] reported that the use of a PAC in 5735 critically ill patients was associated with an apparent lack of benefit and led to increased mortality and increased utilization of resources. The inevitable backlash followed, and at times it was shrill. Editorials with titles such as "Death by pulmonary artery flow-directed catheter,"[86] "Swan

song for the Swan-Ganz catheter?"[87] and "Is it time to pull the pulmonary artery catheter?"[88] appeared in leading journals. They were prompted largely by uncontrolled studies that suggested that mortality, the length of intensive care, and hospital costs were greater when a pulmonary catheter was used in a variety of clinical settings in various heterogeneous patient populations. In 1997, the SCCM tried to address this uncertainty by issuing a Consensus Statement,[89] which did little to address the confusion, as there were no randomized controlled trials (RCTs) to base those recommendations on. The first RCTs started appearing in 2002. In carefully controlled studies, the "routine" use of PACs in various populations, high-risk surgical patients,[65] patients with shock and acute respiratory distress,[60,61] critically ill patients,[59] and patients with congestive heart failure,[72] there was no improvement in outcomes. This led to a rapid and precipitous decline in the use of PACs across all types of ICUs in the United States.[53,90] Of course, this raises questions about maintaining ongoing competence in procedural skills and implications for clinical care and training of newer generations of cardiologists and intensivists.

As the use of the PAC declined and its use presumably more selective, a 2013 Cochrane review of 13 studies with a total of 5686 ICU patients showed that use of a PAC did not alter the mortality, general ICU or hospital LOS, or cost for adult patients in intensive care. The quality of evidence was high for mortality and LOS but low for cost analysis. The investigators made another important point: that newer, less-invasive hemodynamic monitoring tools need to be validated against the PAC before clinical use in critically ill patients.[91]

The fact is that the PAC, which is essentially a diagnostic tool, has been judged by clinical outcomes, standards that are meant to determine the efficacy of therapeutics. Indeed, few other diagnostic tools have been subject to such rigorous and perhaps misdirected scrutiny.

Although PACs are invasive, rendering them more prone to complications, both observed and unseen, they are diagnostic tools at best, and when considered in that context, provide data not easily obtained by other means. As early as 1990, Iberti and his group at Mount Sinai[92] had shown that there was a significant deficit in physicians' knowledge and understanding of PAC data. For example, only 59.5% of attending physicians could correctly identify the PCWP waveform. One cannot condemn chest radiographs or electrocardiograms as deficient if expert interpretation of these tests is lacking. In the scenario of clinical ambiguity for a pathophysiologically complex and critically ill patient, the clinician must first use the necessary tools to garner information, and then use this information to make an informed decision. To attribute clinical outcomes to a diagnostic decision in this setting is not warranted. Certainly, indiscriminate use of any invasive test in the wrong setting is undesirable, and may pose unnecessary risk. Clearly, "routine PA catheterization" lacks fundamental grounding in that no diagnostic test should be performed "routinely" without an appropriate context, even a simple venous blood sample.

With respect to risk, even when used in the appropriate population, clinicians should ensure that catheters are placed, used, and maintained optimally and that known pitfalls are avoided to minimize the risk. Avoidance of pitfalls includes not only PAC specific factors, but also increasing the reliance on operator independent data points such as mixed venous oxygen saturation as well as correlation with other laboratory markers of organ perfusion. Prompt removal of PACs after procurement of data also limits risk by minimizing the duration of invasive exposure. Additionally, expertise in obtaining and interpreting the waveforms and a firm fundamental understanding of the data derived will allow clinicians to make the most of data garnered following PAC placement. Even an uncomplicated catheter placement is rendered useless if data gathering or interpretation is faulty.

With respect to a multitude of less invasive hemodynamic tools, the PAC has been used in many more patients and clinical scenarios and subjected to more RCTs than any of these tools.

The plethora of existing data suggesting that "routine" PA catheterization in ICUs is not beneficial is likely multifactorial: poor patient selection, inability to identify and interpret data, untoward invasive risk, and the lack of effective therapies for the condition studied. As Richard and colleagues[60] correctly observed "Even if the purpose of monitoring with PAC is ultimately to save lives, it would be unrealistic to believe that the prognosis of patients could be improved by its presence alone."

A reasonable approach to the selective use of the PA catheter would be to

1. Understand the pitfalls and optimize procedural and interpretive handling, thus minimizing risk
2. Deploy only with appropriate patient selection and clinical scenario, thus maximizing potential benefit
3. Use only as long as necessary, remove as soon as possible
4. Correlate with nonoperator-dependent, highly sensitive variables such as SvO_2

5. Follow trends rather than focus solely on absolute values
6. Limit insertion and use by teams that have special training or expertise in performing and interpreting hemodynamic monitoring, just as we do with echocardiography or ventilators, for example
7. Continue research to better understand patient selection and define appropriate indications

CURRENT INDICATIONS FOR PA CATHETERIZATION

In light of the preceding, it becomes clear that in the hands of an operator who is fully aware of the many pitfalls and complications of the PAC and highly experienced in the synthesis and interpretation of data obtained from the PAC, it can be a valuable diagnostic tool. In the hands of such an operator, there is no diagnostic intervention that has been applied as widely, performed as easily, and subject to such intense scrutiny as the PAC. There is no demonstrated mortality benefit in applying this diagnostic tool "routinely" to large

---

Box 2
Indications for PA catheterization

Not indicated as routine in high-risk cardiac and noncardiac patients

Indicated in patients with cardiogenic shock during supportive therapy

Indicated in patients with discordant right and left ventricular failure

Indicated in patients with severe chronic heart failure requiring inotropic, vasopressor, and vasodilator therapy

Indicated in patients with suspected "pseudosepsis" (high cardiac output, low systemic vascular resistance, elevated right atrial and pulmonary capillary wedge pressures)

Indicated in some patients with potentially reversible systolic heart failure, such as fulminant myocarditis and peripartum cardiomyopathy

Indicated for the hemodynamic differential diagnosis of pulmonary hypertension

Indicated to assess response to therapy in patients with precapillary and mixed types of pulmonary hypertension

Indicated for the transplantation workup

Adapted from Chatterjee K. The Swan-Ganz catheters: past, present, and future. A viewpoint. Circulation 2009;119(1):147–52; with permission.

heterogeneous populations of critically ill patients, nor is there increased mortality or length of stay.

It is also abundantly clear that in current clinical practice, no assessment of pulmonary hypertension or management of advanced heart failure or evaluation for heart transplant proceeds without PA catheterization. In most other scenarios, despite all that has been written, patient selection and tailored therapy is still an art and is highly operator dependant. Indications that are relevant to the use of the PAC in cardiac critical care are listed in **Box 2**.

SUMMARY

The PAC has come a full circle. Devised by cardiologists to probe the inner workings of the heart, it has inspired much research and clinical use. Over time, evidence has developed that harm could result if it is not used judiciously. Nevertheless, it remains a simple diagnostic intervention, done at the bedside with proven utility in cardiac critical care. Many technologies seek to supplant the PAC, but none has been subjected to as much clinical use and scrutiny. It is paramount that the user be intimately familiar with the pitfalls, the dangers of misinterpretation, and the potential complications of this device. More importantly, thoughtful patient selection and judicious use of this device can mitigate any possible harm and maximize utility.

REFERENCES

1. Bernard GR, Sopko G, Cerra F, et al. Pulmonary artery catheterization and clinical outcomes: National Heart, Lung, and Blood Institute and Food and Drug Administration Workshop Report. Consensus Statement. JAMA 2000;283(19):2568–72.
2. Nossaman BD, Scruggs BA, Nossaman VE, et al. History of right heart catheterization: 100 years of experimentation and methodology development. Cardiol Rev 2010;18(2):94–101.
3. Cournand A. Cardiac catheterization; development of the technique, its contributions to experimental medicine, and its initial applications in man. Acta Med Scand Suppl 1975;579:3–32.
4. Cournand A. Historical details of Claude Bernard's invention of a technique for measuring the temperature and the pressure of the blood within the cavities of the heart. Trans N Y Acad Sci 1980;39:1–14.
5. Chaveau A, Marey EJ. Memoires de L'Academie Inmperial de Medicine. Appareils et Experiences Cardiographiques 1863.
6. Forssmann W. Die Sondierung des Rechten Herzens. Klin Wochenschr 1929;8(45):2085–7.
7. Berry D. Pioneers in cardiology. Werner Forssmann-sowing the seeds for selective cardiac catheterization procedures in the twentieth century. Eur Heart J 2009;30(11):1296–7.
8. Forssmann-Falck R. Werner Forssmann: a pioneer of cardiology. Am J Cardiol 1997;79(5):651–60.
9. Mueller RL, Sanborn TA. The history of interventional cardiology: cardiac catheterization, angioplasty, and related interventions. Am Heart J 1995;129(1):146–72.
10. Cournand A, Lauson HD, Bloomfield RA, et al. Recording of right heart pressures in man. Exp Biol Med 1944;55(1):34–6.
11. Cournand A, Riley RL, Breed ES, et al. Measurement of cardiac output in man using the technique of catheterization of the right auricle or ventricle. J Clin Invest 1945;24(1):106–16.
12. Cournand A, Ranges HA. Catheterization of the right auricle in man. Exp Biol Med 1941;46(3):462–6.
13. Berseus S, Lagerlof H, Werko L. A comparison between the direct Fick and the Grollman methods for determination of the cardiac output in man. Acta Med Scand Suppl 1950;239:258.
14. Hamilton WF, Riley RL, Attyah AM, et al. Comparison of the Fick and dye injection methods of measuring the cardiac output in man. Am J Physiol 1948;153(2):309–21.
15. Richard D. Cardiac output by the catheterization technique, in various clinical conditions. Fed Proc 1945;4:215–20.
16. Bloomfield RA, Lauson HD, Cournand A, et al. Recording of right heart pressures in normal subjects and in patients with chronic pulmonary disease and various types of cardio-circulatory disease. J Clin Invest 1946;25(4):639–64.
17. Raju TN. The Nobel chronicles. 1956: Werner Forssmann (1904-79); Andre Frederic Cournand (1895-1988); and Dickinson Woodruff Richards, Jr (1895-1973). Lancet 1999;353(9167):1891.
18. Hellems HK, Haynes FW, Dexter L. Pulmonary capillary pressure in man. J Appl Physiol 1949;2(1):24–9.
19. Lategola M, Rahn H. A self-guiding catheter for cardiac and pulmonary arterial catheterization and occlusion. Proc Soc Exp Biol Med 1953;84(3):667–8.
20. Bradley RD. Diagnostic right-heart catheterisation with miniature catheters in severely ill patients. Lancet 1964;2(7366):941–2.
21. Fife WP, Lee BS. Construction and use of self-guiding, right heart and pulmonary artery catheter. J Appl Physiol 1965;20:148–9.
22. Scheinman MM, Abbott JA, Rapaport E. Clinical uses of a flow-directed right heart catheter. Arch Intern Med 1969;124(1):19–24.
23. Swan HJ. The pulmonary artery catheter in anesthesia practice. 1970. Anesthesiology 2005;103(4):890–3.
24. Swan HJ, Ganz W, Forrester J, et al. Catheterization of the heart in man with use of a flow-directed

balloon-tipped catheter. N Engl J Med 1970;283(9): 447–51.

25. Forrester JS, Ganz W, Diamond G, et al. Thermodilution cardiac output determination with a single flow-directed catheter. Am Heart J 1972;83(3): 306–11.

26. Chatterjee K, Swan HJ, Ganz W, et al. Use of a balloon-tipped flotation electrode catheter for cardiac mounting. Am J Cardiol 1975;36(1):56–61.

27. Vincent JL. The pulmonary artery catheter. J Clin Monit Comput 2012;26(5):341–5.

28. West JB, Dollery CT, Naimark A. Distribution of blood flow in isolated lung; relation to vascular and alveolar pressures. J Appl Physiol 1964;19:713–24.

29. Komadina KH, Schenk DA, LaVeau P, et al. Interobserver variability in the interpretation of pulmonary artery catheter pressure tracings. Chest 1991; 100(6):1647–54.

30. Falicov RE, Resnekov L. Relationship of the pulmonary artery end-diastolic pressure to the left ventricular end-diastolic and mean filling pressures in patients with and without left ventricular dysfunction. Circulation 1970;42(1):65–73.

31. Rahimtoola SH, Loeb HS, Ehsani A, et al. Relationship of pulmonary artery to left ventricular diastolic pressures in acute myocardial infarction. Circulation 1972;46(2):283–90.

32. Scheinman M, Evans GT, Weiss A, et al. Relationship between pulmonary artery end-diastolic pressure and left ventricular filling pressure in patients in shock. Circulation 1973;47(2):317–24.

33. Mangano DT. Monitoring pulmonary arterial pressure in coronary-artery disease. Anesthesiology 1980;53(5):364–70.

34. Sarin CL, Yalav E, Clement AJ, et al. The necessity for measurement of left atrial pressure after cardiac valve surgery. Thorax 1970;25(2):185–9.

35. Bell H, Stubbs D, Pugh D. Reliability of central venous pressure as an indicator of left atrial pressure. A study in patients with mitral valve disease. Chest 1971;59(2):169–73.

36. Killu K, Oropello JM, Manasia AR, et al. Effect of lower limb compression devices on thermodilution cardiac output measurement. Crit Care Med 2007;35(5):1307–11.

37. Paarmann H, Groesdonk HV, Sedemund-Adib B, et al. Lack of agreement between pulmonary arterial thermodilution cardiac output and the pressure recording analytical method in postoperative cardiac surgery patients. Br J Anaesth 2011;106(4):475–81.

38. Mutoh T, Kazumata K, Ishikawa T, et al. Performance of bedside transpulmonary thermodilution monitoring for goal-directed hemodynamic management after subarachnoid hemorrhage. Stroke 2009;40(7):2368–74.

39. Diwan A, McCulloch M, Lawrie GM, et al. Doppler estimation of left ventricular filling pressures in patients with mitral valve disease. Circulation 2005;111(24):3281–9.

40. Oh JK. Echocardiography as a noninvasive Swan-Ganz catheter. Circulation 2005;111(24):3192–4.

41. Feissel M, Michard F, Faller JP, et al. The respiratory variation in inferior vena cava diameter as a guide to fluid therapy. Intensive Care Med 2004; 30(9):1834–7.

42. Thom O, Taylor DM, Wolfe RE, et al. Comparison of a supra-sternal cardiac output monitor (USCOM) with the pulmonary artery catheter. Br J Anaesth 2009;103(6):800–4.

43. Lopes PC, Sousa MG, Camacho AA, et al. Comparison between two methods for cardiac output measurement in propofol-anesthetized dogs: thermodilution and Doppler. Vet Anaesth Analg 2010; 37(5):401–8.

44. Crexells C, Chatterjee K, Forrester JS, et al. Optimal level of filling pressure in the left side of the heart in acute myocardial infarction. N Engl J Med 1973;289(24):1263–6.

45. Forrester JS, Diamond G, Chatterjee K, et al. Medical therapy of acute myocardial infarction by application of hemodynamic subsets (first of two parts). N Engl J Med 1976;295(24):1356–62.

46. Forrester JS, Diamond G, Chatterjee K, et al. Medical therapy of acute myocardial infarction by application of hemodynamic subsets (second of two parts). N Engl J Med 1976;295(25):1404–13.

47. Dikshit K, Vyden JK, Forrester JS, et al. Renal and extrarenal hemodynamic effects of furosemide in congestive heart failure after acute myocardial infarction. N Engl J Med 1973;288(21):1087–90.

48. Walinsky P, Chatterjee K, Forrester J, et al. Enhanced left ventricular performance with phentolamine in acute myocardial infarction. Am J Cardiol 1974;33(1):37–41.

49. Chatterjee K, Swan HJ, Kaushik VS, et al. Effects of vasodilator therapy for severe pump failure in acute myocardial infarction on short-term and late prognosis. Circulation 1976;53(5):797–802.

50. Abrams E, Forrester JS, Chatterjee K, et al. Variability in response to norepinephrine in acute myocardial infarction. Am J Cardiol 1973;32(7):919–23.

51. Ommen SR, Nishimura RA, Appleton CP, et al. Clinical utility of Doppler echocardiography and tissue Doppler imaging in the estimation of left ventricular filling pressures: a comparative simultaneous Doppler-catheterization study. Circulation 2000; 102(15):1788–94.

52. Ruisi CP, Goldberg RJ, Kennelly BM, et al. Pulmonary artery catheterization in patients with acute coronary syndromes. Am Heart J 2009;158(2): 170–6.

53. Wiener RS, Welch HG. Trends in the use of the pulmonary artery catheter in the United States, 1993-2004. JAMA 2007;298(4):423–9.

54. Cohen MG, Kelly RV, Kong DF, et al. Pulmonary artery catheterization in acute coronary syndromes: insights from the GUSTO IIb and GUSTO III trials. Am J Med 2005;118(5):482–8.

55. Gore JM, Goldberg RJ, Spodick DH, et al. A community-wide assessment of the use of pulmonary artery catheters in patients with acute myocardial infarction. Chest 1987;92(4):721–7.

56. Zion MM, Balkin J, Rosenmann D, et al. Use of pulmonary artery catheters in patients with acute myocardial infarction. Analysis of experience in 5,841 patients in the SPRINT Registry. SPRINT Study Group. Chest 1990;98(6):1331–5.

57. Goldstein JA. Pathophysiology and management of right heart ischemia. J Am Coll Cardiol 2002; 40(5):841–53.

58. Connors AF Jr, Speroff T, Dawson NV, et al. The effectiveness of right heart catheterization in the initial care of critically ill patients. SUPPORT Investigators. JAMA 1996;276(11):889–97.

59. Rhodes A, Cusack RJ, Newman PJ, et al. A randomised, controlled trial of the pulmonary artery catheter in critically ill patients. Intensive Care Med 2002;28(3):256–64.

60. Richard C, Warszawski J, Anguel N, et al. Early use of the pulmonary artery catheter and outcomes in patients with shock and acute respiratory distress syndrome: a randomized controlled trial. JAMA 2003;290(20):2713–20.

61. National Heart, Lung, and Blood Institute Acute Respiratory Distress Syndrome (ARDS) Clinical Trials Network, Wheeler AP, Bernard GR. Pulmonary-artery versus central venous catheter to guide treatment of acute lung injury. N Engl J Med 2006;354(21):2213–24.

62. Clermont G, Kong L, Weissfeld LA, et al. The effect of pulmonary artery catheter use on costs and long-term outcomes of acute lung injury. PloS One 2011;6(7):e22512.

63. Shoemaker WC, Appel PL, Kram HB, et al. Prospective trial of supranormal values of survivors as therapeutic goals in high-risk surgical patients. Chest 1988;94(6):1176–86.

64. Boyd O, Grounds RM, Bennett ED. A randomized clinical trial of the effect of deliberate perioperative increase of oxygen delivery on mortality in high-risk surgical patients. JAMA 1993;270(22): 2699–707.

65. Sandham JD, Hull RD, Brant RF, et al. A randomized, controlled trial of the use of pulmonary-artery catheters in high-risk surgical patients. N Engl J Med 2003;348(1):5–14.

66. Schwann NM, Hillel Z, Hoeft A, et al. Lack of effectiveness of the pulmonary artery catheter in cardiac surgery. Anesth Analg 2011;113(5):994–1002.

67. Lenkin AI, Kirov MY, Kuzkov VV, et al. Comparison of goal-directed hemodynamic optimization using pulmonary artery catheter and transpulmonary thermodilution in combined valve repair: a randomized clinical trial. Crit Care Res Pract 2012;2012: 821218.

68. Steimle AE, Stevenson LW, Chelimsky-Fallick C, et al. Sustained hemodynamic efficacy of therapy tailored to reduce filling pressures in survivors with advanced heart failure. Circulation 1997; 96(4):1165–72.

69. Stevenson LW, Tillisch JH. Maintenance of cardiac output with normal filling pressures in patients with dilated heart failure. Circulation 1986;74(6): 1303–8.

70. Franciosa JA, Wilen M, Ziesche S, et al. Survival in men with severe chronic left ventricular failure due to either coronary heart disease or idiopathic dilated cardiomyopathy. Am J Cardiol 1983;51(5): 831–6.

71. Unverferth DV, Magorien RD, Moeschberger ML, et al. Factors influencing the one-year mortality of dilated cardiomyopathy. Am J Cardiol 1984;54(1): 147–52.

72. Binanay C, Califf RM, Hasselblad V, et al. Evaluation study of congestive heart failure and pulmonary artery catheterization effectiveness: the ESCAPE trial. JAMA 2005;294(13):1625–33.

73. Galie N, Hoeper MM, Humbert M, et al. Guidelines for the diagnosis and treatment of pulmonary hypertension. Eur Respir J 2009;34(6):1219–63.

74. Chatterjee K, De Marco T, Alpert JS. Pulmonary hypertension: hemodynamic diagnosis and management. Arch Intern Med 2002;162(17): 1925–33.

75. McGee DC, Gould MK. Preventing complications of central venous catheterization. N Engl J Med 2003;348(12):1123–33.

76. Evans DC, Doraiswamy VA, Prosciak MP, et al. Complications associated with pulmonary artery catheters: a comprehensive clinical review. Scand J Surg 2009;98(4):199–208.

77. Iberti TJ, Benjamin E, Gruppi L, et al. Ventricular arrhythmias during pulmonary artery catheterization in the intensive care unit. Prospective study. Am J Med 1985;78(3):451–4.

78. Sprung CL, Pozen RG, Rozanski JJ, et al. Advanced ventricular arrhythmias during bedside pulmonary artery catheterization. Am J Med 1982; 72(2):203–8.

79. Morris D, Mulvihill D, Lew WY. Risk of developing complete heart block during bedside pulmonary artery catheterization in patients with left bundle-branch block. Arch Intern Med 1987;147(11): 2005–10.

80. Arnaout S, Diab K, Al-Kutoubi A, et al. Rupture of the chordae of the tricuspid valve after knotting of the pulmonary artery catheter. Chest 2001;120(5): 1742–4.

81. Damen J, Bolton D. A prospective analysis of 1,400 pulmonary artery catheterizations in patients undergoing cardiac surgery. Acta Anaesthesiol Scand 1986;30(5):386–92.

82. Kearney TJ, Shabot MM. Pulmonary artery rupture associated with the Swan-Ganz catheter. Chest 1995;108(5):1349–52.

83. Bossert T, Gummert JF, Bittner HB, et al. Swan-Ganz catheter-induced severe complications in cardiac surgery: right ventricular perforation, knotting, and rupture of a pulmonary artery. J Card Surg 2006;21(3):292–5.

84. Del Guercio LR, Cohn JD. Monitoring operative risk in the elderly. JAMA 1980;243(13):1350–5.

85. Marino PL. The ICU Book. 2nd edition. Philadelphia: Lippincott Williams and Wilkins; 1997. p. 154.

86. Robin ED. Death by pulmonary artery flow-directed catheter. Time for a moratorium? Chest 1987;92(4): 727–31.

87. Soni N. Swan song for the Swan-Ganz catheter? BMJ 1996;313(7060):763–4.

88. Dalen JE, Bone RC. Is it time to pull the pulmonary artery catheter? JAMA 1996;276(11):916–8.

89. Pulmonary Artery Catheter Consensus Conference: consensus statement. New Horiz 1997;5(3):175–94.

90. Leibowitz AB, Oropello JM. The pulmonary artery catheter in anesthesia practice in 2007: an historical overview with emphasis on the past 6 years. Semin Cardiothorac Vasc Anesth 2007;11(3): 162–76.

91. Rajaram SS, Desai NK, Kalra A, et al. Pulmonary artery catheters for adult patients in intensive care. Cochrane Database Syst Rev 2013;(2):CD003408.

92. Iberti TJ, Fischer EP, Leibowitz AB, et al. A multicenter study of physicians' knowledge of the pulmonary artery catheter. Pulmonary Artery Catheter Study Group. JAMA 1990;264(22): 2928–32.

Cardiogenic Shock

Howard A. Cooper, MD[a],*, Julio A. Panza, MD[b]

KEYWORDS

- Cardiogenic shock • Acute myocardial infarction • Prognosis • Reperfusion • Inflammation
- Intra-aortic balloon pump • Left ventricular assist device • Extracorporeal membrane oxygenation

KEY POINTS

- Cardiogenic shock is a final common pathway defined by a marked reduction in cardiac output and inadequate end-organ perfusion, which can result from an array of cardiac insults.
- Cardiogenic shock is a systemic disease involving a vicious cycle of inflammation, ischemia, and progressive myocardial dysfunction, which often results in death.
- Cardiogenic shock is the leading cause of death from acute myocardial infarction; urgent revascularization favorably impacts mortality.
- Cardiogenic shock is a life-threatening emergency that requires intensive monitoring accompanied by aggressive hemodynamic support with vasopressors, inotropes, and/or mechanical circulatory support.
- Novel therapeutic strategies are required to reduce the unacceptably high mortality rates currently associated with cardiogenic shock.

INTRODUCTION

Cardiogenic shock (CS) is a dramatic and highly lethal condition that has long presented a challenge to those who care for patients in the cardiac intensive care unit (CICU). CS represents the final common pathway of a large number of pathologic conditions, leading to a marked impairment of cardiac output and consequently a state of inadequate end-organ perfusion. As a result, a vicious cycle of inflammation, ischemia, and progressive myocardial dysfunction ensues, which often results in death. Despite decades of study, the mortality rate associated with CS remains stubbornly high. Indeed, recent studies have called into question the role of interventions previously believed to be of significant benefit. Nevertheless, an expanding understanding of the pathophysiology of this condition, and the availability of increasingly sophisticated pharmacologic and mechanical therapies, are likely to result in substantially improved outcomes for patients with CS in the years ahead.

ETIOLOGY

The cause of CS may be left ventricular (LV) or right ventricular (RV) pump failure, severe valvular regurgitation, or ventricular disruption, alone or in combination (**Box 1**). Although sometimes included as a type of CS, obstructive shock (eg, valvular obstruction, pulmonary embolism, cardiac tamponade) is not discussed in this review. The inciting event precipitating CS may be abrupt in origin, as is the case for acute myocardial infarction (AMI) or fulminant myocarditis, or may be the rapid decompensation of a chronic disorder, such as dilated cardiomyopathy. No large-scale registries of CS exist, and therefore reliable data regarding the relative contribution of these various etiologies are not available. **Fig. 1** displays the experience of our tertiary CICU during 2012.

Disclosures: The authors have nothing to disclose.
[a] Coronary Care Unit, Medstar Heart Institute, Medstar Washington Hospital Center, 110 Irving Street Northwest, Suite NA-1103, Washington, DC 20010, USA; [b] Division of Cardiology, Westchester Medical Center, 100 Woods Road, Valhalla, NY 10595, USA
* Corresponding author.
E-mail address: howard.a.cooper@medstar.net

Cardiol Clin 31 (2013) 567–580
http://dx.doi.org/10.1016/j.ccl.2013.07.009
0733-8651/13/$ – see front matter © 2013 Elsevier Inc. All rights reserved.

Box 1
Etiologies of cardiogenic shock

1. Left ventricular pump failure
   a. Acute myocardial infarction (STEMI, non-STEMI)
   b. Acute myocarditis
   c. Tako-tsubo cardiomyopathy
   d. Cardiac contusion
   e. End-stage cardiomyopathy
   f. Prolonged cardiopulmonary bypass
   g. Septic shock with severe myocardial depression
2. Right ventricular pump failure
   a. Right ventricular infarction
   b. End-stage pulmonary hypertension
3. Acute valvular regurgitation
   a. Ischemic mitral regurgitation
   b. Papillary muscle rupture
   c. Myxomatous degeneration of the mitral valve with rupture of chordae tendinae
   d. Infective endocarditis
   e. Aortic dissection
   f. Trauma
4. Ventricular disruption
   a. Ventricular septal rupture
   b. Free wall rupture

INCIDENCE

Because of the wide spectrum of causes of CS, the true incidence of this condition is unknown; however, the most common cause of CS remains AMI, for which the incidence has been well described. CS occurs in 5% to 8% of patients hospitalized with AMI, and is more common among patients presenting with ST-segment elevation myocardial infarction (STEMI) than among those with non-STEMI.[1] The incidence of CS complicating AMI remained stable for many years, but recently appears to have decreased in parallel with the adoption of primary percutaneous coronary intervention (PCI) for STEMI. For example, in a large population-based registry of acute coronary syndromes, the overall incidence of CS fell from 12.9% in 1997 to 5.5% in 2006.[2] Importantly, only a minority of patients with AMI with CS arrive at the hospital with an established clinical syndrome of organ hypoperfusion. In most (>70%) cases, shock develops following hospital admission.[3,4]

OUTCOMES

Although the mortality rate associated with CS likely varies depending on the etiology, systematic data on outcomes are available only for CS resulting from AMI. CS is the most common cause of death in patients hospitalized with AMI, and short-term mortality rates have been slow to improve. Earlier studies reported mortality rates as high as 80%.[5] In-hospital mortality in the SHould we emergently revascularize Occluded Coronaries for CS (SHOCK) Trial Registry was 60%, similar to the 59.4% rate reported from the Global Registry of Acute Coronary Events (GRACE) registry.[6,7] In some recent reports, however, in-hospital mortality rates of less than 50% have been achieved.[2,8,9] In our CICU, we treated 438 patients with post-MI CS from 2006 to 2012, with an in-hospital mortality rate of 37%. Importantly, several studies have demonstrated that among

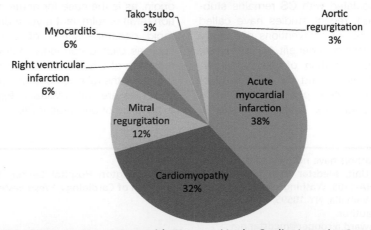

Fig. 1. Etiology of CS in 34 consecutive patients with CS treated in the Cardiac Intensive Care Unit of the Medstar Washington Hospital Center in 2012.

CS survivors, long-term outcomes are quite favorable.[10–12]

PATHOPHYSIOLOGY

Investigations into the pathophysiology of CS in the early twentieth century concluded, in general, that "shock… is largely, and probably solely, a manifestation of heart failure."[13] However, even then, the possibility that mechanisms other than pump dysfunction contributed to the shock state was seriously considered. Indeed, Boyer wrote in 1944 that "…it is still conceivable that peripheral mechanisms play a contributory role."[13] Over the ensuing decades, a clearer understanding of the complex interplay between forces local and systemic, mechanical and biochemical, has begun to emerge.

A more contemporary understanding of CS considers it to be the final common pathway of a number of derangements that affect the entire circulatory system (**Fig. 2**). CS is initiated by a severe reduction in cardiac output, lowering perfusion of the coronary arteries, which may already be compromised by atherosclerotic lesions. This leads to ischemia, further worsening of myocardial performance, and hence the perpetuation of a vicious cycle within the heart. Further myocardial necrosis and/or stunning may result from distal embolization and/or reperfusion injury when fibrinolytics therapy or primary PCI is undertaken, or from reocclusion of the infarct artery. Right ventricular failure may be the primary cause of CS, but more commonly is a contributing factor.

As a response to this central circulatory derangement, compensatory neurohumoral responses occur, including activation of the sympathetic and angiotensin-renin systems. These may temporarily increase contractility and induce peripheral vasoconstriction in an attempt to maintain central blood pressure and sustain flow to vital organs. However, the ultimate result is worsening myocardial ischemia, further peripheral organ hypoperfusion, and an increase in the risk of ventricular arrhythmias. Catecholamines (intrinsic or pharmacologic) increase myocardial oxygen

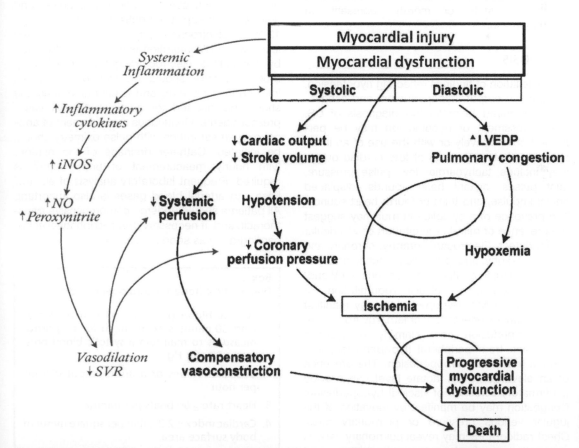

Fig. 2. Modern paradigm of CS in acute myocardial infarction. LVEDP, left ventricular end-diastolic pressure. (*From* Antman EM, Braunwald E. Acute myocardial infarction. In: Braunwald E, Fauci A, Kasper D, et al, editors. Harrison's Principles of Internal Medicine. 15th edition. New York: McGraw-Hill; 2001. p. 1395; with permission.)

demand and may also be directly myocardiotoxic. Neurohumoral activation leads to salt and water retention, resulting in pulmonary edema, worsening hypoxia, and further ischemia. When these compensatory mechanisms are overwhelmed, anaerobic metabolism and lactic acidosis ensue, further depressing myocardial function.[14]

Inflammatory mediators, including interleukin-6 (IL-6) and tumor necrosis factor-alpha (TNF-α), are frequently elevated in CS and have a negative inotropic effect. In addition, cytokines lead to the production of high levels of nitric oxide (NO) through induction of inducible nitric oxide synthase (iNOS). This may result in a state of inappropriate vasodilation, worsening hypotension, and lactic acidosis.[1] Consistent with these observations, approximately 20% of patients in the SHOCK trial demonstrated findings characteristic of the systemic inflammatory response syndrome, with low systemic vascular resistance, fever, leukocytosis, and elevated inflammatory markers, such as C-reactive protein.[15] However, despite intensive investigation, it remains unclear whether these mechanisms are important contributors to the shock state or merely represent an epiphenomenon.[1]

DIAGNOSIS

A constellation of findings reflecting hypotension, low cardiac output, hypoperfusion, and congestion is required to make the diagnosis of CS. The assessment of hypotension may be performed noninvasively or with the use of an intra-arterial catheter. Findings of low cardiac output may include tachycardia, low pulse pressure, faint pulses, distant heart sounds, displaced apical impulse, and third or fourth heart sounds. The presence of a systolic murmur may suggest the presence of mitral regurgitation or ventricular septal defect. Electrocardiography, coronary and LV angiography, and, particularly, echocardiography are useful to confirm the presence of LV and/or RV dysfunction, valvular regurgitation, or cardiac disruption. Hypoperfusion may manifest as agitation, disorientation, or lethargy from cerebral hypoperfusion; cool, clammy, or cyanotic extremities from peripheral hypoperfusion; and oliguria from renal hypoperfusion. The presence of an elevated serum lactate level can provide confirmatory evidence of visceral hypoperfusion. Congestion may be manifest by elevation of the jugular venous pressure or pulmonary rales. Chest radiography may reveal pulmonary venous congestion or frank pulmonary edema, and serum natriuretic peptide levels are generally elevated.

Various sets of diagnostic criteria for CS have been proposed, each of which relies on invasive hemodynamic measurements obtained from a pulmonary artery catheter (PAC), in addition to clinical findings. There is no consensus as to which of these invasive criteria represent the diagnostic "gold standard," but the criteria used for entry into the SHOCK trial are generally accepted (**Box 2**).

GENERAL CONSIDERATIONS, MONITORING, AND THERAPY
General Considerations

CS is a life-threatening emergency. Hence, once the diagnosis of CS is established, the clinician must immediately seek to understand the cause of the clinical condition as well as initiate therapy before irreversible injury to vital organs ensues. Meticulous patient monitoring in a cardiac intensive care unit is essential, as rapid changes often occur throughout the clinical course. Frequent clinical assessment should be performed by an expert team composed of, at a minimum, a cardiac intensivist, cardiac critical care nurse, and respiratory therapist. All patients should undergo 12-lead electrocardiography (with right-sided leads when RV infarction is suspected), followed by continuous electrocardiographic monitoring. Blood pressure should be monitored with an intra-arterial catheter, and a central venous line should be inserted for administration of vasopressor agents. Continuous measurement of arterial oxygen saturation with pulse oximetry should be initiated. Catheter drainage of the bladder with hourly measurement of urine output is required. Frequent laboratory analysis of electrolytes and arterial blood gases is also important. All patients should undergo comprehensive transthoracic and, if necessary, transesophageal echocardiography as soon as feasible.

Box 2
Diagnostic criteria for cardiogenic shock

1. Systolic blood pressure <90 mm Hg for at least 30 minutes or the need for supportive measures to maintain a systolic blood pressure ≥90 mm Hg

2. Cool extremities *or* a urine output <30 mL per hour

3. Heart rate ≥60 beats per minute

4. Cardiac index ≤2.2 L/min per square meter of body surface area

5. Pulmonary capillary occlusion pressure ≥15 mm Hg

Hemodynamic Monitoring

The role of invasive hemodynamic monitoring with a PAC in patients with CS is uncertain. No clinical trial has yet established a clinical benefit with the use of this modality in this clinical setting. Less invasive or noninvasive alternatives, such as trans-pulmonary thermodilution, pulse contour analysis, thoracic electrical bioimpedance, and bedside Doppler echocardiography are being used with increasing frequency.[16] Nevertheless, monitoring with a PAC may serve multiple important functions in the setting of CS (**Box 3**), and most authorities continue to recommend the insertion of a PAC in patients with CS.[17] When a PAC is used, clinical judgment is essential to avoid potentially cata-strophic complications (eg, pulmonary artery rupture).

Initial Therapy

Limited initial fluid resuscitation is reasonable un-less frank pulmonary edema is present. The main-tenance of adequate oxygenation and airway protection is essential, and mechanical intubation is frequently required. Care should be taken to avoid oxygen toxicity and unnecessarily high levels of positive end-expiratory pressure. Moderate hy-perventilation may assist in correcting acidemia. Hypokalemia and hypomagnesemia predispose patients to ventricular arrhythmia and should be aggressively corrected. If sustained atrial or ven-tricular arrhythmias are present, prompt electrical cardioversion should be performed. Amiodarone

---

Box 3
Role of the pulmonary artery catheter in cardiogenic shock

- Eliminate diagnostic uncertainty
- Distinguish among various hemodynamic profiles
  - Left ventricular failure: high PAOP, low car-diac output, high SVR
  - Right ventricular failure: high RA pressure and a ratio of right atrial/PAOP >0.8
  - Mitral regurgitation: large v-wave in the PAOP tracing
  - Ventricular septal rupture: significant step-up in oxygen saturation between the RA and the pulmonary artery
- Guide fluid and inotropic therapy
- Provide prognostic data (eg, cardiac power)

Abbreviations: PAOP, pulmonary artery occlusion pres-sure; RA, right atrium; SVR, systemic vascular resis-tance.

---

is useful to prevent arrhythmia recurrence. Inap-propriate bradycardia, which can be due to excess vagotonia, heart block, or drug effects, should be corrected pharmacologically or with temporary transvenous pacing. Narcotic analgesics in mod-erate doses are useful to limit pain and anxiety, as well as reduce preload, afterload, and sympa-thetic activity. Diuretics can be used to decrease filling pressures and relieve pulmonary congestion. Beta blockers and calcium channel blockers should be avoided, as they have negative inotropic properties and may worsen shock.[18] Marked hy-perglycemia (and any hypoglycemia) should be avoided, and an insulin infusion may be required.

Reperfusion

When the etiology of CS is AMI, rapid relief of ischemia is essential. Standard, guideline-recommended medical therapy should be initiated, with the exception that medications that lower blood pressure (beta blockers, nitrates) should be omitted. In the setting of STEMI, fibrinolytic ther-apy has been shown to reduce the incidence of CS; however, no study has demonstrated a bene-ficial effect of fibrinolytic therapy on mortality once CS is established.[12,19,20]

The landmark SHOCK trial randomized 302 pa-tients with CS complicating STEMI to either initial medical stabilization or emergency revasculariza-tion. Medical therapy included administration of fibrinolytic therapy and the insertion of an intra-aortic balloon pump (IABP) in most patients. Pa-tients in the revascularization arm underwent angioplasty or coronary artery bypass graft (CABG) surgery as soon as possible and within 6 hours of randomization. The primary end point was all-cause mortality at 30 days, and was not significantly different in the medical therapy and revascularization groups (56.0% vs 46.7%, P = .11). However, mortality was significantly reduced in the revascularization group at 6 months and 1 year by an absolute 13% at both time points.[3] Based on these results, emergency revas-cularization in suitable patients with CS is recom-mended, irrespective of time delay.[17]

The use of CABG surgery for CS was first re-ported in 1972.[21] In the SHOCK trial, one-third of the patients in the randomized early revasculariza-tion arm were treated with a surgical approach. Outcomes were similar to those treated with PCI.[3] However, rates of CABG surgery in the setting of CS are decreasing because of inherent time delays, increasingly favorable results with PCI, and the hesitancy of many surgeons to oper-ate on patients with high operative mortality in the era of public reporting of surgical outcomes.[9,14] In the recent Intraaortic Balloon Pump in CS (IABP-SHOCK II) trial (see later in this article), only 3% of patients with CS in the setting of AMI underwent immediate CABG surgery.[9]

Pharmacologic Therapy

The major goals of pharmacologic therapy in CS are to maintain adequate arterial pressure and cardiac output to allow for adequate tissue perfusion and thereby maintain tissue viability. Unfortunately, both inotropes and vasopressors, although frequently required, increase myocardial oxygen demand and have other adverse effects on the failing heart. Not surprisingly, higher vasopressor doses are associated with worse outcomes, likely due to both more severe hemodynamic derangement as well as direct toxic effects.[22] Therefore, the lowest possible doses should be used, and frequent adjustments should be made based on measured hemodynamic parameters.

Randomized trial data informing the choice of vasoactive agents in CS are extremely limited. A recent multicenter trial randomized 1679 patients with shock of any cause to initial treatment with either dopamine or norepinephrine in a double-blind fashion. In the overall trial, there was no significant difference in mortality at 28 days. In a subgroup of 280 patients with CS, mortality was significantly higher among patients treated with dopamine; however, there was no significant interaction between treatment effect and shock subgroup, so this may be a chance finding within a small subgroup.[23] The American College of Cardiology Foundation/American Heart Association (ACCF/AHA) guidelines no longer recommend the use of any particular agent(s), although they do note that the use of dopamine may be associated with excess hazard.[17] Therefore, until further trial data become available, treatment decisions must be based on clinical experience and individual hemodynamic profiles. **Table 1** includes the pharmacologic effects of commonly used

Table 1
Vasoactive agents in cardiogenic shock

Vasoactive Agent	Mechanism of Action	Preferred Use
Dobutamine	Beta-1 agonist	To increase cardiac output in an unstable patient when blood pressure is not critically low (systolic blood pressure ≥100 mm Hg).
Milrinone	Phosphodiesterase-3 inhibitor	To increase cardiac output in a patient who is not critically unstable and the blood pressure is not critically low.
Dopamine	Low dose: Dopamine receptor agonist Beta-1 agonist High dose: Alpha agonist	To increase cardiac output and blood pressure when the heart rate is not extremely high (≥100–110 beats per minute).
Norepinephrine	Alpha agonist Limited beta-1 agonist	To increase blood pressure and cardiac output when the blood pressure is critically low (systolic blood pressure <90 mm Hg) and/or the heart rate is extremely high (>110 beats per minute).
Epinephrine	Alpha agonist Beta-1 agonist Beta-2 agonist	To increase heart rate, contractility, and blood pressure in extremely critical situations (usually near cardiac arrest).
Isoproterenol	Beta-1 agonist Beta-2 agonist	To increase heart rate when the blood pressure is not compromised (systolic blood pressure ≥120 mm Hg).
Phenylephrine	Alpha agonist	To increase blood pressure when it is critically low (systolic blood pressure <90 mm Hg) and myocardial contractility is not compromised. Not recommended in cardiogenic shock.

inotropic and vasopressor agents, as well as our recommendations regarding the clinical situations in which each of these may be used preferentially.

IABP

The IABP is the most widely used form of mechanical hemodynamic support in patients with CS. Introduced in the 1960s, the IABP consists of a balloon inserted into the descending aorta between the arch vessels and the renal arteries (**Fig. 3**A). The balloon inflates after cardiac ejection and deflates before the onset of the following systole. Balloon inflation displaces blood proximally (toward the heart), increasing coronary perfusion pressure and raising diastolic aortic pressure. Deflation of the balloon during systole reduces end-diastolic pressure and LV afterload. IABP use is associated with hemodynamic improvement, increased perfusion of vital organs, maintenance of infarct artery patency, and reduction in myocardial oxygen consumption.[24] However, results of recent observational studies have been mixed with regard to the clinical benefit of

IABP.[25] Therefore, recommendations regarding the use of IABP in CS were recently downgraded from Class I ("is recommended") to Class IIa ("can be useful") in the ACCF/AHA guidelines and to Class IIb ("may be considered") in the European Society of Cardiology guidelines.[17,25]

After both of these guideline updates, however, the results of the IABP-SHOCK II trial were published. This multicenter randomized trial assigned 600 patients with CS complicating AMI to treatment with or without IABP. All patients were expected to undergo early revascularization and receive modern medical therapy. At 30 days, mortality was similar among patients in the IABP group and those in the control group (39.7% and 41.3%, $P = .69$). No subgroup could be identified in which IABP reduced short-term mortality. Fortunately, peripheral ischemic and bleeding complications were uncommon and not different between the groups. Potential limitations of the trial include a relatively small sample size, lower-than-expected mortality in the control group, and a 10% crossover rate to IABP in the control group.[9] The impact of these results on clinical practice and

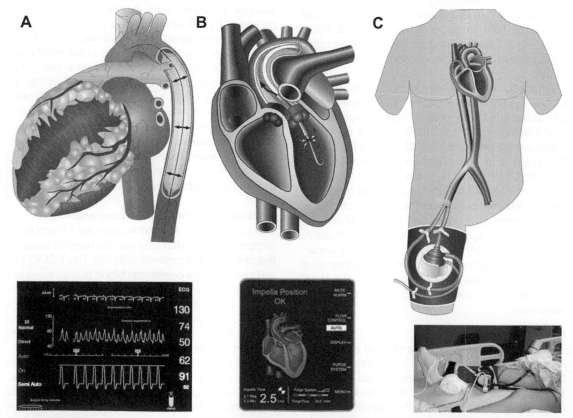

Fig. 3. Schematic representation of selected mechanical circulatory support devices. (*A*) Intra-aortic balloon pump. (*B*) Impella Recover 2.5. (*C*) TandemHeart. (*From* Desai NR, Bhatt DL. Evaluating percutaneous support for cardiogenic shock: data shock and sticker shock. Eur Heart J 2009;30:2073–5; with permission.)

authoritative guidelines is yet to be determined. Given the ease of implantation and the excellent safety profile of the IABP, however, it is likely that its use in CS will remain substantial. However, these disappointing results provide greater impetus to evaluate other forms of mechanical support in patients with refractory CS.

Advanced Mechanical Circulatory Support

Percutaneous LV assist devices

In patients with CS who are refractory to standard therapy, it has been hypothesized that devices that provide greater mechanical circulatory support may lead to better clinical outcomes. Currently, 2 short-term percutaneously implanted ventricular assist devices (pVADs) are available that can be deployed in the catheterization laboratory. These are the TandemHeart (CardiacAssist, Inc, Pittsburgh, PA) and the Impella Recover 2.5 (Abiomed, Aachen, Germany) (see **Fig. 3**B, C).

TandemHeart

The TandemHeart consists of an external centrifugal blood pump, a 21-French inflow cannula placed into the left atrium via transseptal puncture, and a 17-French outflow cannula inserted into the femoral artery. This system provides 4 to 5 L per minute of flow to support the failing LV. Risks include leg ischemia and potentially catastrophic displacement of the inflow cannula into the right atrium.

Initial trials confirmed the hemodynamic efficacy of the TandemHeart system. For example, Thiele and colleagues[26] showed an improvement in cardiac index from 1.7 ± 0.3 L/min to 2.4 ± 0.6 L/min, mean arterial pressure from 63 ± 8 mm Hg to 80 ± 9 mm Hg, and pulmonary artery occlusion pressure (PAOP) from 21 ± 4 mm Hg to 14 ± 4 mm Hg in 18 patients. A later report from the Texas Heart Institute described the clinical course of 117 patients with refractory CS in whom the TandemHeart system was implanted. Patients were at extremely high risk, and half had undergone cardiopulmonary resuscitation before or at the time of device implantation. Survival to hospital discharge was 60% (50% in the STEMI subgroup).[27]

Impella recover 2.5

The Impella Recover 2.5 consists of a catheter-based 12-French pump motor inserted via the femoral artery and positioned across the aortic valve. The pump pulls blood from the LV through an inlet area near the tip of the catheter, and expels blood into the proximal ascending aorta, providing up to 2.5 L/min of flow (see **Fig. 3**). Risks include leg ischemia and displacement of the catheter out of the LV. The device cannot be used in patients with aortic stenosis, aortic regurgitation, or a mechanical prosthetic aortic valve.

Several small, early studies demonstrated significant hemodynamic improvements with the Impella Recover 2.5 system. For example, Meyns and colleagues[28] reported on 16 patients with CS treated with this device. Improvements in cardiac output (4.1 ± 1.3 L/min to 5.9 ± 1.9 L/min), mean arterial pressure (57.4 ± 13 mm Hg to 80.6 ± 17 mm Hg), and PAOP (29 ± 10 mm Hg to 18 ± 7 mm Hg) were seen after 6 hours of support. More recently, a report from a prospective European registry in 120 consecutive patients showed that plasma lactate decreased from 5.8 ± 5.0 mmol/L on admission to 2.5 ± 2.6 mmol/L at 48 hours.[29]

Randomized trials of pVADs

Notwithstanding encouraging preliminary studies and clear improvements in hemodynamics with each of these pVADs, randomized controlled trials versus IABP are required to prove a clinical benefit in the setting of CS. Three such trials have been conducted to date (2 with the TandemHeart and 1 with the Impella Recover 2.5).[30–32] A meta-analysis of these trials included a total of 100 patients. The pVADs provided superior hemodynamic support when compared with IABP. However, 30-day survival was similar in the pVAD and IABP groups (55% vs 57%, relative risk 1.06, 95% confidence interval 0.68–1.66, $P = .8$). In addition, the IABP had a better safety profile, whereas the pVADs were associated with higher equipment costs.[33] Based on these disappointing results, the current ACCF/AHA guidelines provide only a IIb recommendation ("may be considered") for the use of alternative LV assist devices for patients with refractory CS.[17]

Extracorporeal membrane oxygenation

Veno-arterial (V-A) extracorporeal membrane oxygenation (ECMO) also can be used to support the circulation in patients with CS. The ECMO circuit consists of a centrifugal blood pump, a heater, and a membrane oxygenator. ECMO can be deployed centrally via a sternotomy, or much more rapidly via percutaneously inserted cannulae placed in the right atrium (via the femoral vein) and the descending aorta (via the femoral artery). Flow of approximately 4 L/min can be established quickly and maintained for up to several weeks. Pulmonary support for hypoxic patients is also provided. Complications include limb ischemia, a systemic inflammatory response, and bleeding.

The use of V-A ECMO provides rapid hemodynamic stabilization and resolution of organ dysfunction due to hypoperfusion. Patients presenting with cardiac arrest can be allowed time to demonstrate neurologic recovery. This period of support can be used to bridge a patient to myocardial recovery, LV assist device implantation, or cardiac transplantation. For example, Tang and colleagues[34] recently reported their experience with 21 consecutive patients with CS following AMI, all of whom failed initial therapy with an IABP or Impella Recover 2.5. ECMO support was maintained for 9.0 ± 7.5 days (range 1–25 days). Two patients were bridged to LVAD and subsequent transplantation, whereas 14 were able to be weaned from ECMO. Survival at 30 days was a remarkable 76%. This and other reports suggest that ECMO may be a reasonable management option for patients with refractory CS, but to date, compelling clinical evidence is lacking and no randomized trials have been conducted.

CentriMag

The CentriMag VAD (Thoratec, Pleasanton, CA) is a surgically implanted centrifugal pump with a magnetically levitated rotor that can provide up to 10 L/min of blood flow. For LV support, the inlet cannula is placed in the LV apex and the outlet cannula delivers blood to the ascending aorta. The pump is highly reliable, and support durations of up to 3 months have been reported.[35] Left, right, or biventricular support can be established with 1 or 2 CentriMag devices. In a recent multicenter report, 38 patients with CS (14 post-AMI) were supported for 1 to 60 days (mean, 13 days). Survival at 30 days following device removal was 47%. Complications were relatively uncommon, and included bleeding, infection, and neurologic dysfunction.[36] No randomized trials involving CentriMag implantation in patients with CS have yet been conducted.

MECHANICAL COMPLICATIONS OF AMI

Although CS is usually associated with poor LV contractility, there are several special situations in which the cardiac cause of shock is related to a disruption in the heart's anatomy.

Free Wall Rupture

LV free wall rupture is a rare complication of AMI, occurring in 1% to 3% of patients.[6] In the SHOCK trial registry, free wall rupture accounted for 1.4% of cases of CS.[37] Free wall rupture usually presents in catastrophic fashion, with recurrent chest pain followed by pulseless electrical activity and death. However, a minority of patients survive the initial rupture, in which case, salvage is possible if the diagnosis is made rapidly. Most commonly, bedside echocardiography is used, which demonstrates a significant pericardial effusion containing echodense material consistent with blood. The actual rupture site is rarely identified, but contrast echocardiography may reveal passage of contrast into the pericardial space and thereby confirm the diagnosis.[38] Hemodynamic stability can be restored with pericardiocentesis, with or without percutaneous cardiopulmonary support (ie, ECMO).[39,40] Subsequently, prompt surgical repair of the rupture site is essential. A recent report of 25 consecutive patients with postinfarction free wall rupture operated on at a single center demonstrated a remarkable 84% survival at 6 months.[41]

Ventricular Septal Rupture

The incidence of ventricular septal rupture has decreased to less than 1% in the reperfusion era, with the rupture generally occurring within 24 hours of presentation with STEMI.[42–44] The rupture may be apical and simple or posterobasal and complex. Diagnosis is made with echocardiography. Postinfarction ventricular septal rupture produces a sudden left-to-right shunt, which frequently results in profound heart failure or frank CS. Temporization may be approached with vasodilators, inotropes, and IABP support. In medically treated patients, however, mortality rates exceed 90%.[45] Surgical repair, although carrying a very high mortality rate, is associated with improved results. For example, in a recent report on 2876 consecutively operated patients with postinfarction ventricular septal rupture from the Society of Thoracic Surgeons National Database, survival to 30 days was 48.1%.[46] For this reason, emergency surgical repair is currently recommended in the ACCF/AHA guidelines.[17] However, earlier surgical repair is technically more challenging because of the presence of friable tissues and is associated with higher mortality than delayed repair.[46] Therefore, support with percutaneous LVAD or ECMO for several days to allow for tissue healing before surgery may be an alternative approach.[47–49] Recently, successful transcatheter closure using septal occluder devices in selected patients has been reported.[50]

Papillary Muscle Rupture

Papillary muscle rupture leading to acute, severe mitral regurgitation occurs in approximately 1% of patients with AMI and accounted for 6.9% of cases of CS in the SHOCK trial registry.[42,51] This complication is more likely to occur in inferoposterior MI than in anterior MI because of the single blood supply from the posterior descending artery to the posteromedial papillary muscle. The presentation is similar to ventricular septal rupture, and the diagnosis is readily made with echocardiography. Treatment consists of vasodilation, inotropic support, and IABP, followed by urgent mitral valve repair, or more commonly, replacement. In patients undergoing urgent surgical intervention, 30-day survival rates of 61% to 82% have been reported in recent case series.[52,53]

RV INFARCTION

Hemodynamically significant RV infarction occurs as a result of occlusion of the right coronary artery proximal to the acute marginal branches, complicating 10% to 15% of cases of acute inferior STEMI. Acute RV dysfunction leads to decreased LV preload, decreased cardiac output, and, when profound, CS. In the SHOCK trial registry, RV infarction accounted for 2.8% of cases of CS.[6] The diagnosis is suggested clinically by the classic trial of hypotension, clear lung fields, and elevated jugular venous pressure. Although ST segment elevation in the right-sided electrocardiographic leads (V_3R and V_4R) has a high sensitivity for the presence of RV infarction, this finding does not predict the magnitude of RV dysfunction. Echocardiography is much more reliable in this regard.[54]

Following reperfusion therapy, RV preload should be optimized by monitoring the central venous pressure and assessing the response of cardiac output to volume challenges. In RV infarction, cardiac output becomes highly sensitive to both heart rate and atrioventricular synchrony. Therefore, patients with significant bradycardia may require atrially based pacing and tachyarrhythmias should be treated with prompt cardioversion. Hemodynamic support with inotropes, particularly dobutamine, should be initiated if shock persists. The role of IABP in RV infarction is uncertain, but counterpulsation may improve both RV and LV function by augmenting coronary perfusion. Recent reports suggest that temporary percutaneous or surgical right ventricular assist devices (RVADs) may provide a bridge to recovery in severely compromised patients.[55–57] Most patients with RV infarction will have spontaneous recovery of RV function, although this may occur slowly. Therefore, aggressive support to prevent early death and irreversible organ failure often results in favorable long-term outcomes.

FUTURE DIRECTIONS
Comparative Effective Research

Although there are multiple treatment options available for patients with CS, few have been subjected to adequately powered clinical trials, leaving clinicians with little solid evidence on which to base their treatment decisions. Given the very high event rate in this population, definitive comparative effectiveness trials of existing therapies could be performed with relatively small sample sizes. A consortium of high-volume centers, rapidly cycling though a series of focused, pragmatic trials, would likely bring about dramatic progress in this field. Because of the enormous implications of CS for the public health, federal funding of such an effort should be a priority.

Novel Therapies

Anti-inflammatory therapies
In terms of novel therapies for CS, many opportunities present themselves for further investigation. In the sizable subset of patients with a demonstrable systemic inflammatory response, therapies targeting specific inflammatory mediators, such as IL-6 and TNF-α, might prove to be of benefit. Alternatively, more general inhibitors of inflammation could be investigated, in a manner analogous to the role of corticosteroids in septic shock.[58]

NO inhibition
The role of NO overproduction as a result of induction of iNOS by inflammatory stimuli in the setting of CS remains unresolved. However, the Tilarginine Acetate Injection in a Randomized International Study in Unstable Acute Myocardial Infarction Patients with CS (TRIUMPH) trial did not show a benefit of nonselective NO synthase inhibition in a relatively unselected group of patients with CS.[59] Further work characterizing the role of NO in CS is required, but it is possible that earlier initiation of therapy, more selective inhibition of iNOS, or the targeting of therapy to patients with the highest degree of iNOS activation may result in greater therapeutic efficacy.[60]

Therapeutic hypothermia
Therapeutic hypothermia has recently been proposed as a possible systemic treatment for CS.[61] This widely available treatment decreases the metabolic rate and oxygen consumption, limits reperfusion injury in the heart and other organs, and may reduce infarct size.[62] Furthermore, hypothermia reduces the production of multiple proinflammatory cytokines (Fig. 4).[63] In a case series of 10 adult patients with post cardiac surgery CS refractory to medical therapy, moderate hypothermia was associated with improved hemodynamics and an unexpectedly high survival rate.[64] In another study, moderate hypothermia was associated with increased cardiac index and mean arterial pressure in 28 patients with CS following

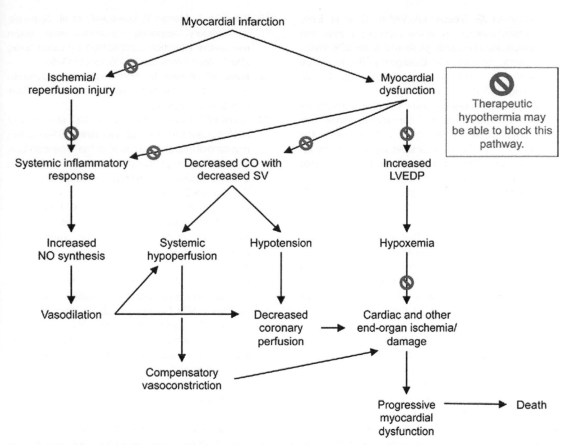

Fig. 4. Pathways potentially affected by therapeutic hypothermia. SV, stroke volume. (*From* Stegman BM, Newby KL, Hochman JS, et al. Post-myocardial infarction cardiogenic shock is a systemic illness in need of systemic treatment: is therapeutic hypothermia one possibility? J Am Coll Cardiol 2012;59:646; with permission.)

cardiac arrest.[65] Further investigation of this therapy in CS is therefore clearly warranted.

Mechanical circulatory support

Recent advances in mechanical circulatory support have been impressive but require further improvement. Surgically implanted systems provide high flow rates but are limited by the invasiveness of the procedure and the significant risk of postoperative complications. Current percutaneous devices are safer and simpler to implant but provide limited flows. Next-generation percutaneously implanted support devices that aim to be simple to implant and maintain, have low complication rates, and provide high flow rates are currently under development.[27]

SUMMARY

CS is a condition in which a marked reduction in cardiac output and inadequate end-organ perfusion results from an array of cardiac insults, the most common of which is AMI. CS is a systemic

disease involving a vicious cycle of inflammation, ischemia, and progressive myocardial dysfunction, which often results in death. This life-threatening emergency requires intensive monitoring accompanied by aggressive hemodynamic support with vasopressors, inotropes, and/or mechanical circulatory support. Other therapies are tailored to the specific pathophysiology, including urgent revascularization for AMI and surgical repair for mechanical disruption. The development of novel therapeutic strategies is urgently required to reduce the unacceptably high mortality rates currently associated with CS.

REFERENCES

1. Reynolds HR, Hochman JS. Cardiogenic shock: current concepts and improving outcomes. Circulation 2008;117:686–97.
2. Jeger RV, Radovanovic D, Hunziker PR, et al. Ten-year trends in the incidence and treatment of cardiogenic shock. Ann Intern Med 2008;149: 618–26.

3. Hochman JS, Sleeper LA, Webb JG, et al. Early revascularization in acute myocardial infarction complicated by cardiogenic shock. SHOCK Investigators. Should We Emergently Revascularize Occluded Coronaries for Cardiogenic Shock. N Engl J Med 1999;341:625–34.

4. Webb JG, Sleeper LA, Buller CE, et al. Implications of the timing of onset of cardiogenic shock after acute myocardial infarction: a report from the SHOCK Trial Registry. SHould we emergently revascularize Occluded Coronaries for cardiogenic shocK? J Am Coll Cardiol 2000;36:1084–90.

5. Hollenberg SM, Kavinsky CJ, Parrillo JE. Cardiogenic shock. Ann Intern Med 1999;131:47–59.

6. Hochman JS, Buller CE, Sleeper LA, et al. Cardiogenic shock complicating acute myocardial infarction—etiologies, management and outcome: a report from the SHOCK Trial Registry. Should we emergently revascularize Occluded Coronaries for cardiogenic shocK? J Am Coll Cardiol 2000;36:1063–70.

7. Awad HH, Anderson FA Jr, Gore JM, et al. Cardiogenic shock complicating acute coronary syndromes: insights from the Global Registry of Acute Coronary Events. Am Heart J 2012;163:963–71.

8. Babaev A, Frederick PD, Pasta DJ, et al. Trends in management and outcomes of patients with acute myocardial infarction complicated by cardiogenic shock. JAMA 2005;294:448–54.

9. Thiele H, Zeymer U, Neumann FJ, et al. Intra-aortic balloon support for myocardial infarction with cardiogenic shock. N Engl J Med 2012;367:1287–96.

10. Singh M, White J, Hasdai D, et al. Long-term outcome and its predictors among patients with ST-segment elevation myocardial infarction complicated by shock: insights from the GUSTO-I trial. J Am Coll Cardiol 2007;50:1752–8.

11. Hochman JS, Sleeper LA, Webb JG, et al. Early revascularization and long-term survival in cardiogenic shock complicating acute myocardial infarction. JAMA 2006;295:2511–5.

12. Holmes DR Jr, Bates ER, Kleiman NS, et al. Contemporary reperfusion therapy for cardiogenic shock: the GUSTO-i trial experience. The GUSTO-I Investigators. Global Utilization of Streptokinase and Tissue Plasminogen Activator for Occluded Coronary Arteries. J Am Coll Cardiol 1995;26:668–74.

13. Boyer N. Cardiogenic shock. N Engl J Med 1944;230:256–60.

14. Bates ER. Cardiogenic shock. In: Jeremias A, Brown D, editors. Cardiac intensive care. Philadelphia: Saunders; 2010. p. 212–24.

15. Kohsaka S, Menon V, Lowe AM, et al. Systemic inflammatory response syndrome after acute myocardial infarction complicated by cardiogenic shock. Arch Intern Med 2005;165:1643–50.

16. Marik PE, Baram M. Noninvasive hemodynamic monitoring in the intensive care unit. Crit Care Clin 2007;23:383–400.

17. O'Gara PT, Kushner FG, Ascheim DD, et al. ACCF/AHA guideline for the management of ST-elevation myocardial infarction: a report of the American College of Cardiology Foundation/American Heart Association Task Force on Practice Guidelines. J Am Coll Cardiol 2013;61:e78–140.

18. Chen ZM, Pan HC, Chen YP, et al. Early intravenous then oral metoprolol in 45,852 patients with acute myocardial infarction: randomised placebo-controlled trial. Lancet 2005;366:1622–32.

19. Effectiveness of intravenous thrombolytic treatment in acute myocardial infarction. Gruppo Italiano per lo Studio della Streptochinasi nell'Infarto Miocardico (GISSI). Lancet 1986;1:397–402.

20. In-hospital mortality and clinical course of 20,891 patients with suspected acute myocardial infarction randomised between alteplase and streptokinase with or without heparin. The International Study Group. Lancet 1990;336:71–5.

21. Dunkman WB, Leinbach RC, Buckley MJ, et al. Clinical and hemodynamic results of intraaortic balloon pumping and surgery for cardiogenic shock. Circulation 1972;46:465–77.

22. Valente S, Lazzeri C, Vecchio S, et al. Predictors of in-hospital mortality after percutaneous coronary intervention for cardiogenic shock. Int J Cardiol 2007;114:176–82.

23. De Backer D, Biston P, Devriendt J, et al. Comparison of dopamine and norepinephrine in the treatment of shock. N Engl J Med 2010;362:779–89.

24. O'Connor CM, Rogers JG. Evidence for overturning the guidelines in cardiogenic shock. N Engl J Med 2012;367:1349–50.

25. Taylor J. ESC guidelines on acute myocardial infarction (STEMI). Eur Heart J 2012;33:2501–2.

26. Thiele H, Lauer B, Hambrecht R, et al. Reversal of cardiogenic shock by percutaneous left atrial-to-femoral arterial bypass assistance. Circulation 2001;104:2917–22.

27. Kar B, Basra SS, Shah NR, et al. Percutaneous circulatory support in cardiogenic shock: interventional bridge to recovery. Circulation 2012;125:1809–17.

28. Meyns B, Dens J, Sergeant P, et al. Initial experiences with the Impella device in patients with cardiogenic shock—Impella support for cardiogenic shock. Thorac Cardiovasc Surg 2003;51:312–7.

29. Lauten A, Engstrom AE, Jung C, et al. Percutaneous left-ventricular support with the Impella-2.5-assist device in acute cardiogenic shock: results of the Impella-EUROSHOCK-registry. Circ Heart Fail 2013;6:23–30.

30. Thiele H, Sick P, Boudriot E, et al. Randomized comparison of intra-aortic balloon support with a percutaneous left ventricular assist device in patients with revascularized acute myocardial infarction complicated by cardiogenic shock. Eur Heart J 2005;26:1276–83.

31. Burkhoff D, Cohen H, Brunckhorst C, et al. A randomized multicenter clinical study to evaluate the safety and efficacy of the TandemHeart percutaneous ventricular assist device versus conventional therapy with intraaortic balloon pumping for treatment of cardiogenic shock. Am Heart J 2006; 152:469.e1–8.

32. Seyfarth M, Sibbing D, Bauer I, et al. A randomized clinical trial to evaluate the safety and efficacy of a percutaneous left ventricular assist device versus intra-aortic balloon pumping for treatment of cardiogenic shock caused by myocardial infarction. J Am Coll Cardiol 2008;52:1584–8.

33. Cheng JM, den Uil CA, Hoeks SE, et al. Percutaneous left ventricular assist devices vs intra-aortic balloon pump counterpulsation for treatment of cardiogenic shock: a meta-analysis of controlled trials. Eur Heart J 2009;30:2102–8.

34. Tang GH, Malekan R, Kai M, et al. Peripheral venoarterial extracorporeal membrane oxygenation improves survival in myocardial infarction with cardiogenic shock. J Thorac Cardiovasc Surg 2013;145:e32–3.

35. Slaughter MS, Tsui SS, El-Banayosy A, et al. Results of a multicenter clinical trial with the Thoratec Implantable Ventricular Assist Device. J Thorac Cardiovasc Surg 2007;133:1573–80.

36. John R, Long JW, Massey HT, et al. Outcomes of a multicenter trial of the Levitronix CentriMag ventricular assist system for short-term circulatory support. J Thorac Cardiovasc Surg 2011;141:932–9.

37. Slater J, Brown RJ, Antonelli TA, et al. Cardiogenic shock due to cardiac free-wall rupture or tamponade after acute myocardial infarction: a report from the SHOCK Trial Registry. Should we emergently revascularize occluded coronaries for cardiogenic shock? J Am Coll Cardiol 2000;36: 1117–22.

38. Mittle S, Makaryus AN, Mangion J. Role of contrast echocardiography in the assessment of myocardial rupture. Echocardiography 2003;20:77–81.

39. Abedi-Valugerdi G, Gabrielsen A, Fux T, et al. Management of left ventricular rupture after myocardial infarction solely with ECMO. Circ Heart Fail 2012;5: e65–7.

40. Anastasiadis K, Antonitsis P, Hadjimiltiades S, et al. Management of left ventricular free wall rupture under extracorporeal membrane oxygenation support. Int J Artif Organs 2009;32:756–8.

41. Zoffoli G, Battaglia F, Venturini A, et al. A novel approach to ventricular rupture: clinical needs and surgical technique. Ann Thorac Surg 2012; 93:1002–3.

42. Gueret P, Khalife K, Jobic Y, et al. Echocardiographic assessment of the incidence of mechanical complications during the early phase of myocardial infarction in the reperfusion era: a French multicentre prospective registry. Arch Cardiovasc Dis 2008;101:41–7.

43. An international randomized trial comparing four thrombolytic strategies for acute myocardial infarction. The GUSTO investigators. N Engl J Med 1993; 329:673–82.

44. Yip HK, Fang CY, Tsai KT, et al. The potential impact of primary percutaneous coronary intervention on ventricular septal rupture complicating acute myocardial infarction. Chest 2004;125: 1622–8.

45. Crenshaw BS, Granger CB, Birnbaum Y, et al. Risk factors, angiographic patterns, and outcomes in patients with ventricular septal defect complicating acute myocardial infarction. GUSTO-I (Global Utilization of Streptokinase and TPA for Occluded Coronary Arteries) Trial Investigators. Circulation 2000; 101:27–32.

46. Arnaoutakis GJ, Zhao Y, George TJ, et al. Surgical repair of ventricular septal defect after myocardial infarction: outcomes from the Society of Thoracic Surgeons National Database. Ann Thorac Surg 2012;94:436–44.

47. Tsai MT, Wu HY, Chan SH, et al. Extracorporeal membrane oxygenation as a bridge to definite surgery in recurrent postinfarction ventricular septal defect. ASAIO J 2012;58:88–9.

48. Rohn V, Spacek M, Belohlavek J, et al. Cardiogenic shock in patient with posterior postinfarction septal rupture—successful treatment with extracorporeal membrane oxygenation (ECMO) as a ventricular assist device. J Cardiovasc Surg 2009;24:435–6.

49. Gregoric ID, Bieniarz MC, Arora H, et al. Percutaneous ventricular assist device support in a patient with a postinfarction ventricular septal defect. Tex Heart Inst J 2008;35:46–9.

50. Assenza GE, McElhinney DB, Valente AM, et al. Transcatheter closure of post-myocardial infarction ventricular septal rupture. Circ Cardiovasc Interv 2012;6:59–67.

51. Thompson CR, Buller CE, Sleeper LA, et al. Cardiogenic shock due to acute severe mitral regurgitation complicating acute myocardial infarction: a

report from the SHOCK Trial Registry. Should we use emergently revascularize Occluded Coronaries in cardiogenic shocK? J Am Coll Cardiol 2000;36:1104–9.

52. Schroeter T, Lehmann S, Misfeld M, et al. Clinical outcome after mitral valve surgery due to ischemic papillary muscle rupture. Ann Thorac Surg 2013; 95:820–4.

53. Russo A, Suri RM, Grigioni F, et al. Clinical outcome after surgical correction of mitral regurgitation due to papillary muscle rupture. Circulation 2008;118: 1528–34.

54. Goldstein JA. Acute right ventricular infarction. Cardiol Clin 2012;30:219–32.

55. Prutkin JM, Strote JA, Stout KK. Percutaneous right ventricular assist device as support for cardiogenic shock due to right ventricular infarction. J Invasive Cardiol 2008;20:E215–6.

56. Marquez TT, D'Cunha J, John R, et al. Mechanical support for acute right ventricular failure: evolving surgical paradigms. J Thorac Cardiovasc Surg 2009;137.e39–40.

57. Kiernan MS, Krishnamurthy B, Kapur NK. Percutaneous right ventricular assist via the internal jugular vein in cardiogenic shock complicating an acute inferior myocardial infarction. J Invasive Cardiol 2010;22:E23–6.

58. Shpektor A. Cardiogenic shock: the role of inflammation. Acute Card Care 2010;12:115–8.

59. Alexander JH, Reynolds HR, Stebbins AL, et al. Effect of tilarginine acetate in patients with acute myocardial infarction and cardiogenic shock: the TRIUMPH randomized controlled trial. JAMA 2007;297:1657–66.

60. Bailey A, Pope TW, Moore SA, et al. The tragedy of TRIUMPH for nitric oxide synthesis inhibition in cardiogenic shock: where do we go from here? Am J Cardiovasc Drugs 2007;7: 337–45.

61. Stegman BM, Newby LK, Hochman JS, et al. Postmyocardial infarction cardiogenic shock is a systemic illness in need of systemic treatment: is therapeutic hypothermia one possibility? J Am Coll Cardiol 2012;59:644–7.

62. Gotberg M, Olivecrona GK, Koul S, et al. A pilot study of rapid cooling by cold saline and endovascular cooling before reperfusion in patients with ST-elevation myocardial infarction. Circ Cardiovasc Interv 2010;3:400–7.

63. Polderman KH. Application of therapeutic hypothermia in the intensive care unit. Opportunities and pitfalls of a promising treatment modality—Part 2: practical aspects and side effects. Intensive Care Med 2004;30:757–69.

64. Yahagi N, Kumon K, Watanabe Y, et al. Value of mild hypothermia in patients who have severe circulatory insufficiency even after intra-aortic balloon pump. J Clin Anesth 1998;10:120–5.

65. Skulec R, Kovarnik T, Dostalova G, et al. Induction of mild hypothermia in cardiac arrest survivors presenting with cardiogenic shock syndrome. Acta Anaesthesiol Scand 2008;52:188–94.

Durable Mechanical Circulatory Support in Advanced Heart Failure
A Critical Care Cardiology Perspective

Anuradha Lala, MD, Mandeep R. Mehra, MD*

KEYWORDS

- Heart failure • Mechanical circulatory support • Device therapy • Transplantation • Recovery

KEY POINTS

- Heart transplantation is often unavailable for most patients with advanced heart failure because of a limited donor supply, so mechanical circulatory support (MCS) is slowly becoming established as a primary standard.
- Selecting appropriate patients for MCS involves meeting a multitude of prespecifications, as one would for transplant evaluation.
- As technology evolves to bring forth more durable, smaller devices, the selection criteria for appropriate recipients of MCS will expand to encompass a broader, less sick population.
- The "Holy Grail" for MCS will be a focus on clinical recovery and explantation of devices rather than the current more narrowly defined indications of device therapy for life or as bridge to transplant.

SCOPE

Heart failure is responsible for more than 1 million hospitalizations annually in the United States, and its estimated costs amount to more than $38 billion.[1–3] Though most patients are hospitalized with acute decompensated heart failure (ADHF) caused by worsening of chronic heart failure, 15% to 20% of ADHF hospitalizations represent new diagnoses of heart failure.[4] The latter often present with pulmonary edema and/or cardiogenic shock, and require cardiac intensive care unit (CICU) care.[5] Of the 80% of patients with chronic heart failure exacerbations, approximately 10% have advanced heart failure.[4]

Patients with advanced heart failure are those with clinically significant circulatory compromise who require consideration of heart transplantation, mechanical circulatory support (MCS), continuous intravenous inotropic therapy, or hospice.[6] Heart transplantation is often unavailable for most patients with advanced heart failure because of a limited donor supply; therefore, MCS is slowly becoming established as a primary standard. The development of smaller, more durable left ventricular assist devices (LVADs) provides a practical and effective form of therapy as a bridge to transplantation (BTT), bridge to candidacy, and destination therapy (DT) for those otherwise not eligible for transplantation. These distinctions are becoming arbitrary however, and may be more appropriately supplanted by the concept of lifetime therapy, with consideration of transplantation when durable device therapy fails.

The authors have nothing to disclose.
Department of Medicine, Division of Cardiology, Brigham and Women's Hospital, Harvard Medical School, 75 Francis Street, A3, Boston, MA 02115, USA
* Corresponding author.
E-mail address: mmehra.harvard@me.com

Cardiol Clin 31 (2013) 581–593
http://dx.doi.org/10.1016/j.ccl.2013.07.003
0733-8651/13/$ – see front matter © 2013 Elsevier Inc. All rights reserved

cardiology.theclinics.com

EVOLUTION OF THE CORONARY CARE UNIT

With the advent of continuous electrocardiographic monitoring, the first coronary care units (CCU) were formed to decrease postmyocardial infarction arrhythmias and mortality in the 1960s.[7] The institution of CCUs across the globe has swiftly decreased mortality from postmyocardial infarction. A paradigm shift is taking place, however, rendering the term "coronary care unit" no longer relevant because of the dramatically different and varied patient population such units now serve. The modern cardiac intensive care unit (CICU) manages patients with invasive and noninvasive hemodynamic monitoring, mechanical ventilation, renal replacement therapies, therapeutic hypothermia protocols, sepsis, pulmonary hypertension, inotropic support, advanced structural heart disease, and MCS. Cardiac intensivists thus require a working knowledge of the types of MCS devices available and associated complications they are likely to encounter.

CLINICAL PROFILES AND DEVICE SELECTION

The approach to MCS depends on patients' clinical status and the trajectory of their heart failure syndrome. The Interagency Registry for Mechanically Assisted Circulatory Support (INTERMACS) provides a clinical profile categorization of patients with heart failure according to clinical severity and acuity (**Table 1**).[8] Although most mechanical support therapy was initially developed for acute profiles 1 and 2, long-term durable devices are increasingly being implanted in patients with profiles 3 and 4.

The contemporary CICU will be faced with the responsibility of caring for all profiles of these patients, not only for consideration of MCS device implantation but also for the management of their associated long-term complications. Short-term options such as the intra-aortic balloon pump, extracorporeal membrane oxygenation, surgically implanted extracorporeal MCS devices, and percutaneously implanted MCS devices play an important role in the management of those in

Table 1
INTERMACS profiles

INTERMACS Profile	Profile Description	Time Frame for Intervention
Profile 1: Critical cardiogenic shock	Patients with life-threatening hypotension despite rapidly escalating inotropic support "crash and burn"	Within hours
Profile 2: Progressive decline	Patients with declining function despite intravenous inotropic support "Sliding on inotropes." Also describes declining patients unable to tolerate inotropes	Within a few days
Profile 3: Stable but inotrope dependent	Stable on inotropic or temporary circulatory support, with demonstrated failure to wean "dependent stability"	Weeks to a few months
Profile 4: Resting symptoms	Stabilized but experiences daily symptoms of congestion at rest or during activities of daily living. Recurrent advanced heart failure	Weeks to a few months
Profile 5: Exertion intolerant	Comfortable at rest but symptomatic with any exertion. Exertion intolerant	Variable urgency: depends on maintenance of nutrition, organ function, and activity
Profile 6: Exertion limited	No fluid overload at rest, but symptomatic within few minutes of exertion. Exertion limited or "walking wounded"	Variable: depends on maintenance of nutrition, organ function, and activity level
Profile 7: Advanced NYHA III	Living comfortably with limited meaningful activity	Transplantation or circulatory support may not currently be indicated

Abbreviation: NYHA III, New York Heart Association functional class III.
Adapted from Stevenson LW, Pagani FD, Young JB, et al. INTERMACS profiles of advanced heart failure: the current picture. J Heart Lung Transplant 2009;28:535–41; with permission.

cardiogenic shock and INTERMACS profile 1 (**Table 2**). A comprehensive approach to these short-term devices is covered elsewhere.

LONG-TERM CIRCULATORY SUPPORT DEVICES
General Principles

Long-term mechanical circulatory support devices have evolved from first-generation or pulsatile pumps to second-generation pumps with contact bearings/seals to now third-generation rotary pumps without mechanical contact bearings. The first-generation LVADs were large, positive displacement pumps with several moving parts. These devices were limited to patients with a body surface area of 1.5 m² or more, did not require systemic anticoagulation, and were essentially the first MCS devices used in clinical practice. Prototypes include the Novacor LVAS, which was first implanted in 1984 as a BTT (WorldHeart, Salt Lake City, UT), and the HeartMate XVE (also called HeartMate I; Thoratec Corp, Pleasanton, CA). In the Thoratec PVAD (paracorporeal ventricular assist device) and Berlin Heart EXCOR (Berlin Heart AG, Berlin, Germany) systems, the blood pump lies external to the patient. The HeartMate XVE was the most widely used of these first-generation pumps, and mimicked normal human physiology in that following electrical activation of the ventricle, preload in the ventricle was ejected at each beat to the systemic circulation. Unfortunately, these pumps were limited by their large size and high rates of mechanical failure and infection, such that more than 50% of pumps needed to be replaced after 18 months of use.[9]

Because of the aforementioned limitations, a new, second generation of LVADs emerged, which are axial pumps that use continuous rather than pulsatile blood flow. This technology enabled the development of pumps that have a single moving part, nearly one-fifth the size and weight of the first-generation pump. These devices draw blood from the left ventricle continuously via a drainage cannula inserted to the left ventricular apex with the use of a rotary pump, which propels blood to the systemic circulation in a nonphasic flow pattern to the ascending aorta. The speed of this rotary pump (8,000–10,000 rpm) can be adjusted directly to increase or decrease preload, thereby affecting blood pressure and output. Prototypes include the Jarvik 2000 (Jarvik Heart, New York, NY, USA), the MicroMed DeBakey VAD (MicroMed Technologies, Woodlands, TX, USA), and the HeartMate II, the most frequently used second-generation LVAD worldwide (**Fig. 1**). Aspirin in addition to systemic anticoagulation is used in all second-generation LVADs, and does not appear to lead to an increase in bleeding in comparison with first-generation pumps.[10]

Third-generation MCS devices are further miniaturized, and suitable for patients with a wide range of body surface areas. These devices also provide continuous blood flow generated by an axial or centrifugal rotor, and have a single moving part, which spins at rates between 2400 and 3200 rpm. The impeller is suspended within a pump-housing through a combination of passive magnets and hydrodynamic thrust bearings. There are no mechanical bearings or any points of contact between the impeller and its pump-housing (**Fig. 2**). The HeartWare or HVAD pump (HeartWare International, Inc, Framingham, MA), recently approved for BTT, is designed to be implanted in the pericardial space, obviating an abdominal pocket, and is thereby proposed to facilitate ease of implantation and shorten recovery times.[11]

Table 2
Short-term MCS devices

Device	Company	Mechanism	Support	Duration
IABP	Multiple	Counterpulsation	Left heart only	Days
Impella	ABIOMED	Axial flow	Left heart only	Days
TandemHeart	CardiacAssist	Centrifugal	Biventricular	Days
ECMO	Multiple	Cardiopulmonary bypass	Biventricular	Days to weeks
BVS5000, AB5000	ABIOMED	Pulsatile	Right, left, or biventricular	Weeks
Thoratec pVAD	Thoratec	Pulsatile	Right, left, or biventricular	Weeks
CentriMag	Levitronix	Centrifugal	Right, left, or biventricular	Weeks

Abbreviations: ECMO, extracorporeal membrane oxygenation; IABP, intra-aortic balloon pump.
Adapted from Peura JL, Colvin-Adams M, Francis GS, et al. Recommendations for the use of mechanical circulatory support: Device strategies and patient selection: a scientific statement from the American Heart Association. Circulation 2012;126:2650; with permission.

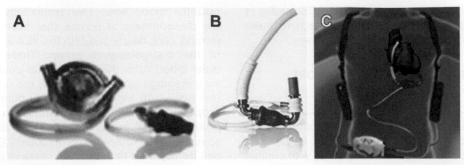

Fig. 1. (*A*) HeartMate XVE (first generation, pulsatile-flow pump) and HeartMate II (second generation, continuous-flow pump). (*B*) HeartMate II left ventricular assist device. (*C*) HeartMate II external equipment. (*Courtesy of* Thoratec, Pleasanton, CA.)

Clinical Trials

The concept of long-term MCS originally emerged as an alternative to transplantation. However, owing to safety concerns and limited durability, the Food and Drug Administration (FDA) largely restricted device use to those patients eligible for cardiac transplantation, forging the concept of BTT. At present there are 8 devices approved by the FDA for long-term MCS as BTT (**Table 3**).[6] Of these, 3 are now approved for the indication of DT. The landmark trial that established DT as an accepted indication for MCS was the REMATCH (Randomized Evaluation of Mechanical Assistance for the Treatment of Congestive Heart Failure) trial, published in 2001. This trial randomized 129 patients ineligible for transplant to medical therapy or MCS with the HeartMate XVE, and demonstrated a 27% absolute and 48% relative risk reduction.[12] This investigation led to a follow-up trial, REMATCH II, which compared the pulsatile-flow HeartMate XVE (52% survival at 1 year) to the continuous-flow HeartMate II (68% survival at 1 year).[10] Compared with the dismal survival rate of 25% for patients medically managed in the 2 trials, the advent of LVADs has demonstrated the greatest magnitude of benefit in advanced heart failure relative to any therapy.

Most recently, patients with the HeartWare device were compared with those implanted contemporaneously with a HeartMate II device via INTERMACS registry data. The primary outcome was survival on the originally implanted device, transplantation, or explantation for ventricular recovery at 180 days. The primary outcome was achieved in 90.7% of the 140 patients who received the HeartWare pump and 90.1% of the 499 patients who received the HeartMate II, establishing pre-specified grounds for noninferiority but not superiority.[13] The results of this trial led to FDA approval of the device in November 2012 for BTT. Although the rates of neurologic events are similar between the two groups, there is speculation that increased thrombotic events are seen with the HeartWare device.[14] The results of the Multi-Center Clinical Trial to Evaluate the HeartWare Ventricular Assist System (VAS) for Destination Therapy for Advanced Heart Failure (ENDURANCE), which compares the HeartMate II and HeartWare devices directly in patients who are not candidates for cardiac transplant are eagerly awaited.

TROUBLESHOOTING AND MANAGEMENT

Once discharged from hospital, long-term complications in patients with MCS involve device malfunction, arrhythmias, volume management, gastrointestinal (GI) bleeding, neurologic events, pump thrombosis, infection, and right heart failure. This section is intended to familiarize the cardiac

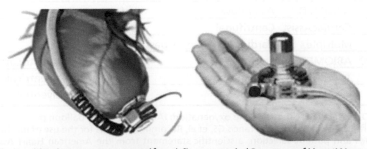

Fig. 2. HeartWare device (third generation, centrifugal-flow pump). (*Courtesy of* HeartWare, Framingham, MA.)

Table 3
Devices for long-term MCS approved by the US Food and Drug Administration

Device	Company	Mechanism	Support	Indications	Portable
Thoratec pVAD	Thoratec	Pulsatile	Right, left, or biventricular	BTT, BTR	Yes
Novacor	World Heart	Pulsatile	Left	BTT, DT	Yes
HeartMate XVE	Thoratec	Pulsatile	Left	BTT, DT	Yes
HeartMate II	Thoratec	Axial, continuous	Left	BTT, DT	Yes
Abiomed TAH	ABIOMED	Pulsatile	Biventricular	BTT, DT	Yes
CardioWest TAH	SynCardia	Pulsatile	Biventricular	BTT	Yes/No
Berlin EXOR Pediatric	Berlin	Pulsatile/pneumatic	Right, left, or biventricular	BTT	No
DeBakey child	MicroMed	Continuous	Left	BTT, BTR	No

Abbreviations: BTR, bridge to recovery; BTT, bridge to transplantation; DT, destination therapy.

Adapted from Peura JL, Colvin-Adams M, Francis GS, et al. Recommendations for the use of mechanical circulatory support: Device strategies and patient selection: a scientific statement from the American Heart Association. Circulation 2012;126:2653; with permission.

intensivist with these commonly encountered issues and to suggest potential therapeutic approaches to management. Perioperative management of MCS devices is not discussed here, this being an aspect managed most commonly in surgical postoperative care units.

Monitoring Device Function

Because continuous-flow LVADs do not contain valves, in the presence of high afterload, low pump speeds, or turning the pump off, blood flow can become retrograde. LVADs also generate substantial negative pressure at the inflow cannula to unload the left ventricle, thereby creating the potential for septal shift or ventricular collapse if pump speeds are too high or patients are preload deplete. The HeartMate II console shows parameters of speed (set by the user and modifiable), power, pulsatility index (PI), and estimated flow, all of which are indicators of appropriate function (**Figs. 3** and **4**).[15]

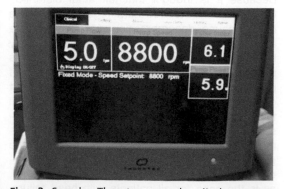

Fig. 3. Sample Thoratec console display screen, showing Pump flow, Pump speed, Pulse index, and Pump power.

Power and flow

At a given speed, power is a direct measure of the current and voltage applied to the motor. The flow is directly related to the power and pump speed. If power values are outside the anticipated physiologic range for a given speed, the flow will be displayed as "+ + +" or "− − −" to represent a calculated flow that is higher or lower than expected. Power also may be increased because of thrombus formation within the rotor, causing an erroneously high flow reading. The minimum flow reading is 3.0 L/min. Increases in volume status or decreases in afterload may cause increased flows. Conversely, an occlusion may decrease flow and correspondingly decrease power.

Pulsatility index (PI)

When the left ventricle contracts, it generates an increase in ventricular pressure and thereby causes an increase in pump flow. These flow increases are measured and averaged over a 15-second interval to produce the PI value displayed on the console. As the speed increases, the level of support from the device increases, causing less generation of increased pressure due to contraction, and therefore will correspond to a decreased PI. Decreased PI may also be observed in scenarios of decreased blood volume or preload depletion. Similarly, if there is an increase in contractility, as may be seen with increases in blood volume, inotropic medications, exercise, or intrinsic myocardial recovery, the PI will increase.

Pump speed

Optimal pump speed is achieved when cardiac index is sufficient (greater than 2.5 L/min/m²), often with the aid of visualizing the left ventricle via

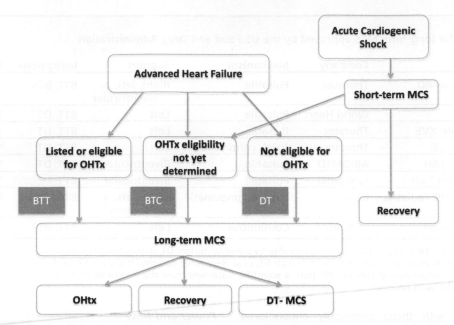

Fig. 4. Device selection flow chart. BTC, bridge to candidacy; BTT, bridge to transplantation; DT, destination therapy; MCS, mechanical circulatory support; OHTx, orthotopic heart transplant.

transthoracic echocardiography. Ideally the left ventricle is decompressed, but not so much so that it is collapsed or that the septum shifts toward the left. Over a period of time, excessive leftward septal shift leads to worsening right heart failure. Allowing for intermittent aortic valve opening and retaining some pulsatility is recommended.[14] The normal speed range is 8800 to 10,000 rpm for the HeartMate II and between 2400 and 3400 rpm for the Heart-Ware. Left ventricular dimensions, septal flattening, degree of aortic regurgitation (if any), mitral regurgitation, and aortic valve opening should be noted and taken into consideration when determining optimal pump speed for each individual patient.

Hypertension and Hypotension

Adequate unloading of the ventricle by the LVAD depends on afterload. Thus the control and maintenance of mean arterial blood pressure (MAP) at less than 90 mm Hg is important to allow for appropriate perfusion as well as to prevent retrograde flow. Specific antihypertensive agents have not been studied in the MCS population. It is generally accepted that one may use angiotensin-converting enzyme inhibitors, angiotensin receptor blockers, hydralazine, nitrates, β-blockers, and dihydropyridine calcium-channel blockers for optimal control of blood pressure. Ideally, neurohormonally directed therapy is used to facilitate myocardial recovery over other agents.

Hypotension in the LVAD patient must be evaluated carefully. The differential diagnosis is broad

and includes dehydration, bleeding, right ventricular dysfunction, tamponade, improper cannula positioning, inadequate pump speed, infection, sepsis, and iatrogenic causes. **Fig. 5** shows an algorithm on considerations of hypotension in the LVAD patient.

Arrhythmias

LVAD patients are at risk for increased morbidity and mortality from atrial and ventricular arrhythmias, primarily because right ventricular filling and function are often compromised, leading to inadequate left ventricular filling, heart failure, syncope, and death. It is well known that the prevalence of atrial arrhythmias increases as symptoms of heart failure worsen in severity.[16] Because it is thought that left atrial distention from congestion and/or mitral regurgitation is the inciting cause, decompression of the left ventricle and, thereby, the left atrium with an LVAD may theoretically decrease this risk. Unfortunately this potential benefit is offset by an increased risk of perioperative atrial arrhythmias as seen in most cardiac surgery,[17] and those with permanent atrial fibrillation are unlikely to have an altered substrate.[18] Thus the management of atrial arrhythmias is not much different than that for the general population. β-Blockers are used in preference to calcium-channel blockers for rate control, as is the case for all patients with heart failure. When poorly tolerated, a rhythm control strategy is favored, using either amiodarone or dofetilide

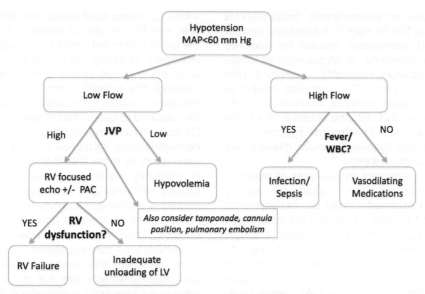

Fig. 5. Evaluation of hypotension in a patient with a left ventricular assist device. JVP, jugular venous pressure; LV, left ventricle; MAP, mean arterial pressure; PAC, pulmonary artery catheter; RV, right ventricle; WBC, white blood cells.

in an attempt to restore sinus rhythm. Ablative therapy is generally reserved for refractory cases.[14] Most patients on LVAD support are on systemic anticoagulation; however, in those with additional risk factors for thromboembolism, higher international normalized ratios (INRs) may be targeted.[18]

The incidence of ventricular arrhythmias after implantation of an MCS device has been reported to be as high as 22% to 52%.[19,20] Mechanisms of ventricular tachycardia (VT) and ventricular fibrillation (VF) in MCS patients include electrolyte abnormalities, "suction events" caused by overdecompression of the left ventricle and/or cannula positioning, irreversible baseline myopathic substrates prior to implantation, and the potential of new reentrant circuits around the inflow cannula in the apex of the left ventricle.[21] Isolated episodes of VT may be well tolerated, terminated with either antitachycardia pacing from an implantable cardioverter-defibrillator (ICD) or with direct cardioversion. Incessant ventricular arrhythmias, however, lead to poor right ventricular and thereby left ventricular filling, resulting in heart failure, emotional trauma, cardiogenic shock, and even sudden cardiac death. Most patients will have an ICD implanted either before MCS implantation or before discharge. Any hemodynamic change that would allow the inflow cannula to come into contact with myocardial structures, particularly the septal wall, can precipitate VT. Such circumstances include bleeding or hypovolemia due to other causes, increased VAD speeds, and improper

angulation of the inflow cannula.[18] On interrogation of the LVAD, one may see low PI numbers indicating ventricular arrhythmias. If a "suction event" is suspected, the VAD speed can be reduced to see if there is improvement, particularly under the guidance of transthoracic echocardiography. Otherwise signs and symptoms of hypovolemia from overdiuresis, bleeding, or dehydration should be investigated. Finally, many patients require antiarrhythmic therapy, most commonly with amiodarone, and need to be followed accordingly.

Bleeding

The incidence of GI bleeding in patients with continuous-flow devices is estimated at 20% or more, based on clinical observations and INTERMACS registry data.[10,22–25] Bleeding can occur anywhere along the GI tract, as patients are on systemic anticoagulation; however, mechanisms of bleeding unique to continuous-flow devices have been the subject of great interest. It is postulated that relatively high nonphysiologic shear stress is imparted on blood components as they move through the device, which promotes von Willebrand Factor (vWF) proteolysis by the metalloprotease ADAMTS13, leading to a decrease in high molecular weight (functional) vWF multimers.[17,25,26] In addition to an observed acquired von Willebrand disease (vWD), patients are also noted to have a predisposition to the development of angiodysplasia. In fact, up to one-third of LVAD patients have GI bleeding episodes related to angiodysplasia or arteriovenous malformations (AVMs) along the GI tract.[27] Inadequate platelet function and hemostasis caused by acquired vWD in the presence of angiodysplasia make these patients more vulnerable to bleeding. One hypothesis as to why AVMs develop relates to the reduced pulse pressure encountered with continuous-flow devices. The absence of a pulse pressure may lead to intestinal hypoperfusion, causing regional hypoxia, vascular dilation, and subsequent angiodysplasia.[28]

As with management of any case of major GI bleeding, anticoagulation should be acutely stopped and reversed if need be. Patients must be supported hemodynamically with intravenous fluids and blood products as needed. It should be noted, however, that in those patients with MCS as a BTT, frequent transfusions leads to an increased chance for human leukocyte antigen (HLA) sensitization, which may make finding a suitable donor organ more difficult, as well affect posttransplant outcomes.[29] A decision to transfuse that is not emergent should therefore be made in consultation with the transplant cardiology team. Reversing high INR values with vitamin K or fresh frozen plasma must be weighed against the risk of pump thrombosis. Once stabilized, a patient with GI bleeding should be evaluated with upper and lower endoscopy in conjunction with the consultation of a gastroenterologist. If this is unrevealing, a capsule endoscopy or balloon enteroscopy should be performed to assess the small bowel.[14] In the setting of persistent bleeding and negative endoscopic evaluation, a tagged red blood scan or angiography can be considered.

In patients with recurrent GI bleeding and no source amenable to therapy, there is very limited, if any, evidence to support the reduction of LVAD pump speed to allow for less shear stress, increased pulsatility, and potential resolution of AVMs.[14] The long-term benefits of octreotide in patients with refractory GI bleeding from small bowel AVMs have been extrapolated for use in the LVAD population.[30] Further studies are needed to determine whether this strategy is effective.

Thrombosis

Although clinically relevant pump thrombosis was noted to be rare in the original HeartMate II trials, in clinical practice the incidence appears to be rising to as much as 10%. Despite the manufacturers' advised INR target of 1.5 to 2.5 (2–3 in clinical trials) in addition to aspirin, the incidence of pump thrombosis is well reported in the literature.[31] Thrombus may grow from smaller deposits

within the pump itself (which can affect flow, power, and PI), or can be consumed directly from the left atrium or left ventricle. Usually the primary indication of pump thrombosis is an increase in power ("power spikes"). PI is also reduced because the pulsatile component of power is decreased relative to the steady component of power required to overcome the burden of thrombus. Clinically, thrombus should also be suspected with hemoglobinuria, increases in lactate dehydrogenase levels to more than 3 times previous levels, or markedly elevated plasma free hemoglobin (usually >40 μmol/L).[15] When clinically suspected, additional anticoagulation may be added with heparin or other intravenous anticoagulants. Thrombolytics have been administered locally or systemically on rare occasions with varying success rates, but this strategy remains uncertain and adverse effects are not trivial, particularly intracranial bleeding complications. If thrombosis persists, definitive therapy remains pump exchange in the operating room.[14,15,31]

Infection

The most common adverse event accounting for 16.2% of all deaths is infection, as observed in the INTERMACS registry, as well as HeartMate BTT and DT clinical trials.[32] Infections in MCS device patients are divided into 3 categories: (1) device-specific, involving the pump, cannula, pocket, or percutaneous driveline; (2) device-related, including infective endocarditis, bacteremia, and mediastinitis; and (3) non–device-related.[33] Patients undergoing MCS implantation are often debilitated from long-standing heart failure and/or cardiogenic shock, with many comorbidities including renal failure, diabetes, malnutrition, and lung disease, conditions all predisposing to infection.[34] An early article by Chinn and colleagues[35] highlights the mainstays of preventing driveline-related infection: (1) immobilization of the percutaneous lead at the exit site is important in preventing disruption of subcutaneous tissue; (2) exit-site care must be executed gently and nontraumatically with meticulous sterile technique, daily or every other day; (3) observation of erythema or increased drainage should prompt investigation and possible hospitalization. Infections may lead to vasodilation and/or sepsis, and may be indicated by increased flows displayed on the monitor. In certain cases of bacteremia, seeding of the device may occur and persist despite intravenous antibiotic therapy, in which case pump exchange may be necessary.

Secondary antibiotic prophylaxis for dental, respiratory, genitourinary, and gastrointestinal procedures has not been studied in the MCS population. The most recent guidelines state antibiotic prophylaxis would be "reasonable and remains at the discretion of the physician."[14]

Device Alarms and "Code" Situations

Health care practitioners responsible for the care of patients with MCS must familiarize themselves with device parameters and their clinical significance. **Fig. 6** summarizes the causes of device alarms and potential interventions.

It is not uncommon for health care practitioners to react to the frequent absence of a pulse in an LVAD patient, prompting the initiation of Adult Cardiac Life Support (ACLS) protocol. It is particularly important in this population to assess the patient first before reacting to alarms on the display or on telemetry. Patients may often tolerate episodes of VT and VF on an LVAD, and will not require cardioversion. When assessing blood pressure, a Doppler machine must be used to obtain a MAP reading. If an arterial line is placed, it is likely to show a diminished pulse pressure of approximately 15 mm Hg or less. A first step in patient assessment should be to auscultate the left upper abdomen for a continuous LVAD hum. If a continuous humming sound is not appreciated, device malfunction should be suspected and acted upon. If a patient is truly clinically unstable, standard ACLS protocols should be practiced, bearing in mind a pulse cannot be used to monitor status

or to dictate appropriate medical therapy. Furthermore, cardiopulmonary resuscitation (CPR) should generally be avoided. Because of the location of the LVAD and its associated connections to myocardial structures, CPR may dislodge components of the device, resulting in fatal bleeding. All emergent situations should involve the urgent consultation of a cardiac surgeon, VAD coordinator, and/or MCS specialized cardiologist. **Fig. 7** illustrates a simplified approach to emergency encounters in VAD patients.

Right Heart Failure and the Need for Biventricular Support

Selecting appropriate patients for successful MCS involves meeting a multitude of prespecifications, as one would in evaluation for cardiac transplant. These criteria include, but are not limited to, acceptable end-organ function, freedom from active malignancy, freedom from toxic habits, and adequate psychosocial support. Right ventricular failure remains the Achilles heel in MCS, and is associated with higher mortality, greater risk of bleeding, longer hospitalization, and higher rate of renal insufficiency.[36,37] Many studies have tried to identify markers for the development of right ventricular failure postimplantation, all of which are generally related to end-organ function including vasopressor requirement, elevated liver function tests, creatinine, and blood urea nitrogen,

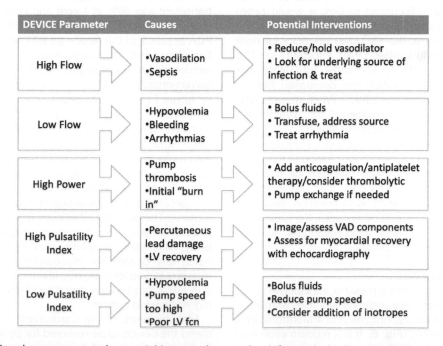

DEVICE Parameter	Causes	Potential Interventions
High Flow	•Vasodilation •Sepsis	• Reduce/hold vasodilator • Look for underlying source of infection & treat
Low Flow	•Hypovolemia •Bleeding •Arrhythmias	• Bolus fluids • Transfuse, address source • Treat arrhythmia
High Power	•Pump thrombosis •Initial "burn in"	• Add anticoagulation/antiplatelet therapy/consider thrombolytic • Pump exchange if needed
High Pulsatility Index	•Percutaneous lead damage •LV recovery	• Image/assess VAD components • Assess for myocardial recovery with echocardiography
Low Pulsatility Index	•Hypovolemia •Pump speed too high •Poor LV fcn	•Bolus fluids •Reduce pump speed •Consider addition of inotropes

Fig. 6. Device alarms: causes and potential interventions. LV fcn, left ventricular function; VAD, ventricular assist device.

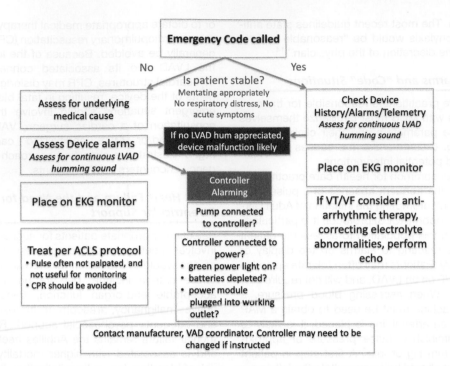

Fig. 7. Approach to emergency encounters in VAD patients. ACLS, Adult Cardiac Life Support; CPR, cardiopulmonary resuscitation; EKG, electrocardiogram; VT/VF, ventricular tachycardia/fibrillation.

as well as a right ventricular stroke work index of less than 450 mm Hg/ml/m² and higher central venous pressure.[38,39] Although the risk of right ventricular failure may also be related to LVAD mechanics itself (discussed earlier), it would seem that the clinical syndrome of right ventricular failure preoperatively is the strongest predictor of right ventricular failure after LVAD implantation. The proportion of patients who suffer right ventricular failure after implantation has decreased but remains at least 5% to 13%.[39] When appropriate, such patients are considered for biventricular MCS as BTT, the mainstay of which has become the CardioWest total artificial heart (TAH) (SynCardia Systems, Inc, Tuscon, AZ). Although the Thoratec paracorporeal VADs can also be used for biventricular support as BTT, their use is limited by large size, higher rates of infection, and poor long-term durability. In other cases, the HeartWare VAD has been used for biventricular support because of its small profile.

Total artificial heart

The SynCardia TAH is a pulsatile, implantable pump that consists of 2 polyurethane ventricles with pneumatically driven diaphragms and 4 Medtronic-Hall tilting disc valves (**Fig. 8**). It is a modern version of the original Jarvik 7, and has since undergone many changes and improvements. Copeland and

colleagues[40,41] published a seminal article in 2004 showing that the device was effective for bridging 79% of patients with inotrope-refractory biventricular failure to heart transplant. Survival after heart transplant was 86% at 1 year and 64% at 5 years, similar to national registry standards, leading to FDA approval of the device as BTT later that year. Experience with the CardioWest TAH is growing, with nearly 1100 completed in early 2013. Implantation is considered for those not only with biventricular failure from cardiomyopathy but also for those with incessant refractory ventricular arrhythmias, complex congenital heart disease, severe allograft failure after cardiac transplantation, and patients with multiple mechanical valves, severe restrictive cardiomyopathy, or mechanical complications from a large myocardial infarction (such in those complicated by ventricular septal rupture or cardiac rupture). The potential advantage of the TAH is that the entire myopathic substrate is removed from the body, eliminating arrhythmic burden. It also eliminates any chance for myocardial recovery and thus is reserved for bridging patients to transplantation. It use may be considered for lifetime therapy in highly selected patients.

Manufacturers of the CardioWest TAH recommend the device to be reserved for patients with a body surface area of 1.7 m² or greater, and a thoracic diameter (anterior vertebral body to

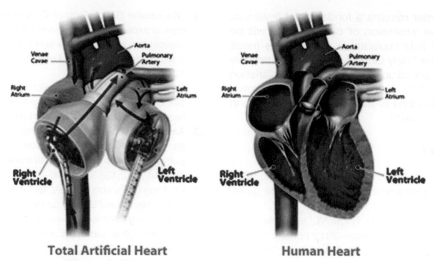

Fig. 8. SynCardia total artificial heart. (*Courtesy of* syncardia.com.)

sternum at 10th thoracic vertebra) of 10 cm or more.[42] The diaphragm of the pump is activated by movement of air from an external driver, allowing for a maximal stroke volume from each ventricle of 70 mL. Drive pressures for the right and left side are adjusted depending the pulmonary and systemic afterload and volume status. Typical drive pressures for the right pump are between 60 and 90 mm Hg, and between 180 and 200 mm Hg on the left side. The TAH rate is set at greater than 120 beats or ejections per minute, and the percentage of time the pump spends in "systole" is set to 45% to 55%. These parameters are configured to allow for full ejection of blood volume and prevention of stasis, and to prevent clinically significant hemolysis.[40,42,43] Systemic anticoagulation is required with an INR target of 2.5 to 3.5, a higher target attributable to the 4 mechanical valves in the TAH unit.

Issues unique to the TAH

Anemia It has been observed that TAH patients have a persistent anemia with hematocrit ranging between 18 and 24, presumably because of a combination of chronic hemolysis, ineffective erythropoiesis, and inflammation (predominant). These patients are noted to have markedly elevated lactate dehydrogenase levels (>1000 units/L), undetectable or low haptoglobin levels, and elevated plasma free hemoglobin, as well as elevated high-sensitivity C-reactive protein and reticulocyte production indices.[43]

Portability The TAH console is heavy, although selected patients can now be transitioned to the Freedom Driver, which is reasonably convenient and highly portable, allowing for discharge to home. Such portability may allow transition from

a BTT-only consideration to DT or lifetime therapy.

ON THE HORIZON

As technology evolves to bring forth more durable, smaller devices, the selection criteria for appropriate recipients of MCS will expand to encompass a broader, less sick population. The National Heart, Lung, and Blood Institute has initiated the Randomized Evaluation of VAD InterVEntion before Inotropic Therapy study, which is a randomized trial comparing LVAD with optimal medical therapy in patients not yet bound to inotropic therapy. This small-scale proof-of-concept trial will serve to establish the safety of durable MCS in noninotropic therapy–bound advanced heart failure, and provide signals for efficacy in this population.

New Devices

Future prospects include a miniaturized LVAD requiring minimally invasive surgery without the need for cardiopulmonary bypass or sternotomy, implanted through the left ventricular apex with a distal cannula in the ascending aorta.[44] Another concept that shows promise and may transform the MCS field is that of partial circulatory support. The Synergy Pocket micropump device (CircuLite, Inc, Saddle Brook, NJ) is placed off-pump via a minithoracotomy, and has an inflow cannula in the left atrium with the outflow in the right subclavian artery, providing 3 L/min of blood flow.[45] Even as devices reduce in size and improve in durability, and clinicians encounter less morbidity, the need to power such devices with a driveline that exits the skin barrier remains a fundamental limitation. As such, the expansion of durable MCS will be limited until fully implantable systems are made available. The "Holy Grail" for MCS will ultimately be a focus on clinical recovery and explanation of devices rather than the current more narrowly defined indications of lifetime device therapy and bridge to transplant.

REFERENCES

1. Lindenfeld J, Albert NM, Boehmer JP, et al. HFSA 2010 comprehensive heart failure practice guideline. J Card Fail 2010;16:e1–194.
2. Go AS, Mozaffarian D, Roger VL, et al. Heart disease and stroke statistics—2013 update: a report from the American Heart Association. Circulation 2013;127:e6–245.
3. Heidenreich PA, Trogdon JG, Khavjou OA, et al. Forecasting the future of cardiovascular disease in the United States: a policy statement from the American Heart Association. Circulation 2011;123:933–44.
4. Joseph SM, Cedars AM, Ewald GA, et al. Acute decompensated heart failure: contemporary medical management. Tex Heart Inst J 2009;36:510–20.
5. O'Connor CM, Stough WG, Gallup DS, et al. Demographics, clinical characteristics, and outcomes of patients hospitalized for decompensated heart failure: observations from the impact-hf registry. J Card Fail 2005;11:200–5.
6. Peura JL, Colvin-Adams M, Francis GS, et al. Recommendations for the use of mechanical circulatory support: device strategies and patient selection: a scientific statement from the American Heart Association. Circulation 2012;126:2648–67.
7. Morrow DA, Fang JC, Fintel DJ, et al. Evolution of critical care cardiology: transformation of the cardiovascular intensive care unit and the emerging need for new medical staffing and training models: a scientific statement from the American Heart Association. Circulation 2012;126:1408–28.
8. Stevenson LW, Pagani FD, Young JB, et al. INTERMACS profiles of advanced heart failure: the current picture. J Heart Lung Transplant 2009;28:535–41.
9. Starling RC, Naka Y, Boyle AJ, et al. Results of the post-U.S. Food and Drug Administration-approval study with a continuous flow left ventricular assist device as a bridge to heart transplantation: a prospective study using the INTERMACS (Interagency Registry for Mechanically Assisted Circulatory Support). J Am Coll Cardiol 2011;57:1890–8.
10. Slaughter MS, Rogers JG, Milano CA, et al. Advanced heart failure treated with continuous-flow left ventricular assist device. N Engl J Med 2009;361:2241–51.
11. Wieselthaler GM, O Driscoll G, Jansz P, et al. Initial clinical experience with a novel left ventricular assist device with a magnetically levitated rotor in a multi-institutional trial. J Heart Lung Transplant 2010;29:1218–25.
12. Rose EA, Gelijns AC, Moskowitz AJ, et al. Long-term use of a left ventricular assist device for end-stage heart failure. N Engl J Med 2001;345:1435–43.
13. Aaronson KD, Slaughter MS, Miller LW, et al. Use of an intrapericardial, continuous-flow, centrifugal pump in patients awaiting heart transplantation. Circulation 2012;125:3191–200.
14. Feldman D, Pamboukian SV, Teuteberg JJ, et al. The 2013 International Society for Heart and Lung Transplantation guidelines for mechanical circulatory support: executive summary. J Heart Lung Transplant 2013;32:157–87.
15. Slaughter MS, Pagani FD, Rogers JG, et al. Clinical management of continuous-flow left ventricular assist devices in advanced heart failure. J Heart Lung Transplant 2010;29:S1–39.
16. Maisel WH, Stevenson LW. Atrial fibrillation in heart failure: epidemiology, pathophysiology, and rationale for therapy. Am J Cardiol 2003;91:2D–8D.
17. Zaman AG, Archbold RA, Helft G, et al. Atrial fibrillation after coronary artery bypass surgery: a model for preoperative risk stratification. Circulation 2000;101:1403–8.
18. Boyle A. Arrhythmias in patients with ventricular assist devices. Curr Opin Cardiol 2012;27:13–8.
19. Cesario DA, Saxon LA, Cao MK, et al. Ventricular tachycardia in the era of ventricular assist devices. J Cardiovasc Electrophysiol 2011;22:359–63.
20. Andersen M, Videbaek R, Boesgaard S, et al. Incidence of ventricular arrhythmias in patients on long-term support with a continuous-flow assist device (HeartMate II). J Heart Lung Transplant 2009;28:733–5.
21. Refaat M, Chemaly E, Lebeche D, et al. Ventricular arrhythmias after left ventricular assist device implantation. Pacing Clin Electrophysiol 2008;31:1246–52.
22. Genovese EA, Dew MA, Teuteberg JJ, et al. Incidence and patterns of adverse event onset during the first 60 days after ventricular assist device implantation. Ann Thorac Surg 2009;88:1162–70.
23. Pagani FD, Miller LW, Russell SD, et al. Extended mechanical circulatory support with a continuous-flow rotary left ventricular assist device. J Am Coll Cardiol 2009;54:312–21.
24. Kirklin JK, Naftel DC, Kormos RL, et al. Fifth INTERMACS annual report: risk factor analysis from more than 6,000 mechanical circulatory support patients. J Heart Lung Transplant 2013;32:141–56.
25. Crow S, Chen D, Milano C, et al. Acquired von Willebrand syndrome in continuous-flow ventricular assist device recipients. Ann Thorac Surg 2010;90:1263–9 [discussion: 1269].

26. Crow S, Milano C, Joyce L, et al. Comparative analysis of von Willebrand factor profiles in pulsatile and continuous left ventricular assist device recipients. ASAIO J 2010;56:441–5.

27. Demirozu ZT, Radovancevic R, Hochman LF, et al. Arteriovenous malformation and gastrointestinal bleeding in patients with the HeartMate II left ventricular assist device. J Heart Lung Transplant 2011;30: 849–53.

28. Miller L. We always need a pulse, or do we?? J Cardiovasc Transl Res 2012;5:296–301.

29. Mehra MR, Uber PA, Uber WE, et al. Allosensitization in heart transplantation: implications and management strategies. Curr Opin Cardiol 2003;18:153–8.

30. Junquera F, Saperas E, Videla S, et al. Long-term efficacy of octreotide in the prevention of recurrent bleeding from gastrointestinal angiodysplasia. Am J Gastroenterol 2007;102:254–60.

31. Boyle AJ, Russell SD, Teuteberg JJ, et al. Low thromboembolism and pump thrombosis with the HeartMate II left ventricular assist device: analysis of outpatient anti-coagulation. J Heart Lung Transplant 2009;28:881–7.

32. Kirklin JK, Naftel DC, Kormos RL, et al. Second INTERMACS annual report: more than 1,000 primary left ventricular assist device implants. J Heart Lung Transplant 2010;29:1–10.

33. International Society for Heart and Lung Transplantation. A 2010 working formulation for the standardization of definitions of infections in patients using ventricular assist devices (VADS). J Heart Lung Transplant 2011;30:375–84.

34. Gordon RJ, Quagliarello B, Lowy FD. Ventricular assist device-related infections. Lancet Infect Dis 2006;6:426–37.

35. Chinn R, Dembitsky W, Eaton L, et al. Multicenter experience: prevention and management of left ventricular assist device infections. ASAIO J 2005;51: 461–70.

36. Miller LW, Guglin M. Patient selection for ventricular assist devices: a moving target. J Am Coll Cardiol 2013;61:1209–21.

37. Dang NC, Topkara VK, Mercando M, et al. Right heart failure after left ventricular assist device implantation in patients with chronic congestive heart failure. J Heart Lung Transplant 2006;25:1–6.

38. Matthews JC, Koelling TM, Pagani FD, et al. The right ventricular failure risk score a pre-operative tool for assessing the risk of right ventricular failure in left ventricular assist device candidates. J Am Coll Cardiol 2008;51:2163–72.

39. Kormos RL, Teuteberg JJ, Pagani FD, et al. Right ventricular failure in patients with the HeartMate II continuous-flow left ventricular assist device: incidence, risk factors, and effect on outcomes. J Thorac Cardiovasc Surg 2010;139:1316–24.

40. Copeland JG, Smith RG, Arabia FA, et al. Cardiac replacement with a total artificial heart as a bridge to transplantation. N Engl J Med 2004; 351:859–67.

41. Copeland JG, Smith RG, Arabia FA, et al. Total artificial heart bridge to transplantation: a 9-year experience with 62 patients. J Heart Lung Transplant 2004;23:823–31.

42. Kasirajan V, Tang DG, Katlaps GJ, et al. The total artificial heart for biventricular heart failure and beyond. Curr Opin Cardiol 2012;27:301–7.

43. Mankad AK, Tang DG, Clark WB, et al. Persistent anemia after implantation of the total artificial heart. J Card Fail 2012;18:433–8.

44. Slaughter MS, Giridharan GA, Tamez D, et al. Transapical miniaturized ventricular assist device: design and initial testing. J Thorac Cardiovasc Surg 2011; 142:668–74.

45. Meyns BP, Simon A, Klotz S, et al. Clinical benefits of partial circulatory support in New York Heart Association Class IIIB and early class IV patients. Eur J Cardiothorac Surg 2011;39:693–8.

Ventricular Arrhythmias
State of the Art

J. William Schleifer, MD[a], Komandoor Srivathsan, MD[b],*

KEYWORDS

- Ventricular tachycardia • Ventricular fibrillation • Antiarrhythmic medications • Catheter ablation
- Electrical storm

KEY POINTS

- Wide complex tachycardia in patients with structural heart disease is most likely ventricular tachycardia (VT), but the 12-lead electrocardiogram should be systematically analyzed for confirmation.
- Direct current cardioversion or infusion of intravenous amiodarone, procainamide, or lidocaine is usually successful for acutely terminating VT.
- A combination of β-blockers and amiodarone is the most effective medical treatment for preventing recurrent VT after implantable cardioverter-defibrillator placement.
- Catheter ablation is an effective treatment of recurrent VT despite antiarrhythmic therapy, but success rates vary depending on the mechanism and substrate of VT.
- Electrical storm that continues despite defibrillation, β-blockade, and antiarrhythmics may respond to general anesthesia, left stellate ganglion blockade, hemodynamic support, or catheter ablation.

INTRODUCTION
Epidemiology of Ventricular Arrhythmias

Sudden cardiac death (SCD) accounts for approximately 300,000 deaths in the United States per year and in most cases is the final result of ventricular tachycardia (VT) or ventricular fibrillation (VF).[1] Ventricular arrhythmias must be recognized and treated promptly because of the high risk of acute mortality. In patients in the cardiac intensive care unit, 8% have episodes of nonsustained VT, 2% develop sustained VT, and 5% are treated for VF.[2] SCD is a significant cause of long-term mortality in ischemic heart disease, accounting for 22% of all causes of death.[3] Nonischemic conditions associated with VT, VF, and SCD include genetic conditions, cardiomyopathies, and idiopathic VT in structurally normal hearts. VT and VF can be challenging to manage, particularly if they recur despite initial therapy. The diversity of pharmacotherapy, devices, catheter ablation techniques, and other interventions increases the complexity of management.

Prognostic Significance

Sustained VT and VF have a high acute mortality and adversely affect long-term prognosis despite treatment. Even asymptomatic nonsustained VT confers higher long-term mortality if programmed stimulation induces sustained VT.[4] VT or VF within 48 hours of the onset of an acute myocardial infarction (MI), although it significantly increases in-hospital mortality, does not adversely affect long-term prognosis.[5] VT or VF immediately after cardiac surgery not only increases in-hospital mortality[6] but also worsens long-term prognosis.[7]

IMMEDIATE CONSIDERATIONS

In patients with suspected VT, rapid but accurate recognition of the rhythm is imperative. Although

Disclosure: The authors have nothing to disclose.
a Division of Cardiovascular Diseases, Mayo Clinic Arizona, 13400 East Shea Boulevard, Scottsdale, AZ 85259, USA;
b Division of Cardiovascular Diseases, Mayo Clinic Hospital, Mayo Clinic Arizona, 5777 East Mayo Boulevard, Phoenix, AZ 85054, USA
* Corresponding author.
E-mail address: srivathsan.komandoor@mayo.edu

treating hemodynamic instability is the first priority in patient care, hemodynamic instability does not confirm the diagnosis of VT. Wide complex tachycardia in patients with a history of coronary artery disease or structural heart disease is most likely VT; even so, the 12-lead electrocardiogram (ECG) must be systematically analyzed to reach the correct diagnosis. Other aspects of evaluating patients with VT are described in **Table 1**.

Noncardiac artifact obscuring a narrow complex rhythm must be excluded. Then, the QRS complexes can be classified as monomorphic (constant in form) or polymorphic (variable in form). Polymorphic VT also requires analysis of the preceding rhythm. In the setting of a prolonged corrected QT interval (QTc), polymorphic VT is consistent with torsades de pointe (TdP)[8] and usually initiates with a short cycle length after a prolonged cardiac cycle.[9]

Several ECG features, summarized in **Fig. 1**, differentiate monomorphic VT from supraventricular tachycardia (SVT) with aberrant conduction. Particularly useful for differentiating VT from SVT with aberrancy are the validated criteria developed by Brugada and colleagues,[10] which are 98.7% sensitive and 96.5% specific for VT and 96% sensitive and 98.7% specific for SVT with aberrancy. **Fig. 2** shows the application of these criteria to an ECG showing VT.

- Absence of an RS complex in the precordial leads: 100% specific for VT
- RS interval (beginning of R to trough of S) greater than 100 milliseconds: 98% specific for VT
- Atrioventricular dissociation: 98% specific for VT
- Apply morphologic criteria to V1 and V6. If both leads are consistent with VT, then VT is diagnosed; otherwise, the rhythm is classified as SVT with aberrancy.

After morphologic criteria are applied, SVT conducting through an accessory pathway remains difficult to distinguish from VT, even with additional criteria.[11] The ECG is also useful for determining the exit site of VT[12] and for distinguishing endocardial from epicardial origin.[13]

NONPHARMACOLOGIC THERAPEUTIC MODALITIES
External Defibrillation and Cardioversion

Early defibrillation with a rectilinear biphasic automatic external defibrillator improves initial success of defibrillation for out-of-hospital VF arrest.[14] Thus, national guidelines recommend early biphasic defibrillation for VF followed by epinephrine and amiodarone administration if the patient is difficult to

---

Table 1
Initial assessment of a patient with VT

Evaluation	Assessment	Goal
Vital signs	Hemodynamic stability	If hemodynamically unstable, treat with urgent DCCV or defibrillation
12-lead ECG	Tachycardia diagnosis	Differentiate VT from SVT with aberrancy; determine VT exit site
History	Symptoms (eg, chest pain indicating ongoing ischemia)	Identify cause and triggers
Current medications	Antiarrhythmics, digoxin, QTc-prolonging medications	Identify pharmacologic contribution to a proarrhythmic state
Family history	Family history of SCD	Determine risk of inherited predisposition to SCD
Physical examination	Canon A waves Murmurs, sternotomy scar	Indicate AV dissociation Indicate existing structural heart disease
Laboratory tests	Electrolytes, creatinine, troponin, thyroid-stimulating hormone, toxicology assays	Identify metabolic, ischemic, or pharmacologic contributions to a proarrhythmic state
Imaging	Chest roentgenography, echocardiography Coronary angiography Computed tomography, magnetic resonance imaging	Indicated in all patients with VT to assess for structural heart disease Indicated if VT occurs secondary to ischemia Indicated in special cases when particular cardiomyopathies are suspected

Abbreviations: A, atrial; AV, atrioventricular; DCCV, direct current cardioversion; QTc, corrected QT interval.

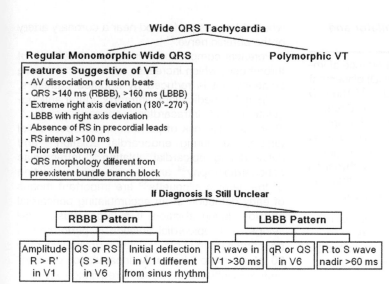

Fig. 1. Criteria for diagnosing a wide QRS complex tachycardia as VT. AV, atrioventricular; LBBB, left bundle branch block; RBBB, right bundle branch block.

defibrillate.[15] In VT, direct current cardioversion (DCCV) must be synchronized, because a shock occurring in a partially repolarized ventricle precipitates VF. In polymorphic VT, defibrillation is required, because synchronization is usually not possible. For comfort, hemodynamically stable conscious patients should be sedated before synchronized DCCV.

- Biphasic waveform defibrillation improves initial success of defibrillation.
- In VT, unsynchronized DCCV can precipitate VF.

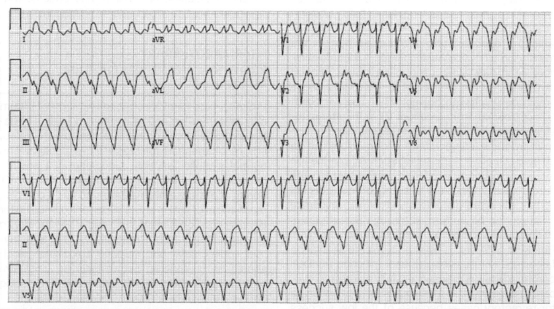

Fig. 2. 12-lead ECG showing monomorphic VT. This ECG shows a regular monomorphic tachycardia with a wide QRS of 160 milliseconds and an atypical QRS morphology in the precordial leads. The Brugada criteria can be applied. Step 1: There is an R wave in V1, so continue to step 2. Step 2: the longest RS interval in a precordial lead is slightly more than 100 milliseconds in V5 and is thus consistent with VT, even although no atrioventricular dissociation (step 3) is visible. Step 4: R is greater than R' in V1, and S is greater than R in V6, meeting morphologic criteria for VT in V1 and V6.

Implantable Cardioverter-Defibrillator and Pacing

Numerous trials have shown the importance of implantable cardioverter-defibrillator (ICD) placement in high-risk patients to prevent SCD.[16–19] The ICD treats but does not prevent recurrent VT. Because ICD shocks cause significant discomfort, inappropriate shocks should be acutely stopped by placing a magnet over the device while awaiting reprogramming. The ICD also can perform antitachycardia pacing, which creates a paced wavefront that collides with the VT wavefront and terminates it.

- ICD implantation significantly reduces mortality from SCD in high-risk patients.
- Inappropriate ICD therapy can be halted by applying a magnet over the device.

Left Cardiac Sympathetic Denervation

Left stellate ganglion resection completely removes sympathetic input to the heart. It effectively prevents VT that recurs despite β-blockade in long QT syndrome (LQTS),[20] catecholaminergic polymorphic VT (CPVT), and other types of VT.[21] Stellate ganglion blockade with lidocaine injection is feasible in unstable patients with electrical storm (ES).[22]

Radiofrequency Catheter Ablation

Catheter ablation techniques are rapidly advancing. VT is mapped by entrainment, pacing, or an electroanatomic system that determines catheter position in a magnetic field.[23] Radiofrequency current ablates the endocardium identified as part of the reentry circuit.[24] Another technique, substrate ablation, identifies slow conduction zones around myocardial scars and isolated potentials; these areas are ablated to prevent VT.[25] The 24-month rate of freedom from recurrent VT or VF after catheter ablation is 48% to 88% in recent trials.[26,27]

VT from the left ventricular endocardium can be ablated via either transseptal access from the left atrium or retrograde arterial access through the aortic valve. If a patient fails endocardial ablation or has an epicardial site of VT origin, epicardial ablation can be performed through percutaneous pericardial access or surgical thoracotomy.[28] Rarely, if both endocardial and epicardial ablation fail or are not possible, ethanol injection in distal coronary arteries may successfully ablate midmyocardial sites; but this technique should be reserved for refractory cases because of the low success rate and risk of complications from the ethanol-induced infarction.[29] Intracardiac echocardiography is integrated with electroanatomic mapping, reducing fluoroscopy time.[30] Cryoablation can be performed to reduce the risk of permanent damage when ablation is performed near a coronary artery or the phrenic nerve.[31]

Potential complications include a 2.8% risk of thrombosis, which increases with more extensive ablations but is reduced by irrigated catheters, antiplatelet medications, intraprocedural anticoagulation, and intracardiac echocardiography.[32] There is a 1% risk of perforation and pericardial tamponade during endocardial ablation[33] and 3.4% during epicardial ablation.[28] Intracardiac echocardiography[34] and fluoroscopic evaluation of the cardiac silhouette[35] are important means of early detection of an accumulating pericardial effusion during ablation. If a large effusion develops, or if epicardial ablation is performed, a pericardial drain is placed until it drains less than 20 mL over 4 to 6 hours. Anticoagulation postprocedure is initiated for patients requiring extensive ablation, patients with atrial fibrillation or severely reduced ejection fraction, or patients who have a hemodynamic support or ventricular assist device (VAD). Antiarrhythmic medications are continued unless the patient experiences marked adverse effects from them. Intensive care unit admission postprocedure is recommended for patients requiring a prolonged procedure (>6 hours), patients requiring an intra-aortic balloon pump or a percutaneous hemodynamic support device such as an Impella (Abiomed, Danvers, MA), patients with a pericardial drain, patients with recurrent VT after unsuccessful ablation, and patients with significant fluid overload after a procedure.

PHARMACOTHERAPY
Intravenous Medications for Acute Management

Procainamide blocks both sodium and potassium channels, slowing and terminating VT. As a negative inotrope, it can cause hypotension; therefore, it is recommended for stable VT in patients with normal systolic function. Lidocaine is a sodium channel blocker that is potentially effective for VT during acute ischemia. Amiodarone has a complex mechanism of action and is superior to lidocaine for treating shock-resistant VF[36] and VT refractory to procainamide.[37] It shows significant long-term thyroid, pulmonary, and hepatic toxicities, which should be considered before initiating long-term oral therapy. **Table 2** lists the recommended dosing and acute adverse effects of these medications.

- Procainamide is preferred for pharmacologic cardioversion of stable VT in patients with normal systolic function.
- Lidocaine is useful for VT during acute ischemia; it does not cause QTc prolongation.

Table 2
Acute and maintenance dosing of intravenous antiarrhythmic medications

Antiarrhythmic	Dosing	Acute Adverse Reactions
Procainamide	Load: 17 mg/kg Maximum rate: 50 mg/min Maintenance: 1–4 mg/min	Hypotension Hold if QRS prolongs >50%
Lidocaine	Load: 1–3 mg/kg Rate: 20–50 mg/min Maintenance: 1–4 mg/min	Reduce dose in heart failure Monitor for neurotoxicity: delirium, seizures, or paresthesias
Amiodarone	Load: 150 mg over 10 min if blood pressure is normal; 300 mg over 19 min if hypotensive Maintenance: 1 mg/min for 6 h, then 0.5 mg/min for 18 h	Caution in cardiogenic shock TdP is rare Use with pacing if patient is severely bradycardic

- Amiodarone is the most effective antiarrhythmic for VT but requires time to load.

Long-Term Oral Therapy

In a randomized controlled trial of sotalol, amiodarone with β-blockers, or β-blockers alone, amiodarone with a β-blocker (metoprolol, carvedilol, or bisoprolol) significantly reduced defibrillator shocks more than sotalol or β-blockers alone.[38] There was no significant mortality difference, and in patients receiving amiodarone, 5% experienced pulmonary adverse events and 5.7% developed thyroid abnormalities. β-Blockers by themselves reduce SCD in patients with MI[39] and improve survival in patients with treated VT or VF.[40]

- A combination of β-blockers and amiodarone is the most successful long-term medical strategy for reducing defibrillator shocks.
- β-blockers improve survival in patients after VT or VF is treated.

Although right ventricular outflow tract (RVOT) and left ventricular outflow tract (LVOT) VT are typically sensitive to diltiazem and verapamil,[41] giving calcium channel blockers acutely during VT when the mechanism of VT is unknown is contraindicated because of the risk of hemodynamic collapse.[15]

Other oral antiarrhythmics may suppress VT that recurs despite treatment with sotalol or amiodarone with β-blockers. Mexiletine is a sodium channel blocker that counteracts the sodium channel gain-of-function mutation in LQTS type 3. Quinidine has a significant side effect profile but may be particularly effective in Brugada syndrome. Flecainide and other class 1C sodium channel blockers are associated with increased mortality in patients with coronary artery disease.[42] However, flecainide can be used in VT associated with structurally normal hearts.[43] Dofetilide and ranolazine are not approved to treat ventricular arrhythmias but have significantly reduced recurrent VT and VF in small studies.[44,45]

VT IN PATIENTS WITH STRUCTURAL HEART DISEASE
VT in Patients with Acute MI

Acute MI significantly increases the risk for VT and VF. Ischemia prolongs the QTc and can trigger polymorphic VT.[46] Acutely, polymorphic VT requires defibrillation, because it is unlikely to allow hemodynamic stability. The patient should then receive urgent coronary reperfusion and other evidence-based therapies for MI. Both lidocaine and amiodarone are used for VT; neither is clearly superior to the other.[47] Lidocaine should not be used prophylactically in patients with MI.[15] Neither long-term antiarrhythmics nor ICD placement are required for VT during acute MI.[5]

VT in Revascularized Patients with Ischemic Cardiomyopathy

Numerous trials show that ICD implantation decreases mortality in patients with ischemic cardiomyopathy at high risk.[16–18] In patients with VT occurring 1 month or more after MI, recurrence can be successfully prevented with catheter ablation before initiation of long-term antiarrhythmics.[27,48]

- Catheter ablation of VT before initiation of long-term antiarrhythmic therapy is reasonable in patients with sustained VT and a previous MI.

VT in Patients with Nonischemic Cardiomyopathy

The mechanisms of VT in nonischemic cardiomyopathy are diverse, including bundle branch reentry, reentry around fibrosis, activation around focal inflammation (as in sarcoidosis), and epicardial involvement. Acutely, VT should be treated with DCCV and amiodarone, because most other antiarrhythmics are negative inotropes. VT with a typical bundle branch block should be evaluated for bundle branch reentry tachycardia, because ablation of the right bundle branch successfully treats bundle branch reentry.[49] Catheter ablation for recurrent VT in patients with dilated cardiomyopathy, arrhythmogenic right ventricular dysplasia (ARVD), hypertrophic cardiomyopathy, or cardiac sarcoidosis is associated with variable success rates.[50–53]

- Catheter ablation of VT in nonischemic cardiomyopathy has variable success rates depending on the mechanism and substrate of VT.

VT in Patients After Cardiac Surgery

VT and VF occur in some patients immediately after coronary artery bypass grafting and valvular surgeries. Sympathetic stimulation, electrolyte abnormalities, ischemia from vein graft closure, atrial dysrhythmias, injury from cannulation, and preexisting substrate all contribute to initiation of VT. Prophylactic amiodarone prevents both atrial arrhythmias and VT,[54] although no mortality benefit has been shown.[55] VT after cardiac surgery increases both in-hospital and long-term mortality,[7] but ICD placement is not indicated.[56]

- Amiodarone prophylaxis reduces postoperative VT and VF.

VT in Patients with VADs

Increasing numbers of patients with advanced heart failure are being supported with VADs. In these patients, VT and VF cause hemodynamic instability from right heart failure, reducing left ventricular preload, which can cause a suction event. Catheter ablation in patients with a VAD is feasible; mapping has shown that VT originates from the scar in 75% of patients and less commonly from the inflow cannula site.[57]

- VT in patients with a VAD comes predominantly from the preexisting substrate rather than from the inflow cannula site.

VT in Patients After Orthotopic Heart Transplantation

VT in orthotopic heart transplant recipients is rare, and acute rejection must be ruled out. β-Blockers should be used cautiously after heart transplantation because of the risk of sinus node dysfunction.[58] Amiodarone, lidocaine, and mexiletine have been used for VT in heart transplant patients.[59]

- Rejection must be ruled out in patients with orthotopic heart transplantation and VT.

VT in Patients with Congenital Heart Disease

Any congenital anomaly involving the ventricles predisposes patients to VT, especially tetralogy of Fallot, transposition of the great arteries, single ventricle, and congenital aortic stenosis. The predominant mechanism is reentry around fibrosis and surgical scar, which is responsive to catheter ablation.[60]

VT IN PATIENTS WITH STRUCTURALLY NORMAL HEARTS
VT in Patients with Brugada Syndrome

Brugada syndrome is diagnosed by coved ST segment increase in leads V1 to V3 either spontaneously or provoked by sodium channel blockade. **Fig. 3** shows an ECG consistent with Brugada syndrome. Impaired sodium channel function prolongs the epicardial action potential, reversing the direction of repolarization and predisposing the ventricle to reentry. Isoproterenol prevents recurrent VT by increasing calcium current and should be titrated to increase the heart rate by 20% and to normalize the ST segments.[61] Quinidine prevents recurrent VF by normalizing the direction of repolarization.[62]

- In patients with Brugada syndrome presenting with VT, isoproterenol infusion should be initiated after DCCV and titrated until the ST segments normalize.

VT in Patients with TdP

TdP is polymorphic VT in the setting of a prolonged QTc in which a premature ventricular depolarization follows a prolonged cardiac cycle, as in **Fig. 4**.[9] TdP can be secondary to electrolyte abnormalities, bradyarrhythmias, or medication effects. After defibrillation, temporarily pacing faster than the intrinsic rate prevents long-short cycles from occurring, and pacing is more successful than isoproterenol and lidocaine in preventing recurrent TdP.[9] Drugs that prolong the QTc must be discontinued, and potassium and magnesium levels must be maintained in normal ranges.

- Pacing prevents recurrent TdP while awaiting clearance of offending medications.

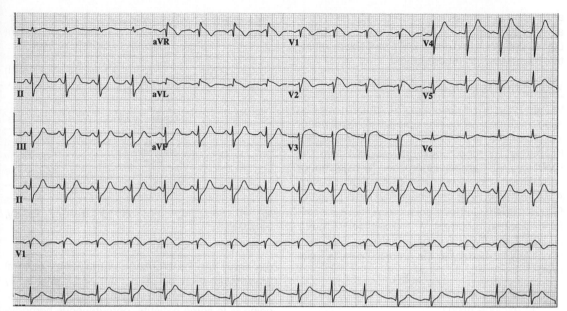

Fig. 3. 12-lead ECG showing coved ST segment elevation in leads V1 to V3 in a patient with Brugada syndrome.

VT in Patients with Congenital LQTS

Congenital LQTS is caused by one of many mutations affecting repolarization. β-Blockers are an essential therapy for most types, and mexiletine is useful in LQTS type 3. Treatment of VT in LQTS requires pacing after DCCV; isoproterenol in patients with LQTS is potentially harmful and can precipitate recurrent VT. Permanent pacemaker placement may be required in LQTS to allow the use of adequate doses of β-blockers.[63]

Left stellate ganglion resection is 91% effective for preventing recurrent VT.[20]

- β-blockade combined with pacing prevents recurrent VT in LQTS.

VT in Patients with CPVT

CPVT occurs when a mutant ryanodine receptor allows calcium to leak into the cytoplasm and cause delayed afterdepolarizations. β-Blockers

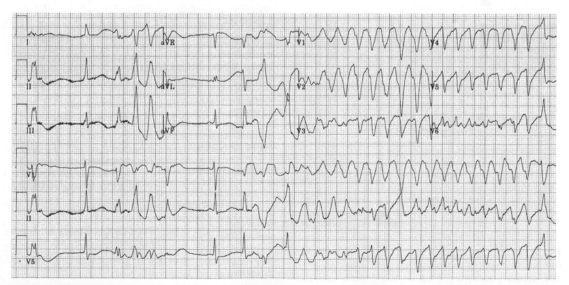

Fig. 4. 12-lead ECG showing the initiation of TdP with a long-short sequence occurring in the setting of a prolonged QT interval.

are essential but may not prevent recurrent VT in all patients, and many patients require an ICD.[64] Left stellate ganglion resection is particularly effective for preventing recurrent VT.[21]

VT in Patients with Idiopathic VT

VT occurring in the absence of structural heart disease, metabolic or pharmacologic provocation, or ion channel dysfunction is considered idiopathic. Idiopathic VT most commonly originates in the RVOT or LVOT and is suppressed by diltiazem or verapamil.[41] Structural heart disease (particularly ARVD causing right ventricular VT) must be carefully excluded. Catheter ablation is often successful in treating recurrent VT. Idiopathic VT rarely causes hemodynamic compromise or SCD and is unlikely to present to the cardiac intensive care unit.

- Patients with RVOT VT should be evaluated to exclude ARVD.

ES

ES is defined as 3 or more episodes of VT or VF within 24 hours; electrical stability deteriorates rapidly, causing high mortality. A diversity of substrates and triggers can cause ES, and no single therapy is effective in all patients. VT refractory to 1 antiarrhythmic may be suppressed by another. After DCCV or defibrillation, amiodarone infusion is typically begun,[36,37] to which a sodium channel blocker can be added if VT recurs. β-Blockade with esmolol, metoprolol, or propranolol can be titrated as blood pressure tolerates. In patients unable to tolerate β-blockade, sympathetic input to

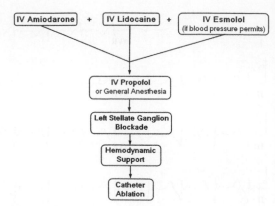

Fig. 6. Therapeutic protocol for treating ES. IV, intravenous.

the heart can be blocked centrally with general anesthesia such as propofol[65] and peripherally with injection of the left stellate ganglion with lidocaine.[22] In some patients, percutaneous hemodynamic support with Impella (Abiomed, Danvers, MA) or TandemHeart (CardiacAssist, Pittsburgh, PA) is necessary.[66] **Fig. 5** shows Impella placement. Catheter ablation is successful for terminating ES in 48% of patients after the first ablation and in 84% after multiple attempts.[67] **Fig. 6** shows an algorithm for treating ES.

SUMMARY

VT and VF commonly occur in the cardiac intensive care unit but have many potential causes. Acutely, synchronized DCCV or pharmacologic cardioversion likely terminate VT, but definitive treatment is complex. Determining the cause, correcting reversible causes, and defining the substrate are the goals of initial evaluation. ICD programming, β-blockers, antiarrhythmics, and catheter ablation should be considered to prevent recurrence. For patients with ES, additional modalities, including general anesthesia, left stellate ganglion blockade, hemodynamic support, and additional catheter ablation, may be considered.

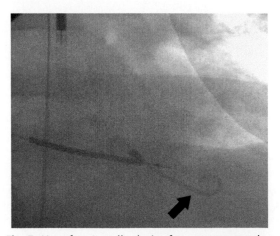

Fig. 5. Use of an Impella device for percutaneous hemodynamic support in a patient with intractable VT. The arrow indicates the tip of the Impella catheter within the left ventricle. A defibrillator lead is also seen in the right ventricular apex.

REFERENCES

1. Myerburg RJ, Kessler KM, Castellanos A. Sudden cardiac death: epidemiology, transient risk, and intervention assessment. Ann Intern Med 1993; 119:1187–97.
2. Ting P, Chua TS, Wong A, et al. Trends in mortality from acute myocardial infarction in the coronary care unit. Ann Acad Med Singapore 2007;36: 974–9.
3. Jokhadar M, Jacobsen SJ, Reeder GS, et al. Sudden death and recurrent ischemic events after

myocardial infarction in the community. Am J Epidemiol 2004;159:1040–6.

4. Buxton AE, Lee KL, DiCarlo L, et al. Electrophysiologic testing to identify patients with coronary artery disease who are at risk for sudden death. N Engl J Med 2000;342:1937–45.

5. Hohnloser SH, Kuck KH, Dorian P, et al. Prophylactic use of an implantable cardioverter-defibrillator after acute myocardial infarction. N Engl J Med 2004;351:2481–8.

6. Pires LA, Hafley GE, Lee KL, et al. Prognostic significance of nonsustained ventricular tachycardia identified postoperatively after coronary artery bypass grafting in patients with left ventricular dysfunction. J Cardiovasc Electrophysiol 2002;13:757–63.

7. El-Chami MF, Sawaya FJ, Kilgo P, et al. Ventricular arrhythmia after cardiac surgery: incidence, predictors, and outcomes. J Am Coll Cardiol 2012;60:2664–71.

8. Krikler DM, Curry PV. Torsade de pointes, an atypical ventricular tachycardia. Br Heart J 1976;38:117–20.

9. Kay GN, Plumb VJ, Arciniegas JG, et al. Torsade de pointes: the long-short initiating sequence and other clinical features: observations in 32 patients. J Am Coll Cardiol 1983;2:806–17.

10. Brugada P, Brugada J, Mont L, et al. A new approach to the differential diagnosis of a regular tachycardia with a wide QRS complex. Circulation 1991;83:1649–59.

11. Steurer G, Gürsoy S, Frey B, et al. The differential diagnosis on the electrocardiogram between ventricular tachycardia and preexcited tachycardia. Clin Cardiol 1994;17:306–8.

12. Segal OR, Chow AW, Wong T, et al. A novel algorithm for determining endocardial VT exit site from 12-lead surface ECG characteristics in human, infarct-related ventricular tachycardia. J Cardiovasc Electrophysiol 2007;18:161–8.

13. Berruezo A, Mont L, Nava S, et al. Electrocardiographic recognition of the epicardial origin of ventricular tachycardias. Circulation 2004;109:1842–7.

14. Morrison LJ, Dorian P, Long J, et al. Out-of-hospital cardiac arrest rectilinear biphasic to monophasic dampened sine defibrillation waveforms with advanced life support intervention trial (ORBIT). Resuscitation 2005;66:149–57.

15. Zipes DP, Camm AJ, Borggrede M, et al. ACC/AHA/ESC 2006 guidelines for management of patients with ventricular arrhythmias and the prevention of sudden cardiac death: a report of the American College of Cardiology/American Heart Association Task Force and the European Society of Cardiology Committee for Practice Guidelines (Writing Committee to Develop Guidelines for Management of Patients with Ventricular Arrhythmias and the Prevention of Sudden Cardiac Death): developed in collaboration with the European Heart Rhythm Association and the Heart Rhythm Society. Circulation 2006;114:e385–484.

16. Moss AJ, Hall J, Cannom DS, et al. Improved survival with an implanted defibrillator in patients with coronary disease at high risk for ventricular arrhythmia. N Engl J Med 1996;335:1933–40.

17. Moss AJ, Zareba W, Hall J, et al. Prophylactic implantation of a defibrillator in patients with myocardial infarction and reduced ejection fraction. N Engl J Med 2002;346:877–83.

18. Bardy GH, Lee KL, Mark DB, et al. Amiodarone or an implantable cardioverter-defibrillator for congestive heart failure. N Engl J Med 2005;352:225–37.

19. Kadis A, Dyer A, Daubert JP, et al. Prophylactic defibrillator implantation in patients with nonischemic dilated cardiomyopathy. N Engl J Med 2004;350:2151–8.

20. Schwartz PJ, Priori SG, Cerrone M, et al. Left cardiac sympathetic denervation in the management of high-risk patients affected by the long-QT syndrome. Circulation 2004;109:1826–33.

21. Coleman MA, Bos M, Johnson JN, et al. Videoscopic left cardiac sympathetic denervation for patients with recurrent ventricular fibrillation/malignant ventricular arrhythmia syndromes besides congenital long-QT syndrome. Circ Arrhythm Electrophysiol 2012;5:782–8.

22. Nademanee K, Taylor R, Bailey WE, et al. Treating electrical storm: sympathetic blockade versus advanced cardiac life support–guided therapy. Circulation 2000;102:742–7.

23. Nademanee K, Kosar EM. A nonfluoroscopic catheter-based mapping technique to ablate focal ventricular tachycardia. Pacing Clin Electrophysiol 1998;21:1442–7.

24. Stevenson WG, Kahn H, Sager P, et al. Identification of reentry circuit sites during catheter mapping and radiofrequency ablation of ventricular tachycardia late after myocardial infarction. Circulation 1993;99:1647–70.

25. Arenal A, Hernandez J, Calvo D, et al. Safety, long-term results, and predictors of recurrence after complete endocardial ventricular tachycardia substrate ablation in patients with previous myocardial infarction. Am J Cardiol 2013;111:499–505.

26. Delacrétaz E, Brenner R, Schaumann A, et al. Catheter ablation of stable ventricular tachycardia before defibrillator implantation in patients with coronary heart disease (VTACH): an on-treatment analysis. J Cardiovasc Electrophysiol 2013;24(5):525–9.

27. Reddy VY, Reynolds MR, Neuzil P, et al. Prophylactic catheter ablation for the prevention of defibrillator therapy. N Engl J Med 2007;357:2657–65.

28. Della Bella P, Brugada J, Zeppenfeld K, et al. Epicardial ablation for ventricular tachycardia: a European multicenter study. Circ Arrhythm Electrophysiol 2011;4:653–9.

29. Tokuda M, Sobieszczyk P, Eisenhauer AC, et al. Transcoronary ethanol ablation for recurrent ventricular tachycardia after failed catheter ablation: an update. Circ Arrhythm Electrophysiol 2011;4: 889–96.

30. Khaykin Y, Skanes A, Whaley B, et al. Real-time integration of 2D intracardiac echocardiography and 3D electroanatomical mapping to guide ventricular tachycardia ablation. Heart Rhythm 2008; 5:1396–402.

31. Di Biase L, Al-Ahamad A, Santeangeli P, et al. Safety and outcomes of cryoablation for ventricular tachyarrhythmias: results from a multicenter experience. Heart Rhythm 2011;8:968–74.

32. Zhou L, Keane D, Reed G, et al. Thromboembolic complications of cardiac radiofrequency catheter ablation: a review of the reported incidence, pathogenesis, and current research directions. J Cardiovasc Electrophysiol 1999;10:611–20.

33. Tokuda M, Kojodjojo P, Epstein LM, et al. Outcomes of cardiac perforation complicating catheter ablation of ventricular arrhythmias. Circ Arrhythm Electrophysiol 2011;4:660–6.

34. Ren JF, Marchlinski FE. Early detection of iatrogenic pericardial effusion: importance of intracardiac echocardiography. JACC Cardiovasc Interv 2010;3:127.

35. Nanthakumar K, Kay GN, Plumb VJ, et al. Decrease in fluoroscopic cardiac silhouette excursion precedes hemodynamic compromise in intraprocedural tamponade. Heart Rhythm 2005;2: 1224–30.

36. Dorian P, Cass D, Schwartz B, et al. Amiodarone as compared with lidocaine for shock-resistant ventricular fibrillation. N Engl J Med 2002;346:884–90.

37. Leak D, Eydt JN. Control of refractory cardiac arrhythmias with amiodarone. Arch Intern Med 1979;139:425–8.

38. Connolly SJ, Dorian P, Roberts RS, et al. Comparison of beta blockers, amiodarone plus beta blockers, or sotalol for prevention of shocks from implantable cardioverter defibrillators: the OPTIC study: a randomized trial. JAMA 2006;295:165–71.

39. Piccini JP, Hranitzky PM, Kilaru R, et al. Relation of mortality to failure to prescribe beta blockers acutely in patients with sustained ventricular tachycardia and ventricular fibrillation following acute myocardial infarction. Am J Cardiol 2008;102:1427–32.

40. Exner DV, Reiffel JA, Epstein AE, et al. Beta-blocker use and survival in patients with ventricular fibrillation or symptomatic ventricular tachycardia: the antiarrhythmics versus implantable defibrillators (AVID) trial. J Am Coll Cardiol 1999;34:325–33.

41. Gill JS, Ward DE, Camm AJ. Comparison of verapamil and diltiazem in the suppression of idiopathic ventricular tachycardia. Pacing Clin Electrophysiol 1992;15:2122–6.

42. Epstein AE, Hallstrom AP, Rogers WJ, et al. Mortality following ventricular arrhythmia suppression by encainide, flecainide, and moricizine after myocardial infarction. JAMA 1993;270:2451–5.

43. Gill JS, Mehta D, Ward DE, et al. Efficacy of flecainide, sotalol, and verapamil in the treatment of right ventricular tachycardia in patients without overt cardiac abnormality. Br Heart J 1992;68:392–7.

44. Baquero GA, Banchis JE, Depalma S, et al. Dofetilide reduces the frequency of ventricular arrhythmias and implantable cardioverter defibrillator therapies. J Cardiovasc Electrophysiol 2012;23: 296–301.

45. Bunch TJ, Mahapatra S, Murdock D, et al. Ranolazine reduces ventricular tachycardia burden and ICD shocks in patients with drug-refractor ICD shocks. Pacing Clin Electrophysiol 2011;34:1600–6.

46. Wolfe CL, Nibley C, Bahndari A, et al. Polymorphous ventricular tachycardia associated with acute myocardial infarction. Circulation 1991;84: 1543–51.

47. Piccini JP, Schulte PJ, Pieper KS, et al. Antiarrhythmic drug therapy for sustained ventricular arrhythmias complicating acute myocardial infarction. Crit Care Med 2011;39:78–83.

48. Kuck KH, Schaumann A, Eckardt L, et al. Catheter ablation of stable ventricular tachycardia before defibrillator implantation in patients with coronary heart disease (VTACH): a multicentre randomized controlled trial. Lancet 2010;375:31–40.

49. Balasundaram R, Rao HB, Kalavakolanu S, et al. Catheter ablation of bundle branch reentrant ventricular tachycardia. Heart Rhythm 2008;5:S68–72.

50. Arya A, Bode K, Piorkowski C, et al. Catheter ablation of electrical storm due to monomorphic ventricular tachycardia in patients with nonischemic cardiomyopathy: acute results and its effect on long-term survival. Pacing Clin Electrophysiol 2010;33:1504–9.

51. Philips B, Madhavan S, James C, et al. Outcomes of catheter ablation of ventricular tachycardia in arrhythmogenic right ventricular dysplasia/cardiomyopathy. Circ Arrhythm Electrophysiol 2012;5: 499–505.

52. Santangeli P, Di Biase L, Lakkireddy D, et al. Radiofrequency catheter ablation of ventricular arrhythmias in patients with hypertrophic cardiomyopathy: safety and feasibility. Heart Rhythm 2010;7: 1036–42.

53. Jefic D, Joel B, Good E, et al. Role of radiofrequency catheter ablation of ventricular tachycardia in cardiac sarcoidosis: report from a multicenter registry. Heart Rhythm 2009;6:189–95.

54. Mitchell LB, Exner DV, Wyse DG, et al. Prophylactic oral amiodarone for the prevention of arrhythmias that begin early after revascularization, valve replacement, or repair. JAMA 2005;294:3093–100.

55. Aasbo JD, Lawrence AT, Krishnan K, et al. Amiodarone prophylaxis reduces major cardiovascular morbidity and length of stay after cardiac surgery: a meta-analysis. Ann Intern Med 2005;143:327–36.

56. Bigger JT. Prophylactic use of implanted cardiac defibrillators in patients at high risk for ventricular arrhythmias after coronary-artery bypass graft surgery. N Engl J Med 1997;337:1569–75.

57. Cantillon DJ, Bianoc C, Wazni OM, et al. Electrophysiologic characteristics and catheter ablation of ventricular tachyarrhythmias among patients with heart failure on ventricular assist device support. Heart Rhythm 2012;9:859–64.

58. Stecker EC, Strelich KR, Chugh SS, et al. Arrhythmias after orthotopic heart transplantation. J Card Fail 2005;11:464–72.

59. Kertesz NJ, Towbin JA, Clunie S, et al. Long-term follow-up of arrhythmias in pediatric orthotopic heart transplant recipients: incidence and correlation with rejection. J Heart Lung Transplant 2003; 22:889–93.

60. Ventura A, Soriano L, Lopez M. Ventricular tachycardia ablation in repaired tetralogy of Fallot. Europace 2011;13:1211.

61. Ohgo T, Okamura H, Noda T, et al. Acute and chronic management in patients with Brugada syndrome associated with electrical storm of ventricular fibrillation. Heart Rhythm 2007;4:695–700.

62. Berne P, Brugada J. Brugada syndrome 2012. Circ J 2012;76:1563–71.

63. Khan IA, Gowda RM. Novel therapeutics for treatment of long-QT syndrome and torsade de pointes. Int J Cardiol 2004;95:1–6.

64. Marks AR. Sudden unexplained death caused by cardiac ryanodine receptor (RyR2) mutations. Mayo Clin Proc 2004;79:1367–71.

65. Mulpuru SK, Patel DV, Wilbur SL, et al. Electrical storm and termination with propofol therapy: a case report. Int J Cardiol 2008;128:e6–8.

66. Abuissa H, Roshan J, Lim B, et al. Use of the Impella microaxial blood pump for ablation of hemodynamically unstable ventricular tachycardia. J Cardiovasc Electrophysiol 2010;21:458–61.

67. Kozeluhova M, Peichl P, Cihak R, et al. Catheter ablation of electrical storm in patients with structural heart disease. Europace 2011;13:109–13.

Cardiac Critical Care After Transcatheter Aortic Valve Replacement

Matthew I. Tomey, MD*, Umesh K. Gidwani, MD*,
Samin K. Sharma, MD

KEYWORDS

- Transcatheter aortic valve replacement • TAVR • Critical care • Complications

KEY POINTS

- Transcatheter aortic valve replacement (TAVR) is a new approach to management of severe aortic stenosis, first described in 2002, that is now available for clinical use in the United States.
- Vulnerability is a defining feature of the initial cohort of patients eligible for TAVR, whose advanced age and comorbidities confer high or extreme surgical risk.
- Patients undergoing TAVR experience acute hemodynamic changes and risk several complications, including hypotension, vascular injury, anemia, stroke, new-onset atrial fibrillation, conduction disturbances and acute kidney injury.
- Critical care after TAVR centers on anticipation, prevention and management of complications. We present our approach to this challenge and identify avenues for future research.

Transcatheter aortic valve replacement (TAVR) has been described as "game changing," providing a novel, less invasive therapeutic option for patients with severe aortic stenosis (AS) whose age and comorbidities make the operative risk of surgical aortic valve replacement (SAVR) high or extreme. Based on the results of the pivotal Placement of Aortic Transcatheter Valves (PARTNER) trial, US Food and Drug Administration (FDA) approval, announcement of coverage by the Centers for Medicare and Medicaid Services in 2012, and after 10 years' experience in Europe, the volume of TAVR procedures in the United States is poised to increase substantially.

Exuberance for adoption of TAVR is balanced by recognition of multisystem complications and a persistently high rate of mortality (24.3% at 1 year and 33.9% at 2 years in PARTNER) only partly attributable to cardiovascular causes.[1] Although this risk reflects, in part, the advanced age and comorbidity that define TAVR candidates, it also highlights the role of care after TAVR, beginning in the intensive care unit (ICU), and our challenge to improve it.

A hybrid of interventional cardiology and cardiac surgery, TAVR demands the collaboration of a heart team, marrying skills from both disciplines, and incorporating multiple additional specialties, including anesthesiology, vascular surgery, and cardiac imaging. This synthesis extends to the ICU, where optimal care after TAVR requires integration of knowledge and experience previously housed separately in cardiothoracic, surgical, medical, and cardiac ICUs. In this respect, care after TAVR epitomizes a paradigm shift in cardiovascular critical care, emphasizing cross-training of

Disclosures: None.
The Zena and Michael A. Wiener Cardiovascular Institute, The Icahn School of Medicine at Mount Sinai, One Gustave L. Levy Place, New York, NY 10029, USA
* Corresponding author. The Zena and Michael A. Wiener Cardiovascular Institute, The Icahn School of Medicine at Mount Sinai, One Gustave L. Levy Place, Box 1030, New York, NY 10029.
E-mail addresses: matthew.tomey@mountsinai.org; umesh.gidwani@mountsinai.org

cardiology.theclinics.com

physicians and nurses and the management of cardiac and surgical problems in the context of complex medical illness.

The objective of critical care after TAVR is to guide patients, often elderly and ill, through a period of acute hemodynamic changes and potential for multisystem complications to maximize chances for survival and functional recovery. In this review, our approach to this challenge is presented, acknowledging limitations to evidence where they exist to prompt future research.

PREPARATION: UNDERSTANDING THE PATIENTS AND THE PROCEDURE
Patients

Patients undergoing TAVR are characterized by advanced age and prevalent comorbidities, including coronary and peripheral artery disease, lung disease, pulmonary hypertension, and cerebrovascular disease. The PARTNER trial, which provides the basis for the initial rollout of TAVR offers a useful preview of the comorbidities and risk profiles of high-risk and extreme-risk patients presenting for TAVR (**Table 1**).[2,3] Many patients assigned to cohort B were believed to be at

extreme risk due to comorbidities not captured by standard risk prediction tools, such as extensive aortic calcification (15.1%), chest wall abnormalities (13.1%), oxygen-dependent respiratory insufficiency (23.5%), or frailty (23.1%).

At present, the indication for TAVR is severe valvular AS, which is consequently a defining feature of the initial cohort of patients undergoing TAVR in the United States. Fixed obstruction to left ventricular outflow at the level of the aortic valve impedes forward flow and subjects the left ventricle to chronic pressure overload and variable degrees of hypertrophy, diastolic, and ultimately systolic dysfunction. Although classically characterized by a high transvalvular pressure gradient (mean, >40 mm Hg), severe AS can present with a low gradient in the presence or absence of left ventricular systolic dysfunction. Augmented myocardial oxygen demand increases susceptibility to ischemia and angina. Reduction in cardiac output, highly sensitive to changes in left ventricular preload, can lead to organ hypoperfusion, and symptoms of lightheadedness and syncope. Increased left ventricular end diastolic pressure leads to pulmonary vascular congestion and dyspnea.

As technical comfort with TAVR increases, both clinical trials and off-label indication creep may shift use to comparatively younger, healthier patients or different valvular lesions,[4] altering the makeup of patients presenting to the ICU. The Society of Thoracic Surgeons/American College of Cardiology Transcatheter Valve Therapy Registry, akin to counterparts in Europe,[5] will provide insight into real-world patient selection, device application, and outcomes.

Procedure

Intensivists should become familiar with the TAVR technique, for which a thorough description, exceeding the scope of this review, has been published.[6] Briefly, TAVR entails transcatheter delivery and implantation of a prosthetic valve within the stenotic native valve.

Prosthesis delivery may be antegrade (via the left ventricle) when vascular access is obtained via the left ventricular apex or the systemic venous system with transseptal puncture, or retrograde when vascular access is obtained via arterial puncture. Potential arterial access sites include the femoral, iliac, axillary, and subclavian arteries, as well as the aorta. Access selection depends on arterial calcification and caliber, as informed by preprocedure imaging.

The first generation of valves includes the Edwards SAPIEN Transcatheter Heart Valve (Edwards Lifesciences, Inc, Irvine, CA), consisting of bovine

Table 1
Age, comorbidities and risk profile in the PARTNER trial

	Cohort A (High Risk)	Cohort B (Extreme Risk)
Estimated 30-d mortality risk after SAVR (%)	15	50
Age (y)	83.6 ± 6.8	83.1 ± 8.6
Society of Thoracic Surgeons score	11.2 ± 5.8	11.8 ± 3.3
Logistic euroSCORE	26.4 ± 17.2	29.3 ± 16.5
Coronary artery disease (%)	74.9	67.6
Peripheral artery disease (%)	43.0	30.3
Cerebrovascular disease (%)	29.3	27.4
Chronic obstructive pulmonary disease (%)	43.4	41.3
Pulmonary hypertension (%)	42.4	42.4
New York Heart Association (NYHA) class III/IV symptoms (%)	94.3	92.2

pericardial tissue with a balloon-expandable stainless steel frame and a polyethylene terephthalate skirt; the related Edwards SAPIEN XT valve, using bovine pericardium and a balloon-expandable cobalt chromium frame; and the Medtronic CoreValve (MCV, Medtronic, Minneapolis, MN), consisting of porcine pericardial tissue with a self-expanding nitinol frame (**Fig. 1**).[7] Several newer valve designs are under investigation to address limitations of first-generation models, in particular, paravalvular aortic regurgitation.

Patients are typically brought to the operating suite in an elective manner, with some having undergone preceding balloon aortic valvuloplasty (BAV) as a temporizing measure before return for TAVR.[8] Preprocedure evaluation includes a battery of testing, including laboratory studies, electrocardiography, chest radiography, echocardiography, coronary angiography, and computed tomography or magnetic resonance angiography.

At a given hospital, TAVR may occur in a catheterization laboratory, surgical operating room, or hybrid of the two, provided capacity to emergently convert to cardiopulmonary bypass is available. The TAVR team involves a team of specialists, including a structural interventionalist and assistants, cardiac surgeon, vascular surgeon, anesthesiologist, cardiac imager, nurses, and technicians.

The procedure is performed under general endotracheal anesthesia. Support lines and tubes typically include a pulmonary arterial catheter, transvenous pacemaker, arterial line, and urinary catheter, along with peripheral venous access. Arterial access may be completely percutaneous or may require cut-down. BAV may be performed before valve delivery. Rapid ventricular pacing is typically performed at the time of valve expansion to minimize cardiac motion and optimize placement. Echocardiography is used during and after TAVR to assess valve positioning and function.

Hemodynamic Changes

Successful replacement of the aortic valve, whether by TAVR or SAVR, yields an acute increase in aortic valve effective orifice area and acute decrease in the mean and peak transaortic pressure gradient. This causes relief of afterload related to left ventricular outflow obstruction but also broader reduction in global left ventricular hemodynamic load, as reflected in significant reduction in valvuloarterial impedance and end-systolic meridional wall stress.[9] The resultant reduction in myocardial oxygen consumption, combined with increased myocardial blood flow, as a result of reduced coronary microvascular compression and increased diastolic perfusion time, contribute to improved myocardial energetics.[10]

Acutely, this hemodynamic change is usually well tolerated, but can be destabilizing. Left ventricular hypertrophy and diastolic dysfunction resulting from compensation for chronic pressure overload can predispose to development of a dynamic intraventricular pressure gradient when valvular obstruction is abruptly relieved, akin to hypertrophic obstructive cardiomyopathy. Patients with small left ventricular end diastolic diameter, high ejection fraction, high ratio of interventricular

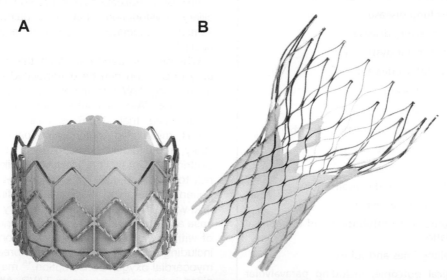

Fig. 1. Transcatheter valves currently in use in the United States. (*A*) Edwards SAPIEN valve (FDA approved). (*B*) Medtronic CoreValve (in phase 3 clinical trials). ([*A*] *Courtesy of* Edwards Lifesciences LLC, Irvine, CA; with permission. [*B*] *Courtesy of* Medtronic, Minneapolis, MN; with permission.)

septum to posterior wall thickness, high valve gradients, and small left ventricular mass are at particular risk.[11] Dubbed "suicide left ventricle,"[12] this phenomenon can lead to hypotension and shock. Endogenous catecholamines and exogenous β-adrenergic agonists exacerbate hypotension by increasing contractility and intraventricular gradients. With volume expansion and temporary use of pure vasopressors, such as phenylephrine or vasopressin, the condition typically resolves over several days.

POSTPROCEDURE COMMUNICATION

Close communication is required between operating and critical care teams (both physicians and nurses) to ensure safe transition of care. Essential elements of handover are listed in **Box 1**. Checklists may be useful to ensure completeness of communication. Whenever possible, ICU staff should meet patients before TAVR to ascertain baseline health status, including neurologic function, and goals of care.

GLOBAL APPROACH TO CRITICAL CARE AFTER TAVR

The role of the intensivist after TAVR is to guide patients through a gauntlet of acute hemodynamic changes and potential complications to optimize

---

Box 1
Key elements of post-TAVR handover

Preprocedure comorbidities

  Prior stroke or neurologic deficits

  Chronic lung disease

  Coronary artery disease

  Left ventricular dysfunction

  Chronic kidney disease

Periprocedural events

  Hypotension

  Arrhythmia and conduction disturbance

  Fluid management

  Bleeding and transfusion

  Vascular access and complications

  Sedation and paralytics

  Difficulties with intubation and mechanical ventilation

  Indwelling lines and tubes

  Technical outcome, including paravalvular regurgitation and requirement for postdilatation

---

the chances for survival and functional recovery. The 3 core elements of post-TAVR critical care are communication, rapid identification and triage of complications, and orderly progression through the ICU.

We advocate a fast-track approach to post-TAVR critical care, paralleling current practice after cardiac surgery (**Fig. 2**). Barring complications, extubation should occur within the first 12 hours after arrival in the ICU, and support lines and tubes should be removed within the first 24 hours. Formal echocardiographic and neurologic assessments are performed 12–24 hours postprocedure. On the second day, diet is advanced and patients are mobilized out of bed and encouraged to ambulate. By the third day, the patient is ready for discharge. To facilitate this, discharge planning should begin by the second ICU day.

MANAGING THE VENTILATOR

We advocate a strategy of early extubation, drawing from trials of fast-track care after cardiac surgery. In a Cochrane systematic review of 25 randomized clinical trials comparing fast-track with conventional care, involving 4118 patients undergoing coronary artery bypass graft surgery (CABG), aortic or mitral valve replacement, early extubation was associated with no significant difference in risks of mortality, myocardial infarction, reintubation or major sepsis, but significant reduction in time to extubation (3.0–10.5 hours vs 3.4–35.1 hours) and ICU length of stay.[13] Additional benefits of early extubation include improved patient comfort, reduced endotracheal tube and ventilator complications (such as vocal fold injury, ciliary dysfunction, cough impairment, and ventilator-associated pneumonia), and reduced costs.[14]

Whether fast-track data from the cardiac surgery population can be extrapolated to patients undergoing TAVR is uncertain, as a fast-track strategy in TAVR has not yet been subjected to a randomized trial. TAVR is less invasive than SAVR, minimizing postoperative pain and tissue injury, and avoiding cardiopulmonary bypass and ventricular dysfunction. However, unlike the low-risk to moderate-risk patients in fast-track trials, patients undergoing TAVR are, by definition, high risk, with a high prevalence of coronary artery disease and chronic lung disease. Deleterious effects of withdrawal of mechanical ventilatory support, including increases in the work of breathing and myocardial oxygen consumption,[15] may be magnified in patients undergoing TAVR. Although we believe early extubation is uniformly desirable, timing of extubation in each case must be

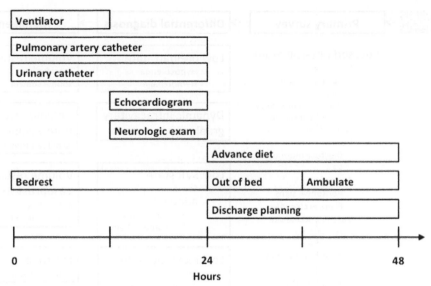

Fig. 2. Post-TAVR care pathway.

individualized. Nurses are integral to this assessment, and protocols for nurse-led early extubation, developed for CABG,[16] may be adaptable to the TAVR setting.

OPTIMIZING NUTRITION

Malnutrition is common among the elderly, and increases in prevalence with increasing frailty and physical dependence.[17] Among adults undergoing cardiac surgery, including aortic valve surgery, surrogate markers for malnutrition, including a low serum albumin level (<2.5 g/dL) and low body mass index (BMI <20 kg/m² or <24 kg/m²), predict postoperative mortality.[18,19] The advanced age, severe AS, multiple comorbidities, and frequent frailty of patients undergoing TAVR suggest that in this highly selected cohort, malnutrition is common. Frailty status, of which malnutrition (measured as serum albumin level) is 1 of 4 components, predicts 1-year mortality after TAVR.[20] It is plausible that malnutrition adversely affects both functional and myocardial recovery after correction of AS.

In the acute care setting, current emphasis is on restarting enteral nutrition as soon as possible after extubation, with a diet tailored to the individual patient. The optimal caloric provision post-TAVR is unknown. Pending further data, a diet containing 120% to 130% of basal energy expenditure (estimated for gender, height, weight, and age), consistent with current practice for patients with congestive heart failure,[21] is reasonable.

Directions for further research include evaluation of the relationship between preprocedure

nutritional status (beyond serum albumin and BMI) and outcomes; description of resting energy expenditure after TAVR using the metabolic cart; and trials of nutritional interventions to improve recovery and functional outcomes after TAVR.

ANTICIPATING, PREVENTING, AND MANAGING COMMON COMPLICATIONS
Hypotension

Hypotension is common after TAVR and mandates rapid evaluation and triage to guide management. A high-quality postprocedure handover prepares the intensivist for differential diagnosis of subsequent hypotension by calling attention to potential mechanisms, such as difficult vascular access (a source of bleeding) or significant paravalvular regurgitation requiring postdilatation (a source of aortic injury). When confronted with acute hypotension in the ICU, our approach, illustrated in **Fig. 3**, begins with a focused physical examination, with particular attention to the vascular examination. If the pulmonary arterial catheter has not yet been removed, its data can be useful to corroborate the findings of the physical examination. Complete blood count and arterial blood gas are essential to identify acute anemia and acidosis. Electrocardiography is used to identify new arrhythmia or signs of myocardial infarction. Echocardiography is useful to reassess valvular and biventricular function, as well as to exclude mechanical complications of TAVR, including tamponade, aortic injury, and ventricular septal defect formation.

As an initial management strategy, fluid resuscitation is appropriate for most cases of acute

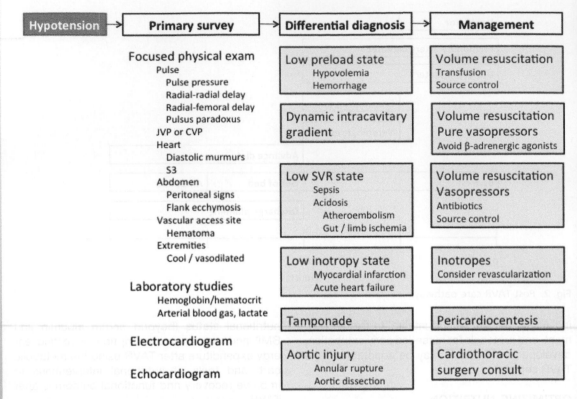

Fig. 3. Approach to hypotension after TAVR.

hypotension after TAVR, coupled with directed management for the source of hypotension (eg, hemostasis for bleeding, revascularization for limb ischemia, antibiotics for infection, pericardiocentesis for tamponade). For patients in whom incipient cardiogenic shock is suspected, as suggested by jugular venous distension, a third heart sound (S3), and cool extremities, invasive hemodynamic monitoring with the pulmonary arterial catheter may be helpful to guide volume management.

Acute Anemia and Vascular Complications

Acute anemia after TAVR represents bleeding until proved otherwise. Bleeding is common; in a series of 943 consecutive patients undergoing TAVR between 2005 and 2011, 20.9% experienced major bleeding and 13.9% had life-threatening bleeding according to Valve Academic Research Consortium (VARC) definitions,[22] of which 23.2% were associated with vascular complications.[23] Furthermore, bleeding is important; requirement for blood transfusion was associated with increased risk of acute kidney injury, major stroke, and mortality at 30 days and 1 year.

We begin our approach to acute anemia with meticulous examination of the vascular access site (**Fig. 4**). Any hematoma should be measured

and marked to facilitate future comparison. If hemostasis cannot be achieved with manual compression, vascular surgical consultation is required. If hematoma is stable or absent, attention should turn to occult sources of bleeding, including the abdomen and retroperitoneum. In this scenario, we advocate early use of abdominal computed tomography, ideally without use of intravenous contrast given proximity to TAVR. Retroperitoneal hemorrhage requires emergent vascular surgery and/or interventional radiology consultation.

With first-generation devices and transfemoral access, major vascular complications have been reported in 5% to 23% of cases.[24] Female gender and small arterial caliber, as demonstrated by preprocedure imaging, confer increased risk. Classification of vascular complications after TAVR is outlined in **Table 2**.

In the absence of vascular complications, blood loss may also occur via the gastrointestinal tract and stool should be examined for frank and occult blood. The combination of acquired deficiency of von Willebrand factor and submucosal angiodysplasias in severe AS, known as Heyde syndrome,[25] may render patients particularly susceptible to gastrointestinal hemorrhage. Rapid improvement in hemostatic abnormalities has been observed in patients after both SAVR and

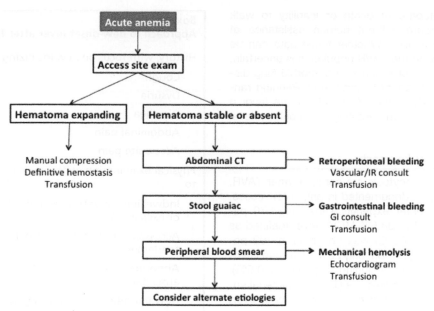

Fig. 4. Approach to acute anemia after TAVR.

BAV,[26,27] and a recent retrospective study suggests that over the long term, TAVR may reduce the risk of recurrent gastrointestinal bleeding.[28] Further research is needed to characterize hemostatic parameters, including von Willebrand factor multimers, after TAVR.

In the absence of evidence of bleeding, alternate causes of anemia should be considered, beginning with examination of the peripheral blood smear. Causes of particular interest for patients undergoing TAVR include disorders of red cell production, including nutritional deficiencies, erythropoietin deficiency (in the setting of comorbid chronic kidney disease), and primary bone marrow disease including myelodysplastic syndromes, as well as disorders of red cell destruction, including mechanical hemolysis (with either native valvular stenosis or prosthetic paravalvular regurgitation). Baseline anemia is common, present in more than 50% of patients before TAVR.

Optimal targets for red blood cell transfusion after TAVR have not been defined. In a recent randomized comparison of liberal versus restrictive transfusion strategies (with hemoglobin cutoffs of 10 g/dL and 8 g/dL, respectively) in elderly patients at high cardiovascular risk undergoing orthopedic surgery, there was no difference in the

Table 2
Vascular complications after TAVR

	Major	Minor
Aortic	Any thoracic aortic dissection	—
Access site or access-related vascular injury[a]	Death	—
	Transfusion >4 units	Transfusion ≥2 but <4 units
	Need for unplanned percutaneous or surgical intervention	Need for compression or thrombin injection therapy
	Irreversible end-organ damage	—
Embolic (noncerebral)	Requiring surgery	Treated by embolectomy/ thrombectomy
	Amputation	—
	Irreversible end-organ damage	—
Other	Left ventricular perforation	—

[a] Examples of vascular injury: dissection, stenosis, perforation, rupture, arteriovenous fistula, pseudoaneurysm, hematoma (including retroperitoneal hemorrhage), irreversible nerve injury, compartment syndrome, failure of percutaneous access site closure device.

primary outcome of death or inability to walk across a room without human assistance at 60-day follow-up.[29] Whether these data can be extrapolated to the TAVR population is uncertain, noting the high prevalence of comorbid lung disease and pulmonary hypertension. Pending randomized study in the TAVR setting, we favor a restrictive approach, targeting a hemoglobin level of 8 g/dL.

Fever and Leukocytosis

Fever and leukocytosis are common after TAVR, but infection is documented in only a few cases. In a single-center experience involving 270 patients (61.6% ES, 38.5% MCV), fever (defined as temperature >37.5°C) was observed in 102 patients (37.8%), of whom only 28 (27.4%) had infections documented, including respiratory (50.5%), urinary (25.0%), access site (14.0%), bacterial endocarditis (3.5%), and bacteremia without overt focus (11.0%).[30]

This infective or inflammatory response is clinically important, with approximately one-third of mortality in the period between 48 hours and 30 days post-TAVR attributed to infection or sepsis in observational series.[31] Why it occurs and how to prevent it are uncertain, and the subject of controversy.[32] Further research is needed to clarify optimal management, including the role of empirical antibiotics. Our approach to evaluation is outlined in **Box 2**.

Stroke and New-Onset Atrial Fibrillation

Stroke, as defined by VARC,[22] occurs in approximately 9% of patients after TAVR, of which 5% are major, 2% are minor, and 3% are transient ischemic attacks.[33] Subclinical cerebral infarction is far more common, evident in most patients on post-TAVR magnetic resonance imaging.[34] In PARTNER, stroke was more common with TAVR than with SAVR.[3]

Intraprocedurally, based on study with transcranial Doppler ultrasonography during transapical TAVR, most strokes occur during BAV, catheter manipulation across the stenotic valve, and valve implantation.[35] This finding is consistent with a hypothesis that most strokes result from embolization of atherosclerotic debris from the aorta and aortic valve.[36] Thrombosis and thromboembolism at the time of valve manipulation may also contribute, noting recent data identifying tissue factor,[37] fibrin, and in vivo fibrin clot formation[38] in stenotic aortic valves. Strategies under investigation to reduce intraprocedural stroke risk include different modalities of anticoagulation, minimization of catheter exchanges and valve

---

Box 2
Approach to new-onset fever after TAVR

History, with focus on new localizing symptoms

    Cough

    Dysuria

    Diarrhea

    Abdominal pain

    Access site pain

Physical examination, with particular attention to

    Indwelling support lines and tubes (remove or exchange)

    Access site erythema, warmth, induration, or tenderness

    Abnormalities of pulmonary percussion and auscultation

    New murmurs of valvular regurgitation

    Abdominal or suprapubic tenderness

    Signs of atheroembolism

Laboratory investigation, with a preliminary survey including

    Blood cultures

    Urinalysis and culture

    Chest radiograph

---

manipulation (such as by foregoing preparatory BAV before prosthesis implantation),[39] and use of embolic protection devices.[40]

The observation that symptom onset is often delayed more than 24 hours after TAVR, rather than immediately, has heightened interest in the mechanisms and modifiable risk factors for postprocedure stroke.[33] Two potential mechanisms include late embolization of valvular or prosthetic debris and thromboembolism related to valvular injury or atrial fibrillation. Current practice favors an antithrombotic strategy of aspirin (indefinitely) plus clopidogrel (to be continued for 1–6 months), but this approach is incompletely tested, and the primacy of antiplatelet versus anticoagulant therapy is subject to controversy.[41]

Choice of antithrombotic therapy is complicated by atrial fibrillation, which is prevalent at baseline and often new onset in the post-TAVR setting. In a series of 138 patients with no known previous atrial fibrillation, new-onset atrial fibrillation (defined as any episode lasting >30 seconds on electrocardiographic monitoring) was observed in 32% of cases.[42] Predictors included left atrial enlargement and transapical access. The mean

CHADS2 score was 3. As is the case outside the TAVR setting, new-onset atrial fibrillation was an important predictor of stroke and systemic embolism (13.6% vs 3.2% at 1 month, $P = .047$ after adjustment), particularly among those not treated immediately with anticoagulant therapy (40% vs 2.9%, $P = .008$). Although these data would seem to favor timely initiation of anticoagulation for new-onset atrial fibrillation, the addition of anticoagulation to dual antiplatelet therapy (so-called triple therapy) is perilous, associated according to recent data with increased risk of bleeding in patients requiring anticoagulation after coronary stenting,[43] and increased risk of death, stroke, embolism, or major bleeding after TAVR in patients in a German registry.[44]

Pending additional trial data, we currently favor the following strategy for antithrombotic therapy after TAVR. For patients with no indication for oral anticoagulation, we prescribe aspirin 81 mg daily indefinitely and clopidogrel 75 mg daily for 1 month, to be continued for up to 6 months in the absence of major bleeding. For patients with baseline or new-onset atrial fibrillation and no indication for dual antiplatelet therapy, we prescribe aspirin 81 mg daily indefinitely and warfarin, titrated to achieve an international normalized ratio of 2.0 to 3.0. For patients with indications for both dual antiplatelet therapy (eg, recent intracoronary stent placement) and anticoagulation, we prescribe clopidogrel 75 mg daily and warfarin. Additional data are needed to help understand the comparative safety and efficacy of dual antiplatelet therapy versus aspirin monotherapy; antiplatelet therapy versus anticoagulant therapy; novel oral anticoagulants; novel antiplatelets; and left atrial appendage exclusion devices in patients after TAVR.

Conduction Disturbances

Expansion of the new valve in the left ventricular outflow tract, adjacent to the left bundle branch, confers a high risk of left bundle branch block (48% and 21% at 1 month) and permanent pacemaker requirement (18% and 4% at 1 month) with MCV and ES, respectively.[45,46] New conduction defects may not be immediately evident, but may emerge in the initial 24 to 48 hours after TAVR. For patients with risk factors for high-grade atrioventricular block, such as MCV implantation or preexisting right bundle branch block, continuous electrocardiographic monitoring is advised for 72 hours after TAVR,[7] and preemptive permanent pacemaker placement may be considered before TAVR. For patients with new conduction defects immediately after TAVR, the appropriate duration of observation with a temporary venous pacemaker is uncertain before implantation of a permanent device. Better prediction tools are needed to discriminate patients who will recover native conduction. Next-generation models with decreased protrusion into the left ventricular outflow tract are designed to reduce the risk of new conduction defects.

Acute Kidney Injury

Acute kidney injury (AKI) is observed in 7% to 12% of patients after TAVR, with reported risk factors including transfusion, hypertension, chronic lung disease, chronic kidney disease, and higher euroSCORE (European System for Cardiac Operative Risk Evaluation).[7] Key potential mechanisms, which may overlap, include prerenal azotemia and ischemic acute tubular necrosis, as may be seen secondary to intraprocedural hypotension or post-TAVR hypovolemia; atheroembolism; contrast-induced nephropathy; allergic interstitial nephritis; and urinary obstruction. When AKI occurs after TAVR, it is associated with increased length of stay, cost, and mortality.[47,48] Although this risk of adverse events likely reflects, in part, covariance of kidney disease with other risk factors for poor outcomes, including microvascular disease, malnutrition, and frailty, AKI can contribute directly to mortality, accounting for 12.5% of non–cardiac-related deaths after TAVR.[49] The cardiovascular intensivist plays a key role in the prevention, identification, and management of AKI after TAVR.

An optimal strategy for prevention of AKI has not been defined specifically for TAVR, but drawing on experience from percutaneous coronary intervention, we favor a strategy of careful periprocedural hydration, minimization of intravenous contrast, and consideration of N-acetylcysteine administration for patients deemed to be at high risk, in particular those with chronic kidney disease.[50]

Surveillance in the ICU setting is facilitated by continuous urine output measurement for the first 24 hours by urinary catheter and daily measurement of blood urea nitrogen, serum creatinine, and electrolytes. The VARC provides a 3-stage classification system for reporting of AKI after TAVR in clinical trials, based on a modification of the RIFLE (Risk, Injury, Failure, Loss, End-stage) classification system.[22] We advocate aggressive investigation for modifiable sources of AKI when serum creatinine increases by more than 50% or 0.3 g/dL greater than baseline or when urine output decreases to less than 0.5 mL/kg/h for 6 hours or more. Basic evaluation should include exclusion of urinary obstruction (via urinary catheter or renal ultrasonography), urine analysis and examination of the urine sediment, and identification and correction of states contributing to renal hypoperfusion and ischemia. Offending nephrotoxins should be withheld. Care is supportive. When AKI leads to severe acidemia or hyperkalemia, hypervolemia, or uremia refractory to medical therapy, suitable vascular access may be required to initiate temporary dialysis.

SUMMARY

TAVR offers a pathway to functional recovery for patients with symptomatic severe AS whose age and comorbidities put safe SAVR out of reach. This pathway begins in the cardiovascular ICU. Next-generation devices, interventional techniques, and pharmacologic strategies under investigation offer promise to improve outcomes and reduce complications after TAVR, including stroke, bleeding, and vascular injury. Additional key advances will come in the arena of post-TAVR critical care. As a model of acute care for patients with a primary cardiac problem and a background of advanced age and multiple comorbidities, post-TAVR critical care will further provide a training ground for the future of cardiovascular intensive care.

REFERENCES

1. Kodali SK, Williams MR, Smith CR, et al. Two-year outcomes after transcatheter or surgical aortic valve replacement. N Engl J Med 2012;366:1686–95.
2. Leon MB, Smith CR, Mack M, et al. Transcatheter aortic-valve implantation for aortic stenosis in patients who cannot undergo surgery. N Engl J Med 2010;363(17):1597–607.
3. Smith CR, Leon MB, Mack MJ, et al. Transcatheter versus surgical aortic-valve replacement in high-risk patients. N Engl J Med 2011;364(23):2187–98.
4. van Mieghem NM, Head SJ, van der Boon RM, et al. The SURTAVI model: proposal for a pragmatic risk stratification for patients with severe aortic stenosis. EuroIntervention 2012;8(2):258–66.
5. Gilard M, Eltchaninoff H, Iung B, et al. Registry of transcatheter aortic-valve implantation in high-risk patients. N Engl J Med 2012;366(18):1705–18.
6. Webb JG, Wood DA. Current status of transcatheter aortic valve replacement. J Am Coll Cardiol 2012;60(6):483–92.
7. Généreux P, Head SJ, Wood DA, et al. Transcatheter aortic valve implantation 10-year anniversary: review of current evidence and clinical implications. Eur Heart J 2012;33:2388–98.
8. Saia F, Marrozzini C, Moretti C, et al. The role of percutaneous balloon aortic valvuloplasty as a bridge for transcatheter aortic valve implantation. EuroIntervention 2011;7(6):723–9.
9. Giannini C, Petronio AS, De Carlo M, et al. The incremental value of valvuloarterial impedance in evaluating the results of transcatheter aortic valve implantation in symptomatic aortic stenosis. J Am Soc Echocardiogr 2012;25:444–53.
10. Rajappan K, Rimoldi OE, Camici PG, et al. Functional changes in coronary microcirculation after valve replacement in patients with aortic stenosis. Circulation 2003;107:3170–5.
11. López Ayerbe J, Evangelista Masip A, Armada Romero E, et al. Predictive factors of abnormal dynamic intraventricular gradient after valve replacement in severe aortic stenosis. Rev Esp Cardiol 2002;55:127–34.
12. Suh WM, Witzke CF, Palacios IF. Suicide left ventricle following transcatheter aortic valve implantation. Catheter Cardiovasc Interv 2010;76:616–20.
13. Zhu F, Lee A, Chee YE. Fast-track cardiac care for adult cardiac surgical patients. Cochrane Database Syst Rev 2012;(10):CD003587.
14. Higgins TL. Pro: early endotracheal extubation is preferable to late extubation in patients following coronary artery surgery. J Cardiothorac Vasc Anesth 1992;6:488–93.
15. Siliciano D. Con: early extubation is not preferable to late extubation in patients undergoing coronary artery surgery. J Cardiothorac Vasc Anesth 1992; 6:494–8.
16. Hawkes C, Foxcroft DR, Yerrell P. Clinical guideline for nurse-led early extubation after coronary artery bypass: an evaluation. J Adv Nurs 2010; 66:2038–49.
17. Visvanathan R, Newbury JW, Chapman I. Malnutrition in older people: screening and management strategies. Aust Fam Physician 2004;33(10):799–805.
18. Engelman DT, Adams DH, Byrne JG, et al. Impact of body mass index and albumin on morbidity and mortality after cardiac surgery. J Thorac Cardiovasc Surg 1999;118:866–73.
19. Thourani VH, Keeling WB, Kligo PD, et al. The impact of body mass index on morbidity and short- and long-term mortality in cardiac valvular surgery. J Thorac Cardiovasc Surg 2011;142(5):1052–61.
20. Green P, Woglom AE, Genereux P, et al. The impact of frailty status on survival after transcatheter aortic valve replacement in older adults with severe aortic stenosis. JACC Cardiovasc Interv 2012;5(9):974–81.
21. Hummell AC. Nutrition for the critically ill cardiac and thoracic patient. In: Cresci G, editor. Nutrition

support for the critically ill patient: a guide to practice. Boca Raton (FL): CRC Press; 2005. p. 519–27.

22. Leon MB, Piazza N, Nikolsky E, et al. Standardized endpoint definitions for transcatheter aortic valve implantation clinical trials: a consensus report from the Valve Academic Research Consortium. J Am Coll Cardiol 2011;57:253–69.

23. Tchetche D, van der Boon RM, Dumontell N, et al. Adverse impact of bleeding and transfusion on the outcome post-transcatheter aortic valve implantation. Am Heart J 2012;164(3):402–9.

24. Genereux P, Head SJ, Van Mieghem NM, et al. Clinical outcomes after transcatheter aortic valve replacement using valve academic research consortium definitions: a weighted meta-analysis of 3,519 patients from 19 studies. J Am Coll Cardiol 2012;59:2317–26.

25. Loscalzo J. From clinical observation to mechanism—Heyde's syndrome. N Engl J Med 2012; 367:1954–6.

26. Vincentelli A, Sesen S, Le Tourneau T, et al. Acquired von Willebrand syndrome in aortic stenosis. N Engl J Med 2003;349:343–9.

27. Bander J, Elmariah S, Aledort LM, et al. Changes in von Willebrand factor-cleaving protease (ADAMTS-13) in patients with aortic stenosis undergoing valve replacement or balloon valvuloplasty. Thromb Haemost 2012;108(1):86–93.

28. Godino C, Lauretta L, Pavon AG, et al. Heyde's syndrome incidence and outcome in patients undergoing transcatheter aortic valve implantation. J Am Coll Cardiol 2013;61(6):687–9.

29. Carson JL, Terrin ML, Noveck H, et al. Liberal or restrictive transfusion in high-risk patients after hip surgery. N Engl J Med 2011;365(26):2453–62.

30. Franzoni I, Latib A, Chieffo A, et al. Fever after TAVI: infection or inflammation? EuroIntervention 2012; 8(Suppl N):351.

31. Van Mieghem NM, van der Boon RM, Nuis RJ, et al. Cause of death after transcatheter aortic valve implantation. Catheter Cardiovasc Interv 2012. http:// dx.doi.org/10.1002/ccd.24597.

32. Onsea K, Agostoni P, Voskuil M, et al. Infective complications after transcatheter aortic valve implantation: results from a single centre. Neth Heart J 2012;20(9):360–4.

33. Nuis RJ, Van Mieghem NM, Schultz CJ, et al. Frequency and causes of stroke during or after transcatheter aortic valve implantation. Am J Cardiol 2012;109(1):1637–43.

34. Ghanem A, Müller A, Nähle CP, et al. Risk and fate of cerebral embolism after transfemoral aortic valve implantation: a prospective pilot study with diffusion-weighted magnetic resonance imaging. J Am Coll Cardiol 2010;55(14):1427–32.

35. Drews T, Pasic M, Buz S, et al. Trancranial Doppler sound detection of cerebral microembolism during

transapical aortic valve implantation. Thorac Cardiovasc Surg 2011;59:237–42.

36. Daneault B, Kirtane AJ, Kodali SK, et al. Stroke associated with surgical or transcatheter treatment of aortic stenosis. J Am Coll Cardiol 2011;58: 2143–50.

37. Natorska J, Marek G, Hlawaty M, et al. Evidence for tissue factor expression in aortic valves in patients with aortic stenosis. Pol Arch Med Wewn 2009; 119(10):636–43.

38. Natorska J, Marek G, Hlawaty M, et al. Fibrin presence within aortic valves in patients with aortic stenosis: association with in vivo thrombin generation and fibrin clot properties. Thromb Haemost 2011; 105(2):254–60.

39. Grube E, Naber C, Abizaid A, et al. Feasibility of transcatheter aortic valve implantation without balloon pre-dilation: a pilot study. JACC Cardiovasc Interv 2011;4(7):751–7.

40. Nietlispach F, Wijesinghe N, Gurvitch R, et al. An embolic deflection device for aortic valve interventions. JACC Cardiovasc Interv 2010;3:1133–8.

41. Rodés-Cabau J, Dauerman HL, Cohen MG, et al. Antithrombotic treatment in transcatheter aortic valve implantation: insights for cerebrovascular and bleeding events. J Am Coll Cardiol 2013. http://dx.doi.org/10.1016/j.jacc.2013.03.029.

42. Amat-Santos IJ, Rodés-Cabau J, Urena M, et al. Incidence, predictive factors, and prognostic value of new-onset atrial fibrillation following transcatheter aortic valve implantation. J Am Coll Cardiol 2012;59(2):178–88.

43. Dewilde WJ, Oirbans T, Verheught FW, et al. Use of clopidogrel with or without aspirin in patients taking oral anticoagulant therapy and undergoing percutaneous coronary intervention: an open-label, randomized, control trial. Lancet 2013;381(9872): 1107–15.

44. Zeymer U, Zahn R, Gerckens U, et al. Antithrombotic therapy after transfemoral aortic valve implantation (TAVI). Potential hazard of triple-therapy [abstract]. Eur Heart J 2011;32(Suppl):900.

45. Piazza N, Onuma Y, Jesserun E, et al. Early and persistent intraventricular conduction abnormalities and requirements for pacemaking after percutaneous replacement of the aortic valve. JACC Cardiovasc Interv 2008;1(3):310–6.

46. Godin M, Eltchaninoff H, Furuta A, et al. Frequency of conduction disturbances after transcatheter implantation of an Edwards Sapien aortic valve prosthesis. Am J Cardiol 2010;106(5):707–12.

47. Kong WY, Yong G, Irish A. Incidence, risk factors and prognosis of acute kidney injury after transcatheter aortic valve implantation. Nephrology (Carlton) 2012;17(5):445–51.

48. Barbash IM, Ben-Dor I, Dvir D, et al. Incidence and predictors of acute kidney injury after transcatheter

aortic valve replacement. Am Heart J 2012;163(6): 1031–6.

49. Wendler O, MacCarthy P. Renal failure after tavi— do we know the full story? J Am Coll Cardiol 2013. http://dx.doi.org/10.1016/j.jacc.2013.04.058.

50. Scheiger MJ, Chambers CE, Davidson CJ, et al. Prevention of contrast induced nephropathy: recommendations for the high risk patient undergoing cardiovascular procedures. Catheter Cardiovasc Interv 2007;69(1):135–40.

Ventilator Management in the Cardiac Intensive Care Unit

Carlos Corredor, MRCP, FRCA,
Sian I. Jaggar, CertMedEd, MD, FRCA*

KEYWORDS

- Mechanical ventilation • Cardiac intensive care unit (CICU) • Cardiopulmonary interactions
- Noninvasive ventilation • Gas exchange • PEEP (positive end expiratory pressure)
- Cardiac dysfunction • Weaning

KEY POINTS

- The number of patients on mechanical ventilation has increased in the modern CICU as a result of increasing complexity and comorbidities in these patients, and a thorough understanding of ventilator management is essential for the practicing cardiac intensivist.
- The heart, lungs, and great blood vessels are contained within the thoracic cavity. Changes in intrathoracic pressure caused by different ventilatory modes (spontaneous or mechanical) have different effects on the determinants of cardiac output and overall cardiac performance.
- Positive end expiratory pressure and continuous positive airway pressure (CPAP) have beneficial effects in terms of the reduction of afterload, myocardial work, and oxygen consumption. Noninvasive mechanical ventilation is an effective and safe option for the management of cardiogenic pulmonary edema.
- The discontinuation of mechanical ventilation may reverse the beneficial effects of positive pressure ventilation in the failing heart. The identification and risk stratification of patients likely to fail weaning is crucial to ensure that interventions can be put in place preemptively.

INTRODUCTION

The role of the cardiac intensive care unit (CICU) has evolved markedly from a purely observational unit dedicated to the monitoring and prompt resuscitation of patients with myocardial infarction to a unit treating an increasingly aging population with complex cardiac conditions and concomitant noncardiac comorbidities.[1]

Patients admitted to the CICU present with a variety of conditions, including complicated myocardial infarction, acute heart failure, refractory arrhythmias, and complications of adult congenital heart disease. Advances in early coronary intervention are reflected in decreasing rates of patients admitted with ST elevation myocardial infarction to the CICU. However, there is an increase in the prevalence of noncardiac critical illness, such as respiratory failure, sepsis, and acute kidney injury.[2]

This new paradigm has led to an increase in the number of patients requiring mechanical ventilation (MV) and with a longer duration of this therapy during their CICU stays. The observational study by Katz and colleagues[1] looked at the characteristics of health care delivery in a coronary care unit at Duke University Hospital. It demonstrated a significant increase in the prevalence of patients requiring prolonged MV (>96 hours) in the 1989–2006 period.

Disclosures: The author has nothing to disclose.
Anaesthesia and Critical Care Department, Royal Brompton Hospital, Sydney Street, London SW3 6NP, UK
* Corresponding author.
E-mail address: s.jaggar@rbht.nhs.uk

Cardiol Clin 31 (2013) 619–636
http://dx.doi.org/10.1016/j.ccl.2013.07.002
0733-8651/13/$ – see front matter © 2013 Elsevier Inc. All rights reserved.

cardiology.theclinics.com

PHYSIOLOGIC BASIS

A review of the physiology of breathing in health, along with cardiopulmonary interactions, is necessary to understand the effects of MV in patients with cardiovascular disease.

Gas exchange takes place between gas in the alveolus and blood. Carbon dioxide diffuses from the blood across the alveolar-capillary membrane and is exhaled; simultaneously, oxygen diffuses down a pressure gradient from the alveolus into the capillary blood. The volume of inhaled gas that participates in gas exchange is termed *alveolar ventilation*. Dead-space ventilation (V_D) is the fraction of inhaled gas that does not participate in gas exchange and together with alveolar ventilation (V_A) makes up total ventilation (V_T): $V_T = V_A + V_D$.

Tidal volume is the volume of gas that is inspired and expired during each breath; it is approximately 7 mL/kg in an adult. The volume of gas that remains in the lungs at the end of a normal expiration is the functional residual capacity (FRC). At FRC, the tendency of the lung tissue to collapse is counterbalanced by the tendency for the chest wall to expand (**Fig. 1**).

In addition, FRC has several important functions; it is a major oxygen store in the body and, thus, maintains a steady arterial P_{O2} buffering the effects of an intermittent tidal delivery of oxygen with each breath. FRC prevents atelectasis by maintaining the lung in a state of partial inflation and by placing the respiratory system in the steep part of its compliance curve, minimizing the work of breathing.

FRC is determined by the compliance of the lung and chest wall. An example commonly encountered in the CICU is in patients with left ventricular failure and pulmonary edema. Alveoli flooded with fluid have diminished compliance and, therefore, reduced FRC. Pulmonary vascular resistance (PVR) is lowest at FRC and increases at both low or large lung volumes.[3]

EFFECT OF SPONTANEOUS BREATHING IN THE CARDIOVASCULAR SYSTEM

The heart, lungs, and great vessels are normally contained within a closed thoracic cavity and interact during each respiratory cycle. The right and left ventricles are connected in series through the pulmonary circulation and, like the great veins and thoracic aorta, are subjected to changes in the intrathoracic pressure. Dynamic mechanical properties of the lung and chest wall, such as compliance and elastance, can, therefore, have an effect on cardiac function.

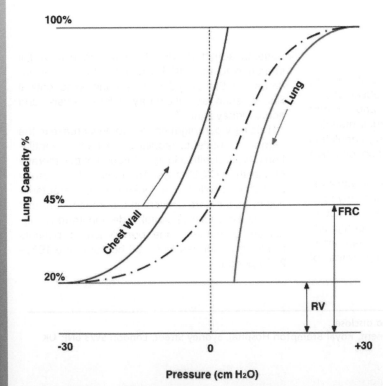

Fig. 1. Lung and chest wall pressure-volume curve. Continuous-line curves are pressure-volume diagrams for lung and chest wall. Dotted-line curve represents pressure-volume curve of the total respiratory system. At FRC, combined pressure of the total system is 0. RV, right ventricular.

Inspiration occurs when inspiratory muscles generate a negative intrapleural pressure creating a pressure gradient, down which gas enters the lung from the atmosphere. The drop in intrapleural pressure expands the lungs but also affects the heart and intrathoracic blood vessels. The muscular cardiac wall is normally subjected to extramural forces (eg, intrathoracic pressure) in addition to intramural stress produced by the pressure inside the cardiac chambers. Transmural pressure equals the intrachamber pressure minus the extramural pressure. Inspiration produces a decrease in the extramural stress applied to the cardiac chambers and, thus, an increase in the transmural pressure. Inspiration increases diastolic filling of the right atrium as a consequence of the favorable pressure gradient created by the difference between the right atrial pressure and the intrathoracic pressure. The increased venous return is reflected in a higher right ventricular end-diastolic volume (RVEDV) (preload) and RV stroke volume. Conversely, during spontaneous inspiration, the left ventricle (LV) experiences a decrease in stroke volume caused by increased afterload. The afterload rises because as intrathoracic pressure decreases the extramural pressure of the LV also decreases and, as explained earlier, results in an increased transmural pressure for the LV. The LV must now generate a higher wall tension (afterload) against the increased transmural pressure.[4,5]

The right and left ventricles share a common septum and circumferential fibers. This anatomic and mechanical relationship makes the ventricles interdependent. Therefore, changes in end diastolic pressure of the RV will have an effect on the LV. The increased venous return and RV volume with inspiration produce a transient shift of the intraventricular septum toward the LV, decreasing LV end diastolic volume. The leftward shift can be particularly pronounced if the PVR is high, with concomitant increase in RV volume.[6] During normal spontaneous breathing, the septum shift is only transient and there is little evidence that this effect is clinically significant.[4,7] The effect of ventricular interdependence can, however, be pronounced in conditions when pleural pressure becomes extremely negative and lungs are overinflated, such as acute severe asthma or in cases of cardiac tamponade. This exaggerated effect of interdependence explains the pulsus paradoxus phenomenon.[8]

The net effect of inspiration is a small decrease in systolic blood pressure explained by the increased afterload of the LV and consequent decreased stroke volume. The decrease in systolic blood pressure is minimized by the increase in RV filling. Systolic blood pressure increases during expiration as the LV afterload returns to baseline and the inspiratory increased venous return reaches it.[4]

During spontaneous ventilation, normally the respiratory apparatus requires less than 5% of the total oxygen delivery (DO_2). However, the metabolic demand for oxygen can reach up to 25% of the total DO_2 in situations of respiratory distress because of the large O_2 requirements of respiratory muscles.[9] Patients with coronary heart disease and limited reserve can, therefore, experience myocardial ischemia with the increase in afterload and myocardial oxygen consumption that occurs with large decreases in intrathoracic pressure during strenuous spontaneous ventilation.[10]

EFFECTS OF INTERMITTENT POSITIVE PRESSURE VENTILATION ON THE CARDIOVASCULAR SYSTEM

The hemodynamic effects of MV can be continuous or occur cyclically during the respiratory cycle. The hemodynamic effects will be affected by the ventilation mode, the presence of spontaneous respiratory effort, and the addition of positive end expiratory pressure (PEEP).

During intermittent positive pressure ventilation (IPPV), the positive pressure delivered to the airway during inspiration is transmitted to the intrapleural space and intrathoracic structures causing different hemodynamic effects. The main mechanisms behind these effects are the following (Fig. 2)[11]:

- Reduced RV preload
- Increased RV afterload
- The effects of ventricular interdependence on LV preload
- Reduced LV afterload

The entirety of cardiac output returning to the right side of the heart depends on a very small pressure gradient. Guyton's circulatory model states that venous return results from the interaction of the main systemic filling pressure, which is the degree of filling of the systemic circulation, the right atrial pressure, and the resistance to venous return.[12]

Initiation of positive pressure ventilation and the associated positive intrathoracic pressure alters both right atrial pressure and the mean circulatory systemic pressure. The venous return decreases, producing a reduction in RVEDV and stroke volume.[13] The decrease in blood flow also reaches the LV after 3 to 4 beats, causing a reduction in LVEDV. RV afterload increases because of the

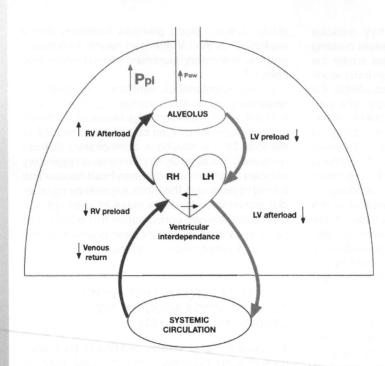

Fig. 2. The hemodynamic effects of positive pressure ventilation. Left side of the heart (LH), airway pressure (Paw), pleural pressure (Ppl), right side of the heart (RH).

effect of positive pressure in the pulmonary vasculature.[14]

Ventricular interdependence is evident when decreased RVEDV, in the presence of an increased transseptal pressure gradient, causes the septum to shift right, resulting in an increased LVEDV and LV stroke volume. The opposite is observed during expiration. Venous inflow transiently increases to the RV as positive pressure on the vessels is released, increasing both RVEDV and stroke volume. The septum shifts left, and there is a reduction in LVEDV and LV stroke volume.[15]

Positive intrapleural pressure decreases LV afterload because of a reduction in LV transmural pressure. Under these conditions, the LV needs to generate less wall tension to eject blood.[16] The reduction in afterload has potential benefits in the presence of left-sided heart failure because it facilitates ventricular emptying and is reflected in reduced myocardial work and oxygen consumption.[17]

The net resulting effect of the aforementioned mechanisms on cardiac output depends on intravascular volume status and myocardial contractility. Failing ventricles, for example, are very sensitive to changes in afterload.[17] Reduction of venous return, and the subsequent reduction in stroke volume and cardiac output that occur during the respiratory cycle, is the predominant mechanism. MV invariably causes a decrease in cardiac output in patients with hypovolemia, and a low-volume status exaggerates the cyclical changes

in venous return and stroke volume. These cyclical changes in stroke volume and in surrogates, such as stroke volume variation or pulse pressure variation, form the bases of functional hemodynamic monitoring as a tool for assessing fluid responsiveness in mechanically ventilated patients.[18]

EFFECT OF PEEP ON THE CARDIOVASCULAR SYSTEM

Maintaining positive airway pressure at the end of expiration can be achieved by the application of positive end expiratory pressure (PEEP) or continuous positive airway pressure (CPAP). The physiological principles behind these two terms are identical. Convention dictates that the term PEEP is used when positive pressure at the end of expiration is applied during a mechanical ventilation breath and CPAP during spontaneous breathing (**Fig. 3**). PEEP is commonly applied as part of a lung protective ventilation strategy. It promotes alveolar recruitment, prevents damage resulting from the cyclical opening and closing of alveolar units (atelectrauma), and improves oxygenation.

The addition of PEEP leads to a continuous increase in airway and intrapleural pressures. Compliance of the lung and chest wall determines the amount of PEEP that is transmitted from the airway to the intrapleural space.[19]

The effects of PEEP are similar to those of positive pressure ventilation, differing only in that they are continuous and not cyclical. The predominant

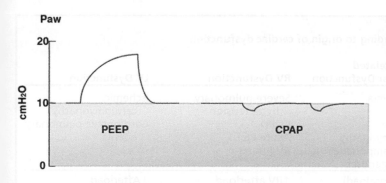

Fig. 3. Airway pressure is maintained at end expiration (shaded area). PEEP (mechanical ventilation) and CPAP (spontaneous breathing)> Paw Airway pressure.

effect of PEEP is that of a reduction in venous return caused by an increase in the resistance to venous return.[20] The reduction in RV venous return, RVEDV, and stroke volume is reflected in a secondary reduction in LV preload.

PEEP and continuous positive airway pressure (CPAP) reduce the afterload of the LV by producing a continuous increase in extramural pressure and, thus, a reduction of the transmural pressure of the LV during the whole respiratory cycle. The reduction in afterload is beneficial in terms of reduction of LV work and oxygen consumption in patients with congestive cardiac failure.[8,21] Indeed, CPAP alone has been demonstrated to achieve respiratory muscle unloading and reduction in afterload without impairing overall cardiac performance and cardiac index (CI).[22]

Noninvasive ventilation is associated with positive physiologic effects in spontaneously breathing patients with congestive heart failure. The reduced LV afterload associated with positive intrapleural pressure produced by CPAP improves CI and systemic oxygen delivery.[23]

Controversy remains surrounding the possible relationship between PEEP and myocardial perfusion and ischemia. Although there is evidence that even clinical levels of PEEP can decrease myocardial blood flow, the overall effect in myocardial oxygen supply is difficult to predict because of the positive effects of PEEP in terms of reduced LV afterload and, thus, oxygen demand.[8]

TYPE OF CARDIAC DYSFUNCTION AND EFFECT OF POSITIVE PRESSURE VENTILATION

As discussed earlier, positive pressure ventilation affects a variety of parameters of cardiac performance variably and can, therefore, have both positive and negative impacts on cardiac function. When IPPV is required, yet likely to induce negative cardiovascular effects, measures should be instituted to minimize these effects (**Table 1**).

INDICATIONS FOR MV IN THE CICU

A primary purpose of mechanical respiratory support is to promote alveolar ventilation and, therefore, carbon dioxide (CO_2) elimination. Additionally, it is also used to correct impaired oxygenation (**Box 1**).

The interface used between the MV device and patients creates an artificial classification. When tracheal intubation is required, the term *invasive ventilation* is used; ventilation is termed *noninvasive ventilation* (NIV) when delivered via a tight-fitting face mask or hood. The boundary between the two terms is blurred in the modern CICU, and they are both now used in a continuum of respiratory support.

There is no single value of arterial P_{CO_2}, P_{O_2}, pH, or oxygen saturation that can predict the need for invasive ventilation.[24] Apnea, severely depressed consciousness level, respiratory arrest, and severe cardiogenic shock are compelling indications for endotracheal intubation and, therefore, invasive MV. However, in other situations, the clinical assessment of underlying disease process and of the overall condition of patients will dictate the most appropriate type of respiratory support.

Esteban and colleagues[25,26] carried out the largest prospective cohort study to date studying the characteristics and outcomes of patients receiving MV in ICUs worldwide. This study demonstrated that acute respiratory failure was by far the most common indication for initiation of MV, accounting for 68.8% of cases studied. Congestive heart failure was the third most common cause of acute respiratory failure (12% of the cases) behind pneumonia (16%) and postoperative respiratory failure (15%).

Congestive cardiac failure can arise from conditions affecting the myocardium, valvular disease, or rhythm disturbances. Regardless of the cause, pulmonary edema is the common denominator that arises from increased left atrial pressure and imbalance in the Starling forces across the

Table 1
Cardiovascular effect of MV according to origin of cardiac dysfunction

	Preload-Related Ventricular Dysfunction	RV Dysfunction	LV Dysfunction
Examples	Hypovolemia Ischemia Restrictive cardiomyopathy Cardiac tamponade Valvular stenoses	Severe pulmonary hypertension COPD Acute PE RV Infarct	Ischemic cardiomyopathy Cardiogenic pulmonary edema
Effect of mandatory ventilation on cardiac function	↓LVEDV (preload) ↓Cardiac output	↑RV afterload ↑RV O$_2$ demand	↓Afterload ↓Myocardial O$_2$ demand ↑Cardiac output
Measures to prevent adverse cardiovascular effects	Fluid loading Minimize airway pressure	Treat hypoxia and acidosis Ensure adequate coronary perfusion Ensure adequate intravascular volume	PEEP/CPAP beneficial

Abbreviations: COPD, chronic obstructive airway diseases; PE, pulmonary embolism.

alveolar-capillary interface (**Fig. 4**). Lung compliance decreases as a result of fluid flooding the alveoli and interstitium, and the additional fluid in the capillary membrane creates a barrier for gas exchange.[27] The resulting ventilation/perfusion mismatch causes hypoxia; the development of stiff, noncompliant lungs leads to an increased work of breathing, ventilatory failure, and CO$_2$ retention. Severe cardiogenic shock or cardiac arrest may compromise the level of consciousness and the ability of patients to maintain a patent airway. Intubation and MV is, therefore, necessary to protect the airway from aspiration in these situations.

Patients admitted to the CICU often have concurrent acute or chronic pulmonary conditions that may compromise oxygenation and/or ventilation and require initiation of positive pressure

Box 1
Common indications for positive pressure ventilation in CICU

- Congestive cardiac failure (cardiogenic pulmonary edema)
- Decreased level of consciousness requiring protection of the airway (eg, severe cardiogenic shock, cardiac arrest)
- Concurrent acute or chronic respiratory disease
- Complications of critical illness (eg, pulmonary embolism, pneumothorax, critical illness induced weakness)

ventilation. Both iatrogenic complications and those inherent to critical illness can develop in the CICU. Critical illness–induced weakness, pulmonary embolism, hospital-acquired pneumonia, and pneumothorax may compromise oxygenation or ventilation and mandate the need for respiratory support.

OXYGENATION CONSIDERATIONS

As previously reviewed, spontaneous respiratory effort (in that it requires oxygen consumption) is a form of exercise. By supporting or taking over completely the work of breathing, respiratory support can minimize this and improve cardiovascular performance.

Oxygenation can be titrated by setting the inspired oxygen concentration (F$_{IO_2}$) and adding PEEP. Other therapeutic options commonly used to improve oxygenation are changing the pattern of ventilation and rescue and advanced oxygenation techniques, such as high-frequency oscillation and extracorporeal membrane oxygenation, which are beyond the scope of this article.

Adequate tissue oxygenation is crucial for maintaining efficient aerobic metabolism and tissue structure and function. Oxygenation is particularly important for highly oxidative organs, such as the heart, especially in the presence of conditions that limit oxygen delivery (eg, coronary disease).

Accepted normal values for Pao$_2$ lie between 80 and 100 mm Hg (10.7–13.3 kPa) and SaO$_2$ greater than 94% while breathing air at sea level.

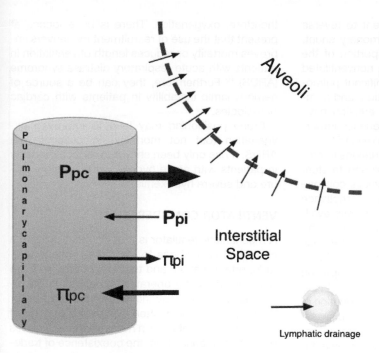

Fig. 4. Starling forces imbalance leading to pulmonary edema of cardiac origin. If left atrial pressure exceeds 20 cm H₂O, pulmonary capillary hydrostatic pressure increases markedly causing net accumulation of fluid in the interstitium and alveolar space. Starling equation: πpc, pulmonary capillary colloid osmotic pressure; πpi, pulmonary interstitium colloid osmotic pressure; K, filtration coefficient endothelium; Ppc, pulmonary capillary hydrostatic pressure; Ppi, pulmonary interstitium hydrostatic pressure; Q, net flow of fluid across pulmonary capillary membrane.

$$Q = K[(Ppc-Ppi)- (\pi pc-\pi pi)$$

Traditionally, these values have been used as cut-off points for the diagnosis of hypoxia and as targets for titration of oxygenation in critical care units.[28]

There is, however, a strong body of evidence suggesting that high concentrations of oxygen are potentially harmful and associated with poor outcomes in certain cardiovascular conditions. Arterial hyperoxia has been associated with undesirable cardiovascular responses, such as reduced stroke volume and cardiac output, increased systemic vascular resistance, coronary artery vasoconstriction, and reduced coronary blood flow.[29]

Two recent systematic reviews called into question the routine use of high-flow oxygen for the treatment of acute myocardial infarction. They found no evidence of oxygen therapy being beneficial in this setting; on the contrary, they found that it may result in greater infarct size and increased mortality.[30,31] Hyperoxia can also be harmful in the context of resuscitation following cardiac arrest. A cohort study of 6326 patients admitted to the ICU following resuscitation from cardiac arrest found arterial hyperoxia (Pao₂ >300 mm Hg/40 kPa) to be independently associated with increased in-hospital mortality compared with either hypoxia (Pao₂ <60 mm Hg/8 kPa) or normoxia.[32]

Optimal oxygen delivery to the tissues (DO₂) is the result of adequate cardiac output and arterial oxygen content.[33] This relationship is described by the following equation:

$$DO_2 \text{ (mL/min)} = CO \text{ (L/min)} \times CaO_2 \times 10$$

where CaO_2 is the total arterial oxygen content (the product of the oxygen bound to hemoglobin plus the oxygen carried in solution) and CO is cardiac output. The multiplier 10 is used because of the different measurement units used for CaO_2 (mL.dL^{-1}) and cardiac output (l. min^{-1}).

Adequate DO₂ ensures that aerobic metabolism is maintained and preserves tissue viability. The aforementioned equation makes clear that manipulating MV parameters only modifies one variable and that ensuring an adequate cardiac output and hemoglobin content are necessary for maintaining a satisfactory oxygen delivery. Together with clinical signs, lactate, base deficit, and mixed venous saturation (SvO₂) and central venous saturation (S$_c$O₂) are commonly used as surrogate markers of adequacy of tissue perfusion. It is, therefore, reasonable to titrate inspired oxygen to the lowest possible levels that meet the oxygen requirement of the tissues and maintain aerobic metabolism.

High F_{IO_2} levels can be insufficient to reverse hypoxemia in the presence of pulmonary shunt. Shunt occurs when a substantial portion of the cardiac output is in contact with a nonventilated area of the lung. Patients with significant pulmonary edema, pneumonic consolidation, and compression of lung tissue by pleural effusion have poor lung compliance and can experience important degrees of shunt causing hypoxemia.[34]

PEEP or CPAP is used in these situations to promote reopening of collapsed alveoli and to stent open the small airways opposing alveolar collapse and atelectasis. PEEP improves lung compliance by increasing the number of alveolar units available for ventilation, increasing the FRC, and reducing the work of breathing.[35,36] PEEP may also protect from ventilator-induced lung injury by preventing damage from the repeated opening and closing of alveolar units (atelectrauma).[37]

There are important caveats to the application of PEEP to patients with cardiovascular disease. PEEP in itself does not reduce lung water in patients with pulmonary edema. Indeed, it may actually increase the water content of the lungs by obstructing lymphatic drainage.[38] The benefit of PEEP/CPAP in the setting of cardiogenic pulmonary edema derives from improvements in lung mechanics and LV performance and not from any effects on lung water. PEEP will only improve tissue oxygenation if any negative effects of positive pressure on cardiac output are considered and counterbalanced (see **Table 1**). As previously reviewed, PEEP can significantly affect ventricular preload; therefore, sufficient intravascular volume must be ensured to maintain an adequate cardiac output.

Other therapeutic options that can be considered to improve oxygenation are increasing the ratio of inspiratory to expiratory time (I/E ratio), recruitment maneuvers, and prone positioning. Under normal circumstances the I/E ratio is set at 1:2, which means that the expiratory time is twice the inspiratory time. Prolonging the inspiratory time increases the I/E ratio and improves oxygenation by increasing the mean airway pressure, generating recruitment of atelectatic alveolar units. However, inspiratory time equal or greater than expiratory time can generate significant gas trapping, decrease in venous return and hemodynamic compromise in patients with compromised cardiovascular function. An inverse ratio of ventilation occurs when the inspiratory time exceeds the expiratory time (eg, 2:1). This scenario can be very uncomfortable for patients and often requires deep sedation and paralysis.[39]

Recruitment maneuvers involve the episodic delivery of high pressure and volume breaths with the aim of increasing the number of open alveoli and, therefore, oxygenation. There is no evidence at present that the use of recruitment maneuvers improves mortality or reduces length of ventilation in patients with acute respiratory distress syndrome (ARDS).[40] Furthermore, they can be a source of hemodynamic instability in patients with cardiac pathologies.

Prone positioning may lead to improved oxygenation (but not mortality) in patients with ARDS. It has only been shown to reduce mortality in patients with acute hypoxemic respiratory failure and severe hypoxemia.[41]

VENTILATOR CONSIDERATIONS

A mechanical ventilator is a device that delivers a controlled flow of gas to the airway. The magnitude, rate, duration, and triggering of the flow are determined by the operator. Advances in microprocessor technology have given the operator nearly limitless, and often confusing, options of flow delivery. Confusion in nomenclature of modes of ventilation arises from the coexistence of trademark names and historical abbreviations that do not always reflect the clinical application of the mode, potentially creating confusion that may adversely affect patient care.[42] Modern definitions of ventilation modes are based on combinations of 3 parameters: control variable, breath sequence, and targeting scheme.[43]

Control can be defined as the variable that the ventilator uses to control inspiration. The variable can be identified according to the relationship between peak inspiratory pressure and to the load experienced by the ventilator. In volume control, the peak pressure changes as the ventilator load changes, while maintaining a constant tidal volume. Pressure control maintains a constant peak inspiratory pressure as the ventilator load changes. In other words, pressure is the independent variable during pressure control, and volume is the independent variable during volume control.

Breath sequence can be
- Continuous mandatory ventilation when the ventilator controls all breaths but may allow patient triggering
- Synchronized intermittent mandatory ventilation (SIMV), which allows patients to take spontaneous breaths between mandatory breaths
- Continuous spontaneous ventilation, when all breaths are spontaneous

Modern ventilators can respond to changes in patients' lung compliance, lung resistance, and respiratory effort. The ventilator response is determined by the targeting or feedback scheme programmed into the device. Feedback schemes range from simple static set points (eg, pressure limit in pressure control) with full operator input to complex dynamic automatic adjustment of set points based on complex algorithms.[42,43]

Common ventilation modes in use today derive from different combinations of these 3 parameters. **Table 2** reviews the characteristics, theoretical benefits, and disadvantages of commonly used ventilation modes.

Although different modes allow more precise control of ventilation and adjustment according to patients' pathology and lung dynamics, there is no evidence of improved patient outcomes associated with the use of a specific invasive ventilation mode.[46,47] Specifically, there have been no controlled trials to date studying the effect of different modes of invasive ventilation in patients with cardiac failure.

There are hemodynamic advantages associated with modes of ventilation that allow spontaneous respiratory activity. They tend to produce lower levels of mean airway pressure and intrapleural pressure for a given minute volume, compared with fully controlled modes of ventilation. Modes such as CPAP, SIMV, bilevel airway pressure, and pressure support ventilation allow for different degrees of spontaneous breaths. This variability has been shown to reduce the deleterious effects in cardiovascular physiology of positive pressure ventilation.[4,48] However, patients with severe cardiogenic shock or LV dysfunction may benefit more from full ventilatory support that abolishes the effect of an increased oxygen consumption associated with spontaneous breathing.[17]

Ultimately, ventilator settings will depend on local experience, type and brand of equipment, and familiarity with the device available in different CICUs. The clinician should choose a setting that ensures effective minute volume ventilation, optimizes the work of breathing, and minimizes hemodynamic adverse effects.

NIV USE IN CONGESTIVE CARDIAC FAILURE AND ACUTE CARDIOGENIC PULMONARY EDEMA

The last 3 decades have seen an increase in the use of NIV for the management of patients with acute cardiogenic pulmonary edema. The term *NIV* has been used by the literature to denote both CPAP ventilation and the true bilevel ventilation mode that provides noninvasive IPPV (NIPPV).

Early interest was sparked by evidence from observational and small randomized studies demonstrating that CPAP improved oxygenation, reduced work of breathing, and increased cardiac output in patients with cardiogenic pulmonary edema.[21–23,49,50] There has been controversy regarding which method of NIV is more effective. Chadda and colleagues[51] performed a physiologic randomized crossover study suggesting that NIPPV was more effective than CPAP in terms of unloading respiratory muscles and improving cardiac performance. However, concern arose that bilevel ventilation was associated with a higher incidence of myocardial ischemia compared with CPAP.[52] To date, this has not been supported by systematic reviews.[38–40]

Results from recent meta analyses and systematic reviews suggest that the early institution of NIV is associated with a reduction in the rates of endotracheal intubation compared with standard medical therapy. NIV (both CPAP and NIPPV) was also associated with a reduction in mortality compared with standard therapy. None of the reviews found NIPPV to be superior to CPAP in terms of outcomes (**Table 3**). The applicability of these findings is limited, however, by the small size of studies included and wide variations in study populations and interventions.[53–56]

The largest multicenter randomized controlled trial to date studying the effect of NIV in acute cardiogenic pulmonary edema was performed by Gray and colleagues[57] in 2008. The trial included 1069 patients with acute cardiogenic pulmonary edema and aimed to establish whether NIV improved survival when compared with standard medical therapy. A secondary outcome assessed the superiority of NIPPV over CPAP. The patients were randomized to 3 intervention groups: standard oxygen therapy, CPAP (5–15 cm of water), and NIPPV (inspiratory pressure of 8–20 cm H_2O and expiratory pressure of 4–10 cm H_2O). No difference was detected in 7-day mortality between patients receiving standard oxygen therapy (9.7%) and patients treated with NIV (9.5% $P = .87$). There was no significant difference in the composite end point of short-term (within 7 days) mortality and intubation between CPAP (11.7%) and NIPPV (11.1% $P = .81$). However, patient-reported dyspnea, tachycardia, hypercapnia, and acidosis were significantly improved in the NIV ventilation groups compared with standard oxygen therapy.

Despite the large number of patients, this article has some limitations. The trial was set in the emergency department, limiting its applicability to patients that develop pulmonary edema during other stages of their hospital stay. There was

Table 2
Common ventilation modes in use today: characteristic, theoretical benefits, and disadvantages

Mode of Ventilation	Other Names	Characteristics/Theoretical Benefits/Disadvantages
Volume Modes		
Assist-control ventilation	CMV with assist	Ventilator delivers preset volume; breaths can be either *assist* or *control* but of the same volume; may induce hyperinflation and respiratory alkalosis at high respiratory rates
SIMV		Mandatory breaths synchronized to coincide with spontaneous inspiration; guaranteed backup rate; cardiac output can decrease in patients with LV dysfunction because of increased afterload with unsupported spontaneous inspiratory efforts
Pressure Modes		
PCV		Ventilator delivers set target pressure at a set respiratory rate; protects from barotrauma; volume delivered subject to lung compliance
PSV		Patients' inspiratory effort assisted to a preset level; patient triggered, pressure limited, and flow cycled
CPAP	EPAP	Pressures set to remain constant during respiratory cycle while patients are allowed to breathe spontaneously
APRV	BiPap	Clinician set to level CPAP and time spent at each level (inspiratory and expiratory time); CPAP or pressure high and release pressure or pressure low; patients can breathe spontaneously at both levels; potential for hemodynamic compromise in preload-dependent conditions
Dual Modes		
PRVC	AutoFlow (Dräger Medical AG & Co. KGaA, Germany) Adaptive pressure control	Closed-loop, pressure-controlled mode; patient or time triggered with tidal volume as the variable selected by operator; maintains a more stable tidal volume as lung compliance varies while protecting from barotrauma
ASV		Delivers pressure-controlled breaths using automatically calculated optimal settings (tidal volume and frequency) based on patients' ideal body weight and percentage of minute volume ventilation; aims to minimize work of breathing while encouraging spontaneous breaths
PAV		Pressure-controlled output by the ventilator is adjusted to perform accordingly to patients' effort; maximizes ventilator-patient synchrony and reduces work of breathing
NAVA		Electrical activity of diaphragm (Edi) is captured, fed back to ventilator, and breath assistance is delivered proportionally and in synchrony with patients' Edi signal[44,45]

Abbreviations: APRV, airway pressure release ventilation; ASV, adaptive support ventilation; BiPap, bilevel airway pressure; CMV, controlled mandatory ventilation; EPAP, expiratory positive airway pressure; NAVA, neutrally adjusted ventilator assist; PAV, proportional assist ventilation; PCV, pressure-controlled ventilation; PRVC, pressure-regulated volume control; PSV, pressure support ventilation.

Data from MacIntyre NR, Branson RD. Mechanical ventilation. 2nd edition. St Louis (MO): Saunders Elsevier; 2009; and Brander L, Leong-Poi H, Beck J, et al. Titration and implementation of neurally adjusted ventilatory assist in critically ill patients. Chest 2009;135(3):695–703.

Table 3
Summary of meta analyses reviewing the effect of NIV in mortality and need for intubation in acute cardiogenic pulmonary edema

Author/Year	No. Studies	No. of Patients	Mortality NIV vs Standard Medical Care (RR [95% CI] P Value)			Mortality CPAP vs NIPPV (Bilevel)		
			NIV Overall	CPAP	NIPPV (Bilevel)	No. of Studies	No. of Patients	RR (95% CI) P Value
Masip et al,[53] 2005	15	783	0.55 (0.40–0.78) P<.001	0.53 (0.35–0.81) P.03	0.80 (0.35–1.05) P.07	6	219	0.90 (0.38–2.16) P.82
Peter et al,[54] 2006	18	877	N/A	0.59 (0.38–0.90) P.015	0.63 (0.37–1.10) P.11	9	406	0.75 (0.40–1.43) P.38
Winck et al,[55] 2006	16	815	N/A	0.13 (0.05–0.22) P.003	0.07 (0.01–0.14) P.08	7	297	0.02 (−0.06–0.10) P.64
Vital et al,[56] 2008	17	930	0.62 (0.45–0.84)	0.58 (0.38–0.88)	0.70 (0.40–1.23)	6	230	1.19 (0.36–3.86)

Author/Year	No. Studies	No. of Patients	Need for Intubation NIV vs Standard Medical Care (RR [95% CI] P Value)			Need of Intubation CPAP vs NIPPV (Bilevel)		
			NIV Overall	CPAP	NIPPV (Bilevel)	No. of Studies	No. of Patients	RR (95% CI) P Value
Masip et al,[53] 2005	15	783	0.43 (0.32–0.57) P<.001	0.40 (0.27–0.58) P<.001	0.48 (0.30–0.76) P.002	6	219	1.45 (0.62–3.38) P.39
Peter et al,[54] 2006	19	928	N/A	0.44 (0.29–0.66) P.0003	0.50 (0.27–0.90) P.02	9	353	0.94 (0.48–1.86) P.86
Winck et al,[55] 2006	16	805	N/A	0.22 (0.10–0.34) P.0004	0.18 (0.04–0.32) P.01	7	299	0.03(−0.04–0.09) P.41
Vital et al,[56] 2008	17	930	0.53 (0.34–0.83)	0.46 (0.32–0.65)	0.68 (0.27–1.73)	7	257	0.92 (0.36–2.32)

Relative risk of death and intubation in NIV overall, CPAP, or NIPPV versus standard medical care and relative risk of death and intubation in CPAP versus NIPPV (bilevel).
NIV encompasses both CPAP and NIPPV.
Abbreviations: CI, confidence interval; N/A, not available; RR, relative risk.
Data from Refs.[53–56]

also significant crossover between the groups, with 56 patients in the standard-oxygen-therapy group being rescued with NIV. This crossover may have produced an artificially low rate of intubation in the standard-oxygen-therapy group.

The cumulative evidence suggests that NIV (both CPAP and NIPPV) are valuable and safe therapeutic options for the management of acute cardiogenic pulmonary edema in the CICU.

WEANING ISSUES IN PATIENTS WITH CARDIOVASCULAR DISEASE

The term *weaning* is used ubiquitously to describe the transition from full ventilatory support to spontaneous and unsupported breathing. *Liberation* and *discontinuation* have been suggested as more appropriate terms because they convey more urgency to the clinician to remove an intervention associated with morbidity and complications.[58]

Once the underlying process mandating ventilatory support has resolved or stabilized, an assessment should be made of the patient's readiness to have ventilation discontinued. This assessment usually takes place during a spontaneous breathing trial (SBT). An SBT requires the patient to breathe completely unassisted (T-piece connected to endotracheal tube) or with low level CPAP and/or inspiratory pressure support. SBTs usually last for 30 min and during this time patients are closely monitored for signs of discomfort, excessive work of breathing and haemodynamic instability (**Fig. 5**).

With discontinuation, the beneficial effects of MV are effectively reversed, with an abrupt transfer from full ventilator support to spontaneous ventilation. This transition has been likened to performing an exercise stress test in patients with an already limited cardiopulmonary reserve.[59] The effects of weaning in the cardiovascular system can be explained in terms of the effect of negative intrathoracic pressure, increase in the work of breathing, and increase in sympathetic tone.[60]

Spontaneous breathing causes a decrease in intrathoracic pressure that is commensurate with the degree of inspiratory effort. This decrease in pressure produces an increased LV afterload and venous return, resulting in increased RVEDV and LVEDV. Failing ventricles are particularly susceptible to afterload and filling pressure changes.[61]

The increased work of breathing related to the spontaneous respiratory muscle activity causes a surge in demand for oxygen delivery. Myocardial oxygen consumption increases as a result of the need for the higher cardiac output that is required to deliver this and the increased wall stress in the

ventricles. Patients with coronary heart disease may experience significant ischemia during weaning that can lead to failure in the discontinuation of MV.[62–65]

There is significant sympathetic activation associated with the transition to spontaneous ventilation. Heart rate and blood pressure increase with noticeable effects in myocardial oxygen demand, and the associated venoconstriction causes an increase in venous return and preload. There is evidence that patients with chronic respiratory failure (eg, chronic obstructive pulmonary disease [COPD]) have more pronounced sympathetic activation with potential significant adverse effects during the weaning process.[66]

The potential adverse cardiovascular consequences of weaning have to be balanced against possible complications arising from MV (**Table 4**). Once the cardiac condition (eg, ischemia, cardiogenic shock) that prompted the initiation of MV has been treated/stabilized, every effort should be made to liberate patients from MV.

The identification and risk stratification of patients likely to fail weaning is crucial to facilitate preemptive interventions to avoid reintubation. Failed extubation is associated with poor patient outcomes and increased duration of hospital stay.[76]

IDENTIFICATION OF PATIENTS AT RISK OF WEANING FAILURE OF CARDIAC ORIGIN

Both clinical characteristics of patients and diagnostic modalities can be used to predict weaning failure in CICU patients. Awareness of this may help prevent such events by altering management strategies (**Table 5**).

Patients with a known history of LV disease, in isolation or in combination with COPD, are at risk of developing pulmonary edema leading to failure to wean.[61,83] Anecdotal evidence suggests that a combination of tachycardia and hypotension is suggestive of cardiac failure during the weaning process.[84]

Increases in pulmonary artery occlusion pressure (PAOP) and decreases in mixed venous oxygen saturation values have been reported in patients that fail discontinuation of MV.[85] However, the use of the pulmonary artery catheter solely for the purpose of monitoring weaning failure is probably not justified in view of its invasiveness and the lack of evidence of benefit associated with monitoring.[86]

Transthoracic echocardiography or transesophageal echocardiography are widely used in the CICU and are less-invasive methods of determining LV filling pressures. The measurement of

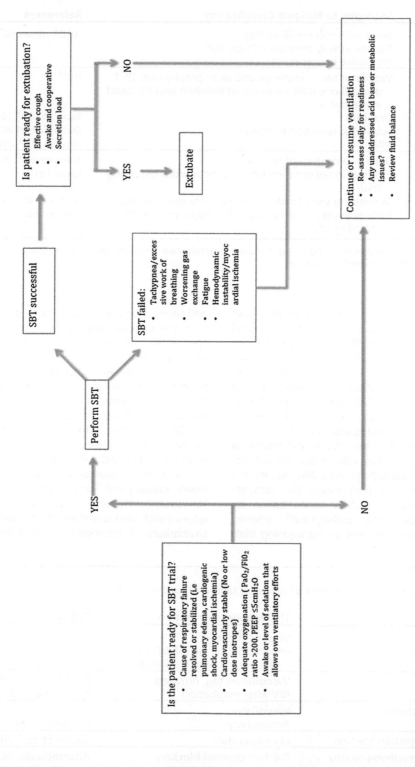

Fig. 5. Sample algorithm for institution of SBT in the CICU.

Table 4
Common complications related to MV in the CICU and evidence-based strategies to reduce their incidence

Complication	Strategies to Mitigate Complication	References
VALI	Small tidal volume (6 mL/kg) Plateau airway pressure <30 cm H_2O Permissive hypercapnia	ARDS network[73]
VAP	Ventilator care bundle (peptic ulcer prophylaxis, DVT prophylaxis, daily cessation of sedation and 30° head elevation) Oral care Subglottic secretion drainage NIV	IHI[74] Mori et al,[67] 2006 Dezfulian et al,[68] 2005 Hess et al,[75] 2005
Prolonged ventilation	Daily interruption of sedation Interruption of sedation before spontaneous breathing trial Minimizing use of sedation in patients receiving MV Early physical and occupational therapy in patients receiving MV	Kress et al,[69] 2000 Girard et al,[70] 2008 Strom et al,[71] 2010 Schweickert et al,[72] 2009

Abbreviations: DVT, deep-vein thrombosis; IHI, Institute for Healthcare Improvement; VAL, ventilator-associated lung injury; VAP, ventilator-associated pneumonia.
Data from Refs.[67–75]

early (E) and late (A) peak diastolic velocities (with Doppler transmitral flow) and tissue Doppler mitral annulus velocities (early [Ea] peak velocity) can help to predict weaning-induced PAOP elevation. Lamia and colleagues[87] found that at the end of a spontaneous ventilation trial, values of E/A greater than 0.95 and E/Ea greater than 8.5 predicted a weaning-induced elevation in PAOP with a sensitivity of 82% and specificity of 91%.

The fluid present in the alveoli and interstitial space during pulmonary edema can be considered a plasma ultrafiltrate (see **Fig. 4**). As the filtered hypo-osmolar fluid leaves the intravascular space, plasma protein concentration increases. Anguel and colleagues[88] tracked changes in plasma proteins during weaning trials and found that a 6% increase in plasma protein from the baseline was 87% sensitive and 95% specific for detecting pulmonary edema–induced by weaning.

Cardiac biomarkers, including B-type natriuretic peptide (BNP) and N-Terminal pro-BNP (NT-pro-BNP), are released by the cardiomyocyte in response to stretch stimuli. Both BNP and NT-pro-BNP have been studied as possible tools for the prediction of weaning failure. Several studies have demonstrated a relationship between an increase in these biomarkers levels and failure to wean consequent on cardiac function.[86,89–92] However, controversy remains surrounding laboratory cutoff values and whether measuring these biomarkers will improve weaning outcomes.

Table 5
Therapeutic options for treatment of weaning failure of cardiac origin

Likely Cause	Therapeutic Intervention	Reference
↑Preload	Diuretic therapy Phosphodiesterase inhibitors (eg, enoximone, milrinone)	Lemaire et al,[61] 1998 Paulus et al,[77] 1994
↑Afterload	Vasodilators (eg, nitrates) NIV after extubation	Routsi et al,[78] 2010 Ferrer et al,[79] 2006
Myocardial ischemia	Vasodilators Angioplasty	 Demoule et al,[80] 2004
Impaired LV ejection fraction	Levosimendan	Sterba et al,[81] 2008
Hypertrophic cardiomyopathy	Calcium channel blockers	Adamopoulos et al,[82] 2005

Data from Refs.[61,77–82]

Finally, elective initiation of NIV immediately following extubation has been shown to reduce the incidence of respiratory failure in patients at risk, including those with underlying cardiac failure.[79]

SUMMARY

Patients admitted to the CICU are of increasing complexity in terms of cardiac conditions and noncardiac comorbidities and, as a consequence, require more and longer duration of ventilatory support. A deep understanding of respiratory physiology and the interactions between the cardiovascular and respiratory systems is essential for managing patients requiring MV in the CICU.

Both NIV and MV requiring an artificial airway are used in the modern CICU in a continuum of respiratory support. Congestive cardiac failure, resulting pulmonary edema, and severe cardiogenic shock are common indications for ventilatory support in the CICU.

A balance between maintaining adequate oxygenation, tissue perfusion, and aerobic metabolism and avoiding the deleterious effects of hyperoxygenation should be considered when titrating oxygen administration. The choice of ventilation modes should be tailored to the specific patient's condition, ensuring effective minute ventilation, reducing the work of breathing and minimizing adverse hemodynamic effects. NIV is a valuable evidence-based therapeutic intervention for the management of patients with acute cardiogenic pulmonary edema.

Discontinuation of MV should be considered as soon as the cardiac pathology that prompted the initiation of respiratory support is stabilized. However, the weaning process can significantly stress the cardiovascular system, and cardiac failure is a common cause of failure to wean. The identification of patients likely to fail and prompt preemptive intervention is crucial for successful weaning and avoiding complications related to prolonged MV.

REFERENCES

1. Katz JN, Shah BR, Volz EM, et al. Evolution of the coronary care unit: clinical characteristics and temporal trends in healthcare delivery and outcomes. Crit Care Med 2010;38(2):375–81.
2. Katz JN, Turer AT, Becker RC. Cardiology and the critical care crisis: a perspective. J Am Coll Cardiol 2007;49(12):1279–82.
3. Steingrub JS, Tidswell M, Higgins TL. Hemodynamic consequences of heart-lung interactions. J Intensive Care Med 2003;18(2):92–9.
4. Duke GJ. Cardiovascular effects of mechanical ventilation. Crit Care Resusc 1999;1(4):388–99.
5. Wise RA, Robotham JL, Summer WR. Effects of spontaneous ventilation on the circulation. Lung 1981;159(4):175–86.
6. Janicki JS, Weber KT. Factors influencing the diastolic pressure-volume relation of the cardiac ventricles. Fed Proc 1980;39(2):133–40.
7. Maughan WL, Kallman CH, Shoukas A. The effect of right ventricular filling on the pressure-volume relationship of ejecting canine left ventricle. Circulation 1981;49(2):382–8.
8. Feihl F, Broccard AF. Interactions between respiration and systemic hemodynamics. Part II: practical implications in critical care. J Intensive Care Med 2009;35(2):198–205.
9. Pinsky MR. Cardiovascular issues in respiratory care. Chest 2005;128(5 Suppl 2):592S–7S.
10. Scharf SM, Bianco JA, Tow DE, et al. The effects of large negative intrathoracic pressure on left ventricular function in patients with coronary artery disease. Circulation 1981;63(4):871–5.
11. Pinsky MR. The effects of mechanical ventilation on the cardiovascular system. Critica 1990;6(3):663–78.
12. Guyton AC, Lindsey AW, Abernathy B, et al. Venous return at various right atrial pressures and the normal venous return curve. Am J Phys 1957;189(3):609–15.
13. Jellinek H, Krenn H, Oczenski W, et al. Influence of positive airway pressure on the pressure gradient for venous return in humans. J Appl Phys 2000;88(3):926–32.
14. Permutt S, Riley RL. Hemodynamics of collapsible vessels with tone: the vascular waterfall. J Appl Phys 1963;18:924–32.
15. Mitchell JR, Whitelaw WA, Sas R, et al. RV filling modulates LV function by direct ventricular interaction during mechanical ventilation. Am J Physiol Heart Circ Physiol 2005;289(2):H549–57.
16. Buda AJ, Pinsky MR, Ingels NB Jr, et al. Effect of intrathoracic pressure on left ventricular performance. N Engl J Med 1979;301(9):453–9.
17. Mathru M, Rao TL, El-Etr AA, et al. Hemodynamic response to changes in ventilatory patterns in patients with normal and poor left ventricular reserve. Crit Care Med 1982;10(7):423–6.
18. Pinsky MR. Heart lung interactions during mechanical ventilation. Curr Opin Crit Care 2012;18(3):256–60.
19. Chapin JC, Downs JB, Douglas ME, et al. Lung expansion, airway pressure transmission, and positive end-expiratory pressure. Arch Surg 1979;114(10):1193–7.
20. Fessler HE, Brower RG, Shapiro EP, et al. Effects of positive end-expiratory pressure and body position on pressure in the thoracic great

veins. Am Rev Respir Dis 1993;148(6 Pt 1): 1657–64.

21. Lenique F, Habis M, Lofaso F, et al. Ventilatory and hemodynamic effects of continuous positive airway pressure in left heart failure. Am J Respir Crit Care Med 1997;155(2):500–5.

22. Naughton MT, Rahman MA, Hara K, et al. Effect of continuous positive airway pressure on intrathoracic and left ventricular transmural pressures in patients with congestive heart failure. Circulation 1995;91(6):1725–31.

23. Baratz DM, Westbrook PR, Shah PK, et al. Effect of nasal continuous positive airway pressure on cardiac output and oxygen delivery in patients with congestive heart failure. Chest 1992;102(5):1397–401.

24. Pierson DJ. Indications for mechanical ventilation in adults with acute respiratory failure. Respir Care 2002;47(3):249–62 [discussion: 262–5].

25. Esteban A, Anzueto A, Frutos F, et al. Characteristics and outcomes in adult patients receiving mechanical ventilation: a 28-day international study. J Am Med Assoc 2002;287(3):345–55.

26. Esteban A, Anzueto A, Alia I, et al. How is mechanical ventilation employed in the intensive care unit? An international utilization review. Am J Respir Crit Care Med 2000;161(5):1450–8.

27. Noble WH, Kay JC, Obdrzalek J. Lung mechanics in hypervolemic pulmonary edema. J Appl Phys 1975;38(4):681–7.

28. O'Driscoll BR, Howard LS, Davison AG. BTS guideline for emergency oxygen use in adult patients. Thorax 2008;63(Suppl 6):vi1–68.

29. Martin DS, Grocott MP. Oxygen therapy in critical illness: precise control of arterial oxygenation and permissive hypoxemia*. Crit Care Med 2013; 41(2):423–32.

30. Wijesinghe M, Perrin K, Ranchord A, et al. Routine use of oxygen in the treatment of myocardial infarction: systematic review. Heart 2009;95(3): 198–202.

31. Cabello JB, Burls A, Emparanza JI, et al. Oxygen therapy for acute myocardial infarction. Cochrane Database Syst Rev 2010;(6):CD007160.

32. Kilgannon JH, Jones AE, Shapiro NI, et al. Association between arterial hyperoxia following resuscitation from cardiac arrest and in-hospital mortality. J Am Med Assoc 2010;303(21):2165–71.

33. Leach RM, Treacher DF. The pulmonary physician in critical care * 2: oxygen delivery and consumption in the critically ill. Thorax 2002;57(2): 170–7.

34. Bein T, Reber A, Stjernstrom H, et al. Ventilation-perfusion ratio in patients with acute respiratory insufficiency. Anaesthesist 1996;45(4):337–42 [in German].

35. Gattinoni L, Pelosi P, Crotti S, et al. Effects of positive end-expiratory pressure on regional distribution of tidal volume and recruitment in adult respiratory distress syndrome. Am J Respir Crit Care Med 1995;151(6):1807–14.

36. Suter PM, Fairley B, Isenberg MD. Optimum end-expiratory airway pressure in patients with acute pulmonary failure. N Engl J Med 1975;292(6): 284–9.

37. Gattinoni L, Caironi P, Cressoni M, et al. Lung recruitment in patients with the acute respiratory distress syndrome. N Engl J Med 2006;354(17): 1775–86.

38. Saul GM, Feeley TW, Mihm FG. Effect of graded administration of PEEP on lung water in noncardiogenic pulmonary edema. Crit Care Med 1982; 10(10):667–9.

39. MacIntyre NR, Branson RD. Mechanical ventilation. 2nd edition. St Louis (MO): Saunders Elsevier; 2009.

40. Hodgson C, Keating JL, Holland AE, et al. Recruitment manoeuvres for adults with acute lung injury receiving mechanical ventilation. Cochrane Database Syst Rev 2009;(2):CD006667.

41. Sud S, Friedrich JO, Taccone P, et al. Prone ventilation reduces mortality in patients with acute respiratory failure and severe hypoxemia: systematic review and meta-analysis. J Intensive Care Med 2010;36(4):585–99.

42. Chatburn RL. Classification of ventilator modes: update and proposal for implementation. Respir Care 2007;52(3):301–23.

43. Hess D. Respiratory care: principles and practice. 2nd edition. Sudbury (MA): Jones & Bartlett Learning; 2012.

44. Sinderby C, Navalesi P, Beck J, et al. Neural control of mechanical ventilation in respiratory failure. Nature 1999;5(12):1433–6.

45. Brander L, Leong-Poi H, Beck J, et al. Titration and implementation of neurally adjusted ventilatory assist in critically ill patients. Chest 2009;135(3): 695–703.

46. Esteban A, Alia I, Gordo F, et al. Prospective randomized trial comparing pressure-controlled ventilation and volume-controlled ventilation in ARDS. For the Spanish Lung Failure Collaborative Group. Chest 2000;117(6):1690–6.

47. Gonzalez M, Arroliga AC, Frutos-Vivar F, et al. Airway pressure release ventilation versus assist-control ventilation: a comparative propensity score and international cohort study. J Intensive Care Med 2010;36(5):817–27.

48. Sternberg R, Sahebjami H. Hemodynamic and oxygen transport characteristics of common ventilatory modes. Chest 1994;105(6):1798–803.

49. Katz JA, Marks JD. Inspiratory work with and without continuous positive airway pressure in patients with acute respiratory failure. Anesthesiology 1985;63(6):598–607.

50. Rasanen J, Heikkila J, Downs J, et al. Continuous positive airway pressure by face mask in acute cardiogenic pulmonary edema. Am J Cardiol 1985;55(4):296–300.

51. Chadda K, Annane D, Hart N, et al. Cardiac and respiratory effects of continuous positive airway pressure and noninvasive ventilation in acute cardiac pulmonary edema. Crit Care Med 2002;30(11):2457–61.

52. Mehta S, Jay GD, Woolard RH, et al. Randomized, prospective trial of bilevel versus continuous positive airway pressure in acute pulmonary edema. Crit Care Med 1997;25(4):620–8.

53. Masip J, Roque M, Sanchez B, et al. Noninvasive ventilation in acute cardiogenic pulmonary edema: systematic review and meta-analysis. J Am Med Assoc 2005;294(24):3124–30.

54. Peter JV, Moran JL, Phillips-Hughes J, et al. Effect of non-invasive positive pressure ventilation (NIPPV) on mortality in patients with acute cardiogenic pulmonary oedema: a meta-analysis. Lancet 2006;367(9517):1155–63.

55. Winck JC, Azevedo LF, Costa-Pereira A, et al. Efficacy and safety of non-invasive ventilation in the treatment of acute cardiogenic pulmonary edema–a systematic review and meta-analysis. Crit Care 2006;10(2):R69.

56. Vital FM, Saconato H, Ladeira MT, et al. Non-invasive positive pressure ventilation (CPAP or bilevel NPPV) for cardiogenic pulmonary edema. Cochrane Database Syst Rev 2008;(3):CD005351.

57. Gray A, Goodacre S, Newby DE, et al. Noninvasive ventilation in acute cardiogenic pulmonary edema. N Engl J Med 2008;359(2):142–51.

58. McConville JF, Kress JP. Weaning patients from the ventilator. N Engl J Med 2012;367(23):2233–9.

59. Pinsky MR. Breathing as exercise: the cardiovascular response to weaning from mechanical ventilation. J Intensive Care Med 2000;26(9):1164–6.

60. Tobin MJ, Jubran A, Hines E Jr. Pathophysiology of failure to wean from mechanical ventilation. Schweiz Med Wochenschr 1994;124(47):2139–45.

61. Lemaire F, Teboul JL, Cinotti L, et al. Acute left ventricular dysfunction during unsuccessful weaning from mechanical ventilation. Anesthesiology 1988; 69(2):171–9.

62. Hurford WE, Lynch KE, Strauss HW, et al. Myocardial perfusion as assessed by thallium-201 scintigraphy during the discontinuation of mechanical ventilation in ventilator-dependent patients. Anesthesiology 1991;74(6):1007–16.

63. Chatila W, Ani S, Guaglianone D, et al. Cardiac ischemia during weaning from mechanical ventilation. Chest 1996;109(6):1577–83.

64. Frazier SK, Brom H, Widener J, et al. Prevalence of myocardial ischemia during mechanical ventilation and weaning and its effects on weaning success. Heart Lung 2006;35(6):363–73.

65. Srivastava S, Chatila W, Amoateng-Adjepong Y, et al. Myocardial ischemia and weaning failure in patients with coronary artery disease: an update. Crit Care Med 1999;27(10):2109–12.

66. Heindl S, Lehnert M, Criée CP, et al. Marked sympathetic activation in patients with chronic respiratory failure. Am J Respir Crit Care Med 2001; 164(4):597–601.

67. Mori H, Hirasawa H, Oda S, et al. Oral care reduces incidence of ventilator-associated pneumonia in ICU populations. J Intensive Care Med 2006;32(2):230–6.

68. Dezfulian C, Shojania K, Collard HR, et al. Subglottic secretion drainage for preventing ventilator-associated pneumonia: a meta-analysis. Am J Med 2005;118(1):11–8.

69. Kress JP, Pohlman AS, O'Connor MF, et al. Daily interruption of sedative infusions in critically ill patients undergoing mechanical ventilation. N Engl J Med 2000;342(20):1471–7.

70. Girard TD, Kress JP, Fuchs BD, et al. Efficacy and safety of a paired sedation and ventilator weaning protocol for mechanically ventilated patients in intensive care (awakening and breathing controlled trial): a randomised controlled trial. Lancet 2008; 371(9607):126–34.

71. Strom T, Martinussen T, Toft P. A protocol of no sedation for critically ill patients receiving mechanical ventilation: a randomised trial. Lancet 2010; 375(9713):475–80.

72. Schweickert WD, Pohlman MC, Pohlman AS, et al. Early physical and occupational therapy in mechanically ventilated, critically ill patients: a randomised controlled trial. Lancet 2009;373(9678):1874–82.

73. Ventilation with lower tidal volumes as compared with traditional tidal volumes for acute lung injury and the acute respiratory distress syndrome. The Acute Respiratory Distress Syndrome Network. N Engl J Med 2000;342(18):1301–8.

74. IHI proposes six patient safety goals to prevent 100,000 annual deaths. Qual Lett Healthc Lead 2005;17(1):11–2, 1.

75. Hess DR. Noninvasive positive-pressure ventilation and ventilator-associated pneumonia. Respir Care 2005;50(7):924–9 [discussion: 929–31].

76. Epstein SK, Ciubotaru RL, Wong JB. Effect of failed extubation on the outcome of mechanical ventilation. Chest 1997;112(1):186–92.

77. Paulus S, Lehot JJ, Bastien O, et al. Enoximone and acute left ventricular failure during weaning from mechanical ventilation after cardiac surgery. Crit Care Med 1994;22(1):74–80.

78. Routsi C, Stanopoulos I, Zakynthinos E, et al. Nitroglycerin can facilitate weaning of difficult-to-wean chronic obstructive pulmonary disease patients: a prospective interventional non-randomized study. Crit Care 2010;14(6):R204.

79. Ferrer M, Valencia M, Nicolas JM, et al. Early noninvasive ventilation averts extubation failure in patients at risk: a randomized trial. Am J Respir Crit Care Med 2006;173(2):164–70.

80. Demoule A, Lefort Y, Lopes ME, et al. Successful weaning from mechanical ventilation after coronary angioplasty. Br J Anaesth 2004;93(2):295–7.

81. Sterba M, Banerjee A, Mudaliar Y. Prospective observational study of levosimendan and weaning of difficult-to-wean ventilator dependent intensive care patients. Crit Care Resusc 2008;10(3): 182–6.

82. Adamopoulos C, Tsagourias M, Arvaniti K, et al. Weaning failure from mechanical ventilation due to hypertrophic obstructive cardiomyopathy. J Intensive Care Med 2005;31(5):734–7.

83. Menzies R, Gibbons W, Goldberg P. Determinants of weaning and survival among patients with COPD who require mechanical ventilation for acute respiratory failure. Chest 1989;95(2):398–405.

84. Teboul JL, Monnet X, Richard C. Weaning failure of cardiac origin: recent advances. Crit Care 2010; 14(2):211.

85. Jubran A, Mathru M, Dries D, et al. Continuous recordings of mixed venous oxygen saturation during weaning from mechanical ventilation and the ramifications thereof. Am J Respir Crit Care Med 1998; 158(6):1763–9.

86. Harvey S, Harrison DA, Singer M, et al. Assessment of the clinical effectiveness of pulmonary artery catheters in management of patients in intensive care (PAC-Man): a randomised controlled trial. Lancet 2005;366(9484):472–7.

87. Lamia B, Maizel J, Ochagavia A, et al. Echocardiographic diagnosis of pulmonary artery occlusion pressure elevation during weaning from mechanical ventilation. Crit Care Med 2009;37(5): 1696–701.

88. Anguel N, Monnet X, Osman D, et al. Increase in plasma protein concentration for diagnosing weaning-induced pulmonary oedema. Intensive Care Med 2008;34(7):1231–8.

89. Mekontso-Dessap A, de Prost N, Girou E, et al. B-type natriuretic peptide and weaning from mechanical ventilation. J Intensive Care Med 2006; 32(10):1529–36.

90. Principi T, Falzetti G, Elisei D, et al. Behavior of B-type natriuretic peptide during mechanical ventilation and spontaneous breathing after extubation. Minerva Anestesiol 2009;75(4):179–83.

91. Abroug F, Ouanes-Besbes L. Detection of acute heart failure in chronic obstructive pulmonary disease patients: role of B-type natriuretic peptide. Curr Opin Crit Care 2008;14(3):340–7.

92. Gerbaud E, Erickson M, Grenouillet-Delacre M, et al. Echocardiographic evaluation and N-terminal pro-brain natriuretic peptide measurement of patients hospitalized for heart failure during weaning from mechanical ventilation. Minerva Anestesiol 2012;78(4):415–25.

Targeted Temperature Management in Survivors of Cardiac Arrest

Ivan Rocha Ferreira Da Silva, MD[a],
Jennifer Ann Frontera, MD[b],*

KEYWORDS

- Mild therapeutic hypothermia • Cardiac arrest survivors • Hypoxic-ischemic brain injury
- Neurologic prognosis

KEY POINTS

- Evidence supports mild therapeutic hypothermia (MTH) as the fifth link of the life chain, with significant decrease in mortality and improvement of neurologic outcomes in cardiac arrest (CA) survivors throughout the last decade.
- Cardiologist and intensivists must be acquainted with the indications and technique because MTH is the only proven neuroprotective therapy for CA survivors.
- Future research will help define current questions, such as the optimal timing, target temperature, and duration of MTH.

INTRODUCTION

Cardiac arrest (CA) is one of the most challenging situations in medicine because it involves not only reinstituting meaningful cardiac activity, but also minimizing secondary neurologic injuries. It is a major public health issue worldwide and a considerable amount of resources are spent in research yearly to understand better pathophysiological mechanisms, as well as therapies, to reduce secondary injuries in survivors. It is estimated that the global incidence of out-of-hospital CA is 82 to 189 cases per 100,000 inhabitants in industrialized countries.[1,2] Data from studies conducted before the widespread use of mild therapeutic hypothermia (MTH) show that only 5% to 20% of CA survivors were discharged from the hospital with good neurologic outcomes.[3–5] Of all the numerous randomized controlled trials (RCTs) that tested therapies to improve neurologic outcome after CA, the

only ones with positive reproducible results were studies using MTH.[6] This article focuses on MTH as the main strategy for post-CA care.

RATIONALE FOR THE USE OF MTH AFTER CA

Hypoxic-ischemic brain injury is a well-known consequence of CA. Brain injury and cardiovascular instability are the major determinants of survival after CA.[7] It is estimated that the cost of care during the first 6 months after a CA for a patient severely disabled or in a vegetative state can be as high as $300,000.[8]

HISTORICAL PERSPECTIVE

The use of hypothermia for clinical purposes has been suggested for thousands of years. Hippocrates advocated the packing of wounded soldiers in snow and ice in 400 BC.[9] Baron Dominique Jean

Disclosures: The authors have nothing to disclose.
[a] Neurocritical Care Unit and Stroke Department, Hospital Copa D'Or, Rio de Janeiro 22031-011, Brazil;
[b] Cerebrovascular Center, Neurological Institute, Cleveland Clinic Lerner College of Medicine, 9500 Euclid Avenue S80, Cleveland, OH 44195, USA
* Corresponding author.
E-mail address: frontej@ccf.org

Cardiol Clin 31 (2013) 637–655
http://dx.doi.org/10.1016/j.ccl.2013.07.010
0733-8651/13/$ – see front matter © 2013 Elsevier Inc. All rights reserved.

Larrey, surgeon-in-chief of the Napoleonic armies, observed that the wounded soldiers lying closer to the campfire died sooner than those in more remote, colder areas did.[10] Clinical interest in hypothermia was revived in the 1930s and 1940s with observations and case reports describing successful resuscitation of drowning victims who were hypothermic.[11] Subsequently, scientific reports of its use after CA[12–14] and in patients with traumatic brain injury[15] were published in the 1950s and 1960s.

In 1964, the legendary anesthesiologist and intensivist Peter Safar[16] recommended in his historic "first ABCs of resuscitation" that hypothermia be used in patients who remain comatose after successful restoration of spontaneous circulation.

At that time, no consensus was reached about the ideal duration and goal temperature, or the ideal candidates for induced hypothermia. Due to adverse effects observed at very low temperatures, and difficulty efficiently and safely inducing and maintaining hypothermia, interest in this treatment modality declined precipitously. Approximately 30 years later, laboratory studies using animal models demonstrated the benefit of mild hypothermia after CA.[17,18] These were followed by several pilot trials of MTH in humans showing improved neurologic function compared with historic controls, as well as safety and feasibility.[19–21] Those studies set the foundation for the seminal RCTs,[22,23] which ushered in a new era in the post-CA care, culminating in 2003 with a statement from the International Liaison Committee on Resuscitation that "unconscious adult patients with spontaneous circulation after out-of-hospital CA should be cooled to 32°C to 34°C for 12 to 24 hours when the initial rhythm was ventricular fibrillation."[24] In 2005, induced hypothermia was included in the American Heart Association chain of survival.[25]

Pathophysiology of Brain Injury in CA

The brain receives approximately 25% of the cardiac output and is a strict aerobic organ with very high demand for glucose and very limited energy storage. Thus, it is extremely vulnerable to ischemic insults. Studies using animal models demonstrated that after 10 minutes of induced brain ischemia brain concentrations of glucose, glycogen, adenosine triphosphate, and phosphocreatine are virtually nonexistent.[26] This is usually followed by loss of transmembrane electrochemical gradients and consequent failure of synaptic transmission,[27] release of glutamate leading to excitotoxic cell death,[28] neuronal necrosis, and apoptosis.[29] Although the restoration of brain perfusion will reestablish energy stores, further injuries can ensue in a process known as reperfusion injury. Some of the studied mechanisms of reperfusion injury include lipid peroxidation, generation of oxygen reactive species, continued glutamate neurotoxicity, activation of calcium-dependent systems, and neuronal damage mediated by inflammatory cells.[30] **Box 1** summarizes some of the known mechanisms of neuronal injury associated with CA.

Protective Effects Associated with MTH

Since the 1950s, animal studies have shown that induced hypothermia can decrease the cerebral blood flow and cerebral metabolic rate of oxygen

---

Box 1
Mechanisms of anoxic-ischemic brain injury

Immediate

1. Cellular energy depletion, with anaerobic metabolism

2. Collapse of transmembrane sodium and potassium gradients

3. Failure of synaptic transmission, axonal conduction, and action potential firing

4. Intracellular acidosis

5. Hypercalcemia

6. Glutamate release, with neuronal hyperexcitability

7. Activation of intracellular enzymatic systems (protein kinase C and B, calcium/calmodulin-dependent protein kinase II, mitogen-activated protein kinases, phospholipase A2, C and D).

8. Mitochondrial dysfunction

9. Reperfusion, with generation of reactive oxygen species and lipid peroxidation

10. Elevated production of nitric oxide and peroxynitrite

11. Blood-brain barrier dysfunction

12. Loss of cerebral autoregulation

Delayed

1. Release of proinflammatory mediators (eg, tumor necrosis factor-α and interleukin-1)

2. Inflammatory cells recruitment

3. Complement activation

4. Caspase activation with apoptosis

5. Coagulation activation

Data from Refs.[27,133–135]

consumption as much as 6% to 7% for each 1°C reduction in brain temperature.[31,32] Recent studies using transcranial Doppler ultrasonography showed a significant decrease in the mean velocities of flow of the middle cerebral artery during MTH, but no changes in jugular venous oxygen saturation, showing a preserved metabolic coupling without further ischemia.[33,34] Additionally, MTH inhibits the release of glutamate and dopamine[35] and induces the release of brain-derived neurotrophic factor,[36] which further inhibits glutamate. A decrease in oxidative stress, free radical generation,[37,38] and cell-death secondary to apoptosis has also been observed.[39] Hypothermia suppresses the inflammatory cascade triggered after CA[40–42] and reduces early hyperemia, delayed hypoperfusion, blood-brain barrier disruption and cerebral edema.[43,44] **Box 2** summarizes the protective mechanisms of MTH.

Box 2
Protective mechanism of therapeutic hypothermia

Early

1. Decrease of cerebral metabolism

2. Decrease in mitochondrial injury and dysfunction

3. Improve ion pump function, decrease intracellular influx of calcium

4. Improve cell membrane leakage, decrease intracellular acidosis

5. Decrease production of reactive oxygen species

6. Decrease formation of cytotoxic edema

Late

1. Decrease of local production of endothelin and thromboxane A2, increase generation of prostaglandins

2. Improve tolerance for ischemia

3. Decrease neuroinflammation

4. Decrease apoptosis

5. Decrease cerebral thermo-pooling

6. Decrease vascular permeability

7. Activation of protective genes

8. Suppression of cortical spreading depression

9. Suppression of seizure activity

10. Decrease coagulation activation and formation of microthrombi

Data from Refs.[71,80]

Hypothermia After CA with Initial Shockable Rhythm

Two landmark studies, published simultaneously in 2002, reported significant improvement of neurologic outcomes using MTH in patients with out-of-hospital CA with ventricular tachycardia or ventricular fibrillation (VT/VF) as the initial arrest rhythm.

The Hypothermia After Cardiac Arrest (HACA) trial was a multicenter European RCT that enrolled 275 survivors of out-of-hospital CA with the initial rhythm of unstable VT or VF.[22] Subjects were randomly assigned to MTH, with a goal temperature of 32° to 34°C for 24 hours using cold air as the cooling method (TheraKool, Kinetic Concepts, Wareham, United Kingdom) versus standard treatment with normothermia. The goal was to reach the target temperature (measured with a bladder probe) within 4 hours after the return of spontaneous circulation (ROSC) and, if necessary, ice packs were used as an adjunct method. After 24 hours at the goal temperature, subjects were passively rewarmed, which was expected to occur over a period of 8 hours. Fifty-five percent of the subjects in the MTH group had a favorable neurologic recovery after 6 months (Cerebral Performance Category score 1 and 2, or ability to work with minor deficit and full independent activities of daily living). This was in contrast to 39% of subjects in the control group (risk ratio for a favorable outcome with hypothermia, 1.40; 95% CI, 1.08–1.81) with an absolute risk reduction of 16% and a number needed to treat to achieve a positive neurologic outcome of six. Additionally, a significant reduction in the rate of death at 6 months in the MTH group was observed (risk ratio for death, 0.74; 95% CI, 0.58–0.95), with an absolute risk reduction of 14% and number needed to treat to avoid one death of seven.

Simultaneously, an Australian trial conducted by Bernard and colleagues[23] enrolled 77 survivors of out-of-hospital CA with an initial rhythm of unstable VT/VF. Subjects enrolled on odd-numbered days received MTH, with a goal temperature of 33°C, for 12 hours, using ice packs as the cooling method. Subjects enrolled on even-numbered days received standard treatment with normothermia. Cooling was started by rescue personnel at the scene of the CA using cold packs (CoolCare, Cheltenham, Victoria, Australia). This was continued in the hospital using ice packs. Body temperature monitoring was performed with a pulmonary artery catheter. After 12 hours, subjects were actively rewarmed for the next 6 hours by external warming with a heated-air blanket, with continued sedation and neuromuscular blockade to suppress shivering. Twenty-one of the 43 subjects (49%) who were treated with MTH survived and had a favorable neurologic recovery (defined as discharged home or to a rehabilitation center) at hospital discharge, compared with 9 of the 34 subjects (26%) treated with normothermia ($P = .05$). The number needed to treat to obtain a favorable neurologic recovery was four. The odds ratio for a good outcome in the hypothermia group compared with the normothermia group, after adjustment by logistic regression for age and time from collapse to ROSC, was 5.25 (95% CI, 1.47 to 18.76; $P = .011$). Though mortality was reduced in the hypothermia group compared with the normothermia group (51% vs 68%), this did not reach statistical significance, likely due to the small sample size in this study.

Hypothermia After CA with Initial Nonshockable Rhythm

In contrast to the studies with VT/VF as the initial rhythm, there are no large RCTs to evaluate the efficacy of MTH in subjects with CA and nonshockable rhythms. Although it would be logical to deduce that the brain injury mechanism could be the same, it is not clear whether other factors influence outcome. Patients with pulseless electric activity or asystole (PEA/asystole) arrest are usually sicker at baseline, and asphyxia and circulatory shock often result in bradycardia or hypotension, or both, before progressing to pulseless CA, during which time additional brain injury may be incurred. Studies from the era before hypothermia showed that subjects with CA and nonshockable rhythms have worse prognosis when compared with VT/VF arrest,[45–48] with the exception of children[46] and subjects with out-of-hospital witnessed CA secondary to a cardiac cause.[49,50]

Some nonrandomized, retrospective and prospective analyses of MTH in nonshockable rhythms have been published. Of these, three studies of out-of-hospital nonshockable rhythm CA found some possible improvement of neurologic outcomes with MTH,[51–53] although one of these showed only a trend for better prognosis but without statistical significance.[53] Another two studies found no benefit of using MTH for out-of-hospital nonshockable rhythm CA.[54,55] The only retrospective study that analyzed in-hospital nonshockable rhythm CA found no benefit for MTH.[56] A meta-analysis including studies before 2010 that tested MTH in nonshockable rhythm CA survivors found that MTH is associated with reduced in-hospital mortality, but no significant neurologic benefit could be found.[57]

Currently, two trials are recruiting subjects to study MTH in nonshockable rhythm CA in-hospital (NCT00886184) and out-of-hospital

(NCT00391469). Until further data are available, MTH does not seem to confer any survival or neurologic benefit to CA survivors who present with a nonshockable rhythm.

APPLICATION OF MTH
Indications

MTH is currently indicated for patients who survive CA with VT/VF as the initial rhythm and who are not able to follow commands after being adequately resuscitated. Its use is strongly supported by the American Heart Association guidelines,[58] the European Resuscitation Council guidelines,[59] and the International Liaison Committee on Resuscitation guidelines.[60] Some centers also use MTH in patients with PEA/asystole as the initial rhythm, although evidence for this practice is limited (see previous discussion). The current data support the use of out-of-hospital CA, although it would be reasonable to treat someone with a witnessed CA secondary to a cardiac cause with VT/VF as the rhythm in the inpatient setting. In addition, the largest trial (HACA) did not include subjects who were resuscitated for more than 60 minutes, which seems a reasonable cutoff, unless the cause for the CA was near-drowning in cold water. Recently, the analysis of a large registry of CA care, including several hospitals in the United States, showed that, compared with patients at hospitals in the quartile with the shortest median resuscitation attempts in nonsurvivors (16 min; interquartile range [IQR] 15–17), those at hospitals in the quartile with the longest attempts (25 min; IQR 25–28) had a higher likelihood of ROSC ($P<.0001$) and survival to discharge ($P<.021$).[61]

Induction

Regardless of the method used to induce MTH, it is extremely important to expedite the process because delays in initiation seem to diminish or even abrogate its beneficial effects in animal models.[62,63] It is suggested that goal core temperature (32°–34°C) should be reached as soon as possible and no more than 8 hours after ROSC. The goal is to reach mild hypothermia because severe cardiac complications are usually encountered with temperatures lower than 30°C.

Several cooling methods, including ice packs and infusion of cold saline, as well as devices (intravascular cooling catheters, nasal cooling, helmets, surface cooling), were tested in small trials. The methods are usually divided in surface cooling (eg, cooling pads, ice packs) or core cooling (eg, intravascular cooling catheters, cold saline infusion). **Table 1** summarizes the most commonly used methods, with their advantages and

Table 1
Most commonly adopted cooling methods

Method	Comments
Core cooling	
Infusion of cold fluids	Usually bolus of 30 ml/kg of normal saline solution at 4°C
	Very rapid method and inexpensive, but no control over temperature goals
	Should not be used as maintenance, but as an induction adjuvant (even in the prehospital setting)
	Studies have shown this volume is well tolerated
Intravascular cooling catheters	Provides quick induction (1.5°–4.5°C) and highly reliable maintenance and rewarming
	Requires invasive procedure with risk of infection, hemorrhage, and venous thrombosis
	Anecdotal evidence suggests less shivering than surface cooling
Surface cooling	
Ice packs	Easy, inexpensive, can provide fairly rapid induction
	No control over temperature goals and overshoot is common
	Should not be used as maintenance, but may be used an induction adjuvant (even in the prehospital setting)
	Risk of severe skin lesions
Water-circulating cooling blankets	Less expensive than other methods, reusable, but inferior to cooling pads or intravascular catheters[67]
	Risk of skin lesions
Cooling pads	Most effective are hydrogel-coated water circulating pads
	Easy to apply, less labor intensive, with fairly fast induction (1.5°–2.0°C) and reliable maintenance and rewarming
	Risk of skin lesions, particularly with prolonged use at a low water temperature
	Cooling pads are reasonably expensive, but avoid risks associated with invasive procedures

disadvantages. To date, there is no evidence to determine the most effective method. A retrospective nonrandomized study with 167 subjects compared surface cooling (using cooling pads) with core cooling (using an intravascular cooling catheter) and found no difference in survival or neurologic outcome between groups.[64] These findings were corroborated by another retrospective study.[65] Evidence does suggest, however, that devices with hydrogel cooling pads are much more effective than conventional cooling blankets.[66,67] Finally, pressure bag infusion of 30 to 40 ml/kg of cold saline or Ringer lactate solution (4°C) can decrease the core body temperature by roughly 1°C per liter of fluid infused.[68–70] Some investigators defend that a combination of core cooling with cold saline infusion with surface cooling might be very effective, possibly with less shivering during induction, although this hypothesis has not been tested in trials to date.[71]

The Neurocritical Care Society Emergency Neurologic Life Support (NCS ENLS) suggests a goal temperature of 32° to 34°C, with the concomitant use of cold saline infusion (4°C, 40 ml/kg intravenous bolus) and a surface or core cooling method for MTH induction.[72]

Maintenance

After core temperature goal is reached, it should be maintained with minimal fluctuations (±0.5°C) for 24 hours. Although one of the main positive RCTs used 12 hours for the maintenance phase, most centers currently adopt 24 hours.[72] A recent small, pilot, randomized trial with 36 subjects suggests that MTH with a target of 32°C may yield better protection than cooling at 34°C, resulting in better short-term and long-term outcomes.[73] **Table 2** summarizes tests commonly ordered during MTH.

Rewarming

The rewarming phase should be as slow and controlled as possible. Animal experiments and human clinical observations suggest that rapid rewarming might lead to loss of many of the benefits and neuroprotective effects of MTH.[74–78] Significant decreases in jugular venous oxygen saturation have been reported during rapid rewarming,[77] as well as isolated brain hyperthermia (with normal core temperature),[75] increases in interleukin 6, and activation of the complement cascade.[79] Rebound cerebral edema and further

Table 2
Tests performed during MTH

Type	Frequency	Comments
Complete blood count, international normalized ratio, activated partial thromboplastin time, fibrinogen	Every 12 h	Watch for DIC, hemolysis, platelet dysfunction
Serum electrolytes (sodium, potassium, phosphorus, magnesium, calcium) and renal function	Every 8 h	Intracellular electrolyte shifts can occur during induction and extracellular shifts during rewarming Monitor for hypokalemia during induction and rebound hyperkalemia during rewarming Replete potassium <3.5 mg/dL Watch for ATN
Arterial blood gases	Every 12 h	Oxygen and carbon dioxide can be overestimated and pH underestimated if not corrected to actual body temperature
Glucose	Every 6 h	Insulin resistance commonly seen
Amylase, lipase, liver function	Every 12 h	Elevation of liver and pancreatic enzymes can occur during MTH, but usually do not represent cell injury
Lactate	Every 8 h	Mild lactic academia can be seen in MTH
Chest radiograph	Daily	Observe for infections and volume overload
EEG	Continuous	Patients should be monitored continuously to detect nonconvulsive status epilepticus
Blood cultures	Every 48 h	Some investigators suggest screening cultures to detect occult bacteremia (MTH induces mild leukopenia and fever cannot be detected)

Abbreviations: ATN, acute tubular necrosis; DIC, disseminated intravascular coagulation.

brain injury are the most feared consequences of rewarming too rapidly.

Some investigators suggest a rewarming rate of 0.2° to 0.5°C per hour in patients after CA and an even slower rate of 0.1° to 0.2°C per hour in patients with primary neurologic conditions, such as traumatic brain injury or stroke.[80] Many cooling devices have feedback mechanisms that permit rewarming at specific speeds. When the target temperature of 36° to 37°C is reached, the cooling device should lock the patient at this normothermic goal for the next 24 to 48 hours because rebound hyperthermia is common, and can be extremely detrimental to the brain.[81] A slower rewarming period can also minimize electrolyte shifts and resistance to insulin changes, normally observed during this phase.

Temperature Monitoring

Monitoring core body temperature during MTH is essential. Noninvasive measurements, such as axillary, oral, tympanic, and temporal temperature, were tested in small studies and are completely unreliable.[71,82,83] According to the NCS ENLS, the preferred route of monitoring temperature in approximate order of preference would be endovascular, esophageal, and bladder or rectal.[72] Intracranial monitoring devices, such as intracranial pressure or brain tissue oxygenation monitors, can offer an exquisite opportunity for reliable brain temperature monitoring, although the device should not be primarily placed for temperature monitoring. Worth mentioning, bladder temperatures in anuric patients might differ considerably from brain temperatures.[84] In the context of anuria, an esophageal, intravascular, or rectal temperature probe is preferred.

COMMONLY ENCOUNTERED PROBLEMS DURING MTH

Table 3 discusses commonly encountered clinical complications during MTH.

Shivering

One of the most problematic challenges when inducing MTH is the triggering of the human body's

Table 3
Most commonly observed physiologic changes and complications during MTH

Physiologic Changes and Complications by Systems	Comments
Cardiovascular	
1. Hypovolemia	Normally secondary to cold diuresis during induction
2. Heart rate	Patients usually develop bradycardia, but matched with decreased body metabolism
	Malignant bradycardia and decreased stroke volumes normally only seen with temperature <30°C (patients should be rewarmed because atropine is usually ineffective)
	Care with use of dexmedetomidine
3. EKG changes	Increase in PR, QT, and QRS intervals
	Arrhythmias normally seen in temperature <30°C (atrial fibrillation and ventricular arrhythmias)
	Rewarming is the most effective treatment in this situation
	Osborn waves normally noted only in cases of severe accidental hypothermia
Renal and electrolytes	Intracellular electrolyte shifts can occur during induction and extracellular shifts during rewarming
	Rapid induction and slow rewarming usually minimize changes
	ATN only observed in case of accidental hypothermia with temperature <28°C
Endocrine	Insulin resistance with hyperglycemia commonly seen
	Goal is normally serum glucose of 140–180 mg/dL
	Insulin requirements may increase during induction and maintenance phases and decrease during rewarming
	Insulin drips are the preferred therapy
Infections	MTH can increase the chances of developing infections, particularly pulmonary infections due to decreased airway ciliary clearance
	Some investigators suggest surveillance blood culture every 48 h, to detect occult bacteremia (MTH induces mild leukopenia and fever cannot be detected)
	Decrease in the temperature used by cooling device to maintain a constant body temperature can be an indirect sign of fever
Blood and coagulation	MTH can induce mild leukopenia, as well as mild coagulation cascade and platelet dysfunction, but without significant clinical impact
	DIC is mostly commonly observed in accidental hypothermia
Thermoregulation:	Shivering markedly increases brain and body metabolism, mitigating most of the protective effects of MTH
	Rapid induction can minimize shivering, and the shivering response is blunted with temperature <34°C (see **Box 3**)
Gastrointestinal	
1. Motility	Patients can develop ileus and delayed gastric emptying
	Effective bowel regimen should be prophylactically prescribed
2. Pancreas and liver	Liver metabolism is markedly decreased and mild increases in liver function enzymes can be observed, but usually of no significance
	Amylase and lipase can also be mildly elevated, but without representing cell injury
	Pancreatitis has been described in patients with severe accidental hypothermia
3. Drug metabolism	Due to liver function decrease, drug metabolism is usually compromised and half-lives of drugs primarily cleared by the enzymatic system may be prolonged
Nutrition	Patients should be fed during MTH, but metabolic requirements should be corrected to body temperature

(continued on next page)

Table 3	
(continued)	
Physiologic Changes and Complications by Systems	**Comments**
Skin	Patients are in high risk for bedsores, due to skin vasoconstriction, immobilization and immune suppression
	Careful observation should be exerted in patients wearing cooling pads
Respiratory and blood gases	Oxygen and carbon dioxide can be overestimated and pH underestimated if blood gas analyses are not corrected to actual body temperature, due to gas solubilization
	Patients in MTH tend to have low actual PCO_2, due to decreased metabolism
	It is controversial whether pH and PCO_2 values management should be guided by corrected arterial blood gases (alpha-stat vs pH-stat theories)
	The authors believe that a combination of corrected arterial blood gases aiming for PCO_2 levels mildly lower than normal (around 35 mm Hg) could avoid cerebral ischemia secondary to extremely low PCO_2 or hyperemia (with increased intracranial pressure) due to high actual PCO_2 levels
Neurologic	Neurologic examination can be extremely blunted during MTH and obscured after rewarming due to decreased drug metabolism
	Patients should be monitored with continuous EEG because nonconvulsive status epilepticus is not rare following anoxic brain injury

Abbreviations: ATN, acute tubular necrosis; DIC, disseminated intravascular coagulation.

thermoregulatory defenses. Shivering and vasoconstriction are physiologic reactions to a decrease in the core body temperature to values lower than the physiologic range. With any minimal decrease of the skin temperature, vasoconstriction ensues. If the core body temperature drops below 35.5, shivering with vigorous muscle contractions to generate heat occurs.[85] Shivering not only decreases the effectiveness of MTH, but can also be harmful because it activates a catecholaminergic response with consequent hypertension, tachycardia, and severe hemodynamic stress. Shivering is associated with increased oxygen consumption and metabolic rate, excess work of breathing, and increased myocardial oxygen consumption.[71,80] In the surgical literature, shivering is strongly associated with cardiac events,[86–89] and animal models of MTH have shown that shivering can negate its neuroprotective effects.[90,91] In a study with neurocritical subjects with traumatic brain injury, shivering was associated with significant lowering of brain tissue oxygenation levels,[92] indicated ischemia and metabolic distress. The Bedside Shivering Assessment Scale (BSAS) is a simple and reliable tool for evaluating the metabolic stress of shivering. It was validated in a study in which it was compared with indirect calorimetry.[93] **Box 3** describes the BSAS.

Most of the autonomic response to a lowering of the core body temperature is derived from hypothalamic centers; however, it is estimated that skin temperature contributes about 20% to

Box 3	
The BSAS	
Score	**Description**
0	None: no shivering noted on palpation of the masseter, neck, or chest wall
1	Mild: shivering localized to the neck and/or thorax only
2	Moderate: shivering involves gross movement of the upper extremities (in addition to neck and thorax)
3	Severe: shivering involves gross movements of the trunk and upper and lower extremities

Adapted from Badjatia N, Strongilis E, Gordon E, et al. Metabolic impact of shivering during therapeutic temperature modulation: the Bedside Shivering Assessment Scale. Stroke 2008;39(12):3243; with permission.

control of vasoconstriction and shivering.[85] All candidates for MTH will be intubated and on mechanical ventilation, so blunting the physiologic responses of the central nervous system to hypothermia with sedation is a natural choice. Propofol is one of the preferred drugs because of its short half-life. Other options include opiates, such as fentanyl infusions or meperidine. The authors typically use meperidine for shivering only in conjunction with continuous electroencephalogram (EEG) monitoring because it has a substantial risk of lowering the seizure threshold. Recently, α2-receptor agonists (dexmedetomidine and clonidine) have received some interest as options for shivering control. Several other drugs with different mechanisms of action have been studied, such as buspirone, nefopam, doxapram, ketanserin, physostigmine, tramadol, ondansetron, and dantrolene, but with mixed results.[85] Magnesium sulfate was shown to lower the shivering threshold in some studies.[78,94–96] Small bolus doses of muscle paralyzers can be used in severe shivering, but repeated or continuous use should be discouraged owing to the risk of development of neuromuscular complications.

Nonpharmacologic approaches can be extremely helpful to combat shivering. Counterwarming of the skin was shown to be feasible and effective in some studies[97–99] because each 4°C increase in mean skin temperature reduces the thresholds for vasoconstriction and shivering by 1°C and 50% of thermal comfort is determined by skin temperature.[85,100] Though skin counterwarming may seem paradoxic, such skin rewarming typically does not affect core body temperature when advanced cooling devices are used.[71,85] Finally, fast induction to goal core temperature might also decrease the incidence of shivering because the shivering response often ceases completely at temperatures below 33.5°C.[15,71,101] **Table 4** summarizes the

Table 4
Most commonly used strategies to combat shivering

Therapy (Frequently Adopted Sequence)	Comments
Fast induction of hypothermia	Shivering tends to be minimized after temperature <35°C is reached
Counterwarming	Fairly effective and safe Use of air-warmed blanket Some hand and feet warming devices have been found to cause thermal burns
Buspirone	Usual dose 30–60 mg po every 8 h Might take 24 h to start acting Contraindicated in cases of severe renal or liver dysfunction Not useful in patients with ileus related to MTH
Magnesium sulfate	Bolus 2–4 g, intravenous, with goal of serum magnesium >2 Continuous drips of 12–16 g/24 h can be used Caution in patients with renal dysfunction Safe in pregnant patients
Meperidine	Bolus of 10–25 mg, intravenous, every 2–3 h Not very sedating Seizures can be observed especially in patients with renal dysfunction
Fentanyl	Bolus of 50–100 μg and drip 25–100 μg/h Watch for hypotension
Dexmedetomidine	Continuous infusion at 0.1–1.4 μg/kg/min May cause hypotension and bradycardia Clonidine is another option with alpha-2 agonism
Propofol	Bolus of 30–50 mg, maintenance drip 20–200 μg/kg/min Watch for hypotension, bradycardia, hypertriglyceridemia, propofol infusion syndrome
Benzodiazepines	Sometimes preferred in patients with hemodynamic instability or seizures
Muscle paralyzers	Very effective, but reserved as last option, due to neuromuscular complications related to prolonged use Bolus administration might decrease incidence of adverse effects Use compromises neurologic examination evaluation

most commonly used drugs and techniques to suppress shivering.

Associated Cardiologic Conditions

Cardiac conditions are the leading primary cause for out-of-hospital CA in the general population; therefore, those patients frequently need further aggressive cardiac care after recovery of spontaneous circulation. Multiple small studies have reported the feasibility and safety of using MTH in patients with cardiogenic shock[102–104] and the application of MTH in combination with emergent percutaneous coronary intervention (PCI),[105–112] as well as the adjunct use of fibrinolytic therapy.[113,114] One multicenter randomized study, Cooling as an Adjunctive Therapy to Percutaneous Intervention in Patients with Acute Myocardial Infarction (COOL-MI), with subjects with acute myocardial ischemia (but no CA) showed that is safe and feasible to perform endovascular core cooling in conjunction with PCI.

Prognostication

The advent of MTH in CA helped improved the neurologic prognosis in survivors, but also created the uncertainty on how to prognosticate outcome in patients who do not follow commands after rewarming. Several studies have tested neurologic examination findings, MRI with diffusion-weighted imaging, somatosensory-evoked potentials (SSEP), EEG, and neuron-specific enolase (NSE) with some interesting results. No definitive guidelines currently exist on how to interpret the test results, but most of the studies have shown that the previous data derived from CA survivors who did not receive MTH do not fully apply to those who receive MTH. The current guidelines of the American Academy of Neurology for prognostication after CA[115] (without MTH) are heavily based on the seminal paper of Levy and colleagues[116] in the early 1980s, which relied on neurologic examination 72 hours after CA. Some current studies with subjects who received MTH showed that the neurologic examination is not a totally reliable tool in this setting. The current experience in most specialized centers indicate that, in addition to the neurologic examination, MRI, EEG, SSEP, and NSE might be interpreted together, with no test alone being more accurate than the others. Moreover, most specialists believe that a longer observation time (at least >72 h but probably >5–7 days) is needed to prognosticate more accurately because some patients can have a remarkable recovery later in the course and elderly patients may take longer to metabolize drugs with central nervous system action because of

decreased liver function secondary to hypothermia. One clear problem with the existing literature regarding outcomes after CA with MTH is that most studies are retrospective, unblinded, and confounded by withdrawal of life-sustaining therapy. A rigorous, prospective, and blinded approach to understanding predictors of outcome is needed. **Table 5** summarizes the most relevant evidence on prognostication after CA and MTH.

CURRENT OUTCOME TRENDS AFTER CA IN THE HYPOTHERMIA ERA

Recent large population studies in the United States showed a consistent trend of decreased mortality after CA in the last decade,[3,117–119] which can be partially attributed to the more widespread use of MTH. Girotra and colleagues[118] analyzed all adults who had an in-hospital CA between 2000 and 2009 at 374 hospitals in the Get with the Guidelines-Resuscitation registry. They reported that risk-adjusted rates of survival to discharge increased from 13.7% in 2000 to 22.3% in 2009 (P<.001), and that rates of clinically significant neurologic disability among survivors decreased over time, with a risk-adjusted rate of 32.9% in 2000 and 28.1% in 2009 (P = .02). Worth mentioning, this study also included subjects with an initial rhythm of PEA/asystole and the exact percentage of subjects who received MTH is not known. The same trend for improved mortality after the implementation of MTH was observed in Dutch, Japanese, and Finnish studies.[120–122] Some studies also indicated an increased use of MTH in the United States and Europe throughout the last decade.[123–127] Some investigators defend that CA survivors should be transferred to CA centers[128] for higher level of care, with some studies showing that it is feasible and might help improve outcomes.[123,125,128–132]

Hyperthermia

Fever after surviving a CA is deleterious and has been shown to impair brain recovery. The exact cause is not fully understood, but evidence shows that activation of inflammatory cytokines occurs after CA, resembling the systemic inflammation seen in septic patients.[111,112] Small studies and case series have disclosed that there is a strong association between poor survival outcomes and a body temperature greater than 37.8°C.[60,113–115] Moreover, fever is directly associated with worse prognosis in stroke and neurocritical patients.[116–121] To date, no RCT has evaluated induced normothermia versus conventional temperature management with the use of antipyretics in CA survivors. The authors suggest an intensive

Table 5
Relevant current evidence on prognostication after CA in patients treated with MTH

Study	Investigators	Conclusion
Retrospective chart review of 37 consecutive adults treated with MTH	Al Thenayan et al,[136] 2008	A motor response better than extension by day 3 was not prognostically reliable after therapeutic induced mild hypothermia for comatose cardiac arrest survivors None of the patients who lost pupillary or corneal reflexes on day 3 or developed myoclonic status epilepticus recovered awareness
Prospective, observational study with 111 subjects treated with MTH	Cronberg et al,[137] 2011	All 17 subjects with NSE levels >33 ng/l failed to recover consciousness In the >33 ng/l NSE group, all 10 studied with MRI had extensive brain injury on diffusion-weighted images, 12/16 lacked cortical responses on SSEP, and all 6 who underwent autopsy had extensive severe histologic damage
Prospective study with 111 subjects treated with MTH	Rossetti et al,[138] 2010	Three clinical variables, assessed within 72 h after CA, showed higher false-positive mortality predictions in MTH compared with the AAN guidelines: incomplete brainstem reflexes recovery (4% vs 0%), myoclonus (7% vs 0%), and absent motor response to pain (24% vs 0%) Unreactive EEG background was incompatible with good long-term neurologic recovery and strongly associated with in-hospital mortality The presence of at least 2 independent predictors out of 4 (incomplete brainstem reflexes, myoclonus, unreactive EEG, and absent cortical SSEP) accurately predicted poor long-term neurologic recovery (positive predictive value = 1.00); EEG reactivity significantly improved the prognostication
Prospective study with 34 subjects treated with MTH	Rossetti et al,[139] 2010	Continuous EEG monitoring showing a nonreactive or discontinuous background during MTH is strongly associated with unfavorable outcome in subjects with coma after CA
Retrospective study with 6 subjects with PSE treated with MTH	Rossetti et al,[140] 2009	Subjects with PSE and preserved brainstem reactions, SSEP and EEG reactivity may have a favorable outcome if their condition is treated as status epilepticus Subjects with nonconvulsive PSE showed a better prognosis than subjects with myoclonic PSE (P = .042)
Multicenter prospective cohort study with 391 subjects treated with MTH	Bouwes et al,[141] 2012	53% had a poor outcome Absent pupillary light responses (FPR 1; 95% CI, 0–7) or absent corneal reflexes (FPR 4; 95% CI, 1–13) 72 h after CPR, and absent SSEPs during hypothermia (FPR 3; 95% CI, 1–7) and after rewarming (FPR 0; 95% CI, 0–18) were reliable predictors Motor scores 72 h after CPR (FPR 10; 95% CI, 6–16) and NSE levels were not reliable predictors

(continued on next page)

Table 5
(continued)

Study	Investigators	Conclusion
Retrospective study with 185 subjects treated with MTH	Leithner et al,[142] 2010	Of 36 subjects with bilateral absent SSEP N20 responses, 35 (97%) had poor outcome One subject had prolonged high amplitude peripheral SSEP, but bilaterally absent N20 3 d after CA and regained consciousness with normal cognitive functions and reproducible N20 responses One subject had minimally detectable N20 at day 3 and recovered consciousness and normal N20 responses on follow-up
Prospective study with 90 subjects treated with MTH	Oksanen et al,[143] 2009	In multiple logistic regression analysis, age, NSE at 48 h, and increase in NSE levels were predictors of poor outcome Cut-off points with 100% specificity in predicting poor outcome were 33 microg/l for NSE at 48 h and a change of 6.4 microg/l from baseline NSE at 24–48 h
Prospective study with 192 subjects (103 hypothermic, 89 nonhypothermic)	Fugate et al,[144] 2010	The absence of pupillary light responses, corneal reflexes, and an extensor or absent motor response at day 3 after CA remained accurate predictors of poor outcome after therapeutic hypothermia (P<.0001 for all) Myoclonic status epilepticus was invariably associated with death (P = .0002) Malignant EEG patterns and global cerebral edema on head computed tomography were associated with death in both hypothermic and normothermic subjects (P<.001) NSE >33 ng/ml levels measured 1–3 d after CA remained associated with poor outcome (P = .017), but had a false-positive rate of 29.3%
Prospective study with 97 subjects who received MTH compared with 133 maintained in normothermia	Steffen et al,[145] 2010	NSE serum levels were significantly lower under MTH compared with normothermia in univariate analysis Recommended cutoff levels for NSE 72 h after ROSC (>33 ng/l) do not reliably predict poor neurologic outcome in CA subjects treated with MTH
Prospective study with 83 subjects treated with MTH	Wijman et al,[146] 2009	Based on MRI: the percentage of brain volume less than an ADC[a] cutoff of 650–700 × 10(-6) mm^2/s best differentiated between survivors and subjects who died or remained vegetative The percentage of brain volume less than ADC 400 to 450 × 10(-6) mm^2/s best distinguished between survivors with good vs impaired neurologic outcome at 6 mo Quantitative DWI at this threshold resulted in a 38% absolute increase in sensitivity for predicting poor outcome compared with the neurologic examination while maintaining 100% specificity

(continued on next page)

Table 5
(continued)

Study	Investigators	Conclusion
Prospective study with 61 subjects treated with MTH	Rossetti et al,[147] 2012	Serum NSE and EEG findings were strongly correlated (Spearman rho = 0.45; $P<.001$) Median NSE peak values were higher in subjects with unreactive EEG background ($P<.001$) and discontinuous patterns ($P = .001$) All subjects with nonreactive EEG died 5 survivors (3 with good outcome) had NSE levels >33 µg/L
Retrospectively analysis of 227 subjects (128 subjects received MTH)	Fugate et al,[148] 2011	Median day of awakening was day 2 for both groups and most (91% hypothermic and 79% nonhypothermic) awakened within 3 d
Retrospective study with 54 subjects treated with MTH	Crepeau et al,[149] 2013	EEG features correlating with poor outcome included seizures, nonreactive background, and epileptiform discharges

Abbreviations: AAN, American Academy of Neurology; ADC, Apparent Diffusion Coefficient; FPR, false-positive ratio; N20, response recorded at 20 ms during SSEP; PSE, postanoxic status epilepticus.
[a] Measures the magnitude of diffusion of water molecules within cerebral tissue; areas with cytotoxic brain injury are darker on an ADC map compared to healthy tissue.
Data from Refs.[136–149].

control, aiming for a core body temperature around 37°C, for at least the first 48 hours after completion of a standard MTH protocol for VF/VT CA.

FUTURE PERSPECTIVES AND ONGOING TRIALS

MTH after CA is still new and, in the near future, some questions still must be answered, such as the optimal goal temperature, duration of MTH, optimal device for MTH, and better ways of prognosticating outcome for these patients. Trials evaluating intra-arrest MTH (NCT00886184) and out-of-hospital initiation of MTH with cold saline (NCT00391469), as well as for in-hospital arrests (NCT00886184), are currently recruiting subjects. Moreover, a trial that will compare surface cooling to core cooling (NCT00827957) and another that will compare MTH at 36°C versus 33°C (NCT01020916) will try to resolve some of the current questions.

SUMMARY

A growing body of evidence supports MTH as the fifth link of the life chain, with significant decrease in mortality and improvement of neurologic outcomes in CA survivors throughout the last decade. The cardiologist and the intensivist must be acquainted with the indications and technique because MTH is, so far, the only proven neuroprotective therapy for CA survivors. Future research

will help better define current questions, such as the optimal timing, target temperature, and duration of MTH.

REFERENCES

1. Rea TD, Pearce RM, Raghunathan TE, et al. Incidence of out-of-hospital cardiac arrest. Am J Cardiol 2004;93(12):1455–60.
2. Sayre MR, Koster RW, Botha M, et al. Part 5: adult basic life support: 2010 international consensus on cardiopulmonary resuscitation and emergency cardiovascular care science with treatment recommendations. Circulation 2010;122(16 Suppl 2): S298–324.
3. Randomized clinical study of thiopental loading in comatose survivors of cardiac arrest. Brain Resuscitation Clinical Trial I Study Group. N Engl J Med 1986;314(7):397–403.
4. Bottiger BW, Grabner C, Bauer H, et al. Long term outcome after out-of-hospital cardiac arrest with physician staffed emergency medical services: the Utstein style applied to a midsized urban/suburban area. Heart 1999;82(6):674–9.
5. Westfal RE, Reissman S, Doering G. Out-of-hospital cardiac arrests: an 8-year New York City experience. Am J Emerg Med 1996;14(4):364–8.
6. Frontera JA. Clinical trials in cardiac arrest and subarachnoid hemorrhage: lessons from the past and ideas for the future. Stroke Res Treat 2013; 2013:263974.
7. Laver S, Farrow C, Turner D, et al. Mode of death after admission to an intensive care unit following

cardiac arrest. Intensive Care Med 2004;30(11): 2126–8.

8. Merchant RM, Becker LB, Abella BS, et al. Cost-effectiveness of therapeutic hypothermia after cardiac arrest. Circ Cardiovasc Qual Outcomes 2009; 2(5):421–8.

9. Rivera-Lara L, Zhang J, Muehlschlegel S. Therapeutic hypothermia for acute neurological injuries. Neurotherapeutics 2012;9(1):73–86.

10. Kochanek PM. Bakken lecture: the brain, the heart, and therapeutic hypothermia. Cleve Clin J Med 2009;76(Suppl 2):S8–12.

11. Polderman KH. Application of therapeutic hypothermia in the ICU: opportunities and pitfalls of a promising treatment modality. Part 1: indications and evidence. Intensive Care Med 2004;30(4):556–75.

12. Benson DW, Williams GR Jr, Spencer FC, et al. The use of hypothermia after cardiac arrest. Anesth Analg 1959;38:423–8.

13. Ravitch MM, Lane R, Safar P, et al. Lightning stroke. Report of a case with recovery after cardiac massage and prolonged artificial respiration. N Engl J Med 1961;264:36–8.

14. Williams GR Jr, Spencer FC. The clinical use of hypothermia following cardiac arrest. Ann Surg 1958; 148(3):462–8.

15. Fay T. Early experiences with local and generalized refrigeration of the human brain. J Neurosurg 1959; 16(3):239–59 [discussion: 259–60].

16. Safar P. Community-wide cardiopulmonary resuscitation. J Iowa Med Soc 1964;54:629–35.

17. Leonov Y, Sterz F, Safar P, et al. Mild cerebral hypothermia during and after cardiac arrest improves neurologic outcome in dogs. J Cereb Blood Flow Metab 1990;10(1):57–70.

18. Sterz F, Safar P, Tisherman S, et al. Mild hypothermic cardiopulmonary resuscitation improves outcome after prolonged cardiac arrest in dogs. Crit Care Med 1991;19(3):379–89.

19. Bernard SA, Jones BM, Horne MK. Clinical trial of induced hypothermia in comatose survivors of out-of-hospital cardiac arrest. Ann Emerg Med 1997;30(2):146–53.

20. Nagao K, Hayashi N, Kanmatsuse K, et al. Cardiopulmonary cerebral resuscitation using emergency cardiopulmonary bypass, coronary reperfusion therapy and mild hypothermia in patients with cardiac arrest outside the hospital. J Am Coll Cardiol 2000;36(3):776–83.

21. Yanagawa Y, Ishihara S, Norio H, et al. Preliminary clinical outcome study of mild resuscitative hypothermia after out-of-hospital cardiopulmonary arrest. Resuscitation 1998;39(1–2):61–6.

22. Hypothermia After Cardiac Arrest Study Group. Mild therapeutic hypothermia to improve the neurologic outcome after cardiac arrest. N Engl J Med 2002;346(8):549–56.

23. Bernard SA, Gray TW, Buist MD, et al. Treatment of comatose survivors of out-of-hospital cardiac arrest with induced hypothermia. N Engl J Med 2002;346(8):557–63.

24. Nolan JP, Morley PT, Vanden Hoek TL, et al. Therapeutic hypothermia after cardiac arrest: an advisory statement by the advanced life support task force of the International Liaison Committee on Resuscitation. Circulation 2003;108(1): 118–21.

25. ECC Committee, Subcommittees and Task Forces of the American Heart Association. 2005 American Heart Association Guidelines for Cardiopulmonary Resuscitation and Emergency Cardiovascular Care. Circulation 2005;112(24 Suppl):IV1–203.

26. Wagner SR, Lanier WL. Metabolism of glucose, glycogen, and high-energy phosphates during complete cerebral ischemia. A comparison of normoglycemic, chronically hyperglycemic diabetic, and acutely hyperglycemic nondiabetic rats. Anesthesiology 1994;81(6):1516–26.

27. Hoesch RE, Koenig MA, Geocadin RG. Coma after global ischemic brain injury: pathophysiology and emerging therapies. Crit Care Clin 2008; 24(1):25–44, vii–viii.

28. Redmond JM, Gillinov AM, Zehr KJ, et al. Glutamate excitotoxicity: a mechanism of neurologic injury associated with hypothermic circulatory arrest. J Thorac Cardiovasc Surg 1994;107(3):776–86 [discussion: 786–7].

29. Nolan JP, Neumar RW, Adrie C, et al. Post-cardiac arrest syndrome: epidemiology, pathophysiology, treatment, and prognostication: a scientific statement from the International Liaison Committee on Resuscitation; the American Heart Association Emergency Cardiovascular Care Committee; the Council on Cardiovascular Surgery and Anesthesia; the Council on Cardiopulmonary, Perioperative, and Critical Care; the Council on Clinical Cardiology; the Council on Stroke (Part II). Int Emerg Nurs 2010;18(1):8–28.

30. Hammer MD, Krieger DW. Hypothermia for acute ischemic stroke: not just another neuroprotectant. Neurologist 2003;9(6):280–9.

31. Alzaga AG, Cerdan M, Varon J. Therapeutic hypothermia. Resuscitation 2006;70(3):369–80.

32. Rosomoff HL, Holaday DA. Cerebral blood flow and cerebral oxygen consumption during hypothermia. Am J Physiol 1954;179(1):85–8.

33. Bisschops LL, Hoedemaekers CW, Simons KS, et al. Preserved metabolic coupling and cerebrovascular reactivity during mild hypothermia after cardiac arrest. Crit Care Med 2010;38(7):1542–7.

34. Bisschops LL, van der Hoeven JG, Hoedemaekers CW. Effects of prolonged mild hypothermia on cerebral blood flow after cardiac arrest. Crit Care Med 2012;40(8):2362–7.

35. Hachimi-Idrissi S, Van Hemelrijck A, Michotte A, et al. Postischemic mild hypothermia reduces neurotransmitter release and astroglial cell proliferation during reperfusion after asphyxial cardiac arrest in rats. Brain Res 2004;1019(1–2):217–25.

36. D'Cruz BJ, Fertig KC, Filiano AJ, et al. Hypothermic reperfusion after cardiac arrest augments brain-derived neurotrophic factor activation. J Cereb Blood Flow Metab 2002;22(7):843–51.

37. Lei B, Cai H, Xu Q, et al. Effect of moderate hypothermia on lipid peroxidation in canine brain tissue after cardiac arrest and resuscitation. Stroke 1994; 25(1):147–52.

38. Maier CM, Sun GH, Cheng D, et al. Effects of mild hypothermia on superoxide anion production, superoxide dismutase expression, and activity following transient focal cerebral ischemia. Neurobiol Dis 2002;11(1):28–42.

39. Eberspacher E, Werner C, Engelhard K, et al. Long-term effects of hypothermia on neuronal cell death and the concentration of apoptotic proteins after incomplete cerebral ischemia and reperfusion in rats. Acta Anaesthesiol Scand 2005; 49(4):477–87.

40. Aibiki M, Maekawa S, Ogura S, et al. Effect of moderate hypothermia on systemic and internal jugular plasma IL-6 levels after traumatic brain injury in humans. J Neurotrauma 1999;16(3):225–32.

41. Kimura A, Sakurada S, Ohkuni H, et al. Moderate hypothermia delays proinflammatory cytokine production of human peripheral blood mononuclear cells. Crit Care Med 2002;30(7):1499–502.

42. Webster CM, Kelly S, Koike MA, et al. Inflammation and NFkappaB activation is decreased by hypothermia following global cerebral ischemia. Neurobiol Dis 2009;33(2):301–12.

43. Karibe H, Zarow GJ, Graham SH, et al. Mild intraischemic hypothermia reduces postischemic hyperperfusion, delayed postischemic hypoperfusion, blood-brain barrier disruption, brain edema, and neuronal damage volume after temporary focal cerebral ischemia in rats. J Cereb Blood Flow Metab 1994;14(4):620–7.

44. Jurkovich GJ, Pitt RM, Curreri PW, et al. Hypothermia prevents increased capillary permeability following ischemia-reperfusion injury. J Surg Res 1988;44(5): 514–21.

45. Meaney PA, Nadkarni VM, Kern KB, et al. Rhythms and outcomes of adult in-hospital cardiac arrest. Crit Care Med 2010;38(1):101–8.

46. Nadkarni VM, Larkin GL, Peberdy MA, et al. First documented rhythm and clinical outcome from in-hospital cardiac arrest among children and adults. JAMA 2006;295(1):50–7.

47. Vayrynen T, Kuisma M, Maatta T, et al. Medical futility in asystolic out-of-hospital cardiac arrest. Acta Anaesthesiol Scand 2008;52(1):81–7.

48. Vayrynen T, Kuisma M, Maatta T, et al. Who survives from out-of-hospital pulseless electrical activity? Resuscitation 2008;76(2):207–13.

49. Stratton SJ, Niemann JT. Outcome from out-of-hospital cardiac arrest caused by nonventricular arrhythmias: contribution of successful resuscitation to overall survivorship supports the current practice of initiating out-of-hospital ACLS. Ann Emerg Med 1998;32(4):448–53.

50. Niemann JT, Stratton SJ, Cruz B, et al. Outcome of out-of-hospital postcountershock asystole and pulseless electrical activity versus primary asystole and pulseless electrical activity. Crit Care Med 2001;29(12):2366–70.

51. Lundbye JB, Rai M, Ramu B, et al. Therapeutic hypothermia is associated with improved neurologic outcome and survival in cardiac arrest survivors of non-shockable rhythms. Resuscitation 2012; 83(2):202–7.

52. Testori C, Sterz F, Behringer W, et al. Mild therapeutic hypothermia is associated with favourable outcome in patients after cardiac arrest with non-shockable rhythms. Resuscitation 2011;82(9): 1162–7.

53. Soga T, Nagao K, Sawano H, et al. Neurological benefit of therapeutic hypothermia following return of spontaneous circulation for out-of-hospital non-shockable cardiac arrest. Circ J 2012;76(11): 2579–85.

54. Dumas F, Grimaldi D, Zuber B, et al. Is hypothermia after cardiac arrest effective in both shockable and nonshockable patients?: insights from a large registry. Circulation 2011;123(8):877–86.

55. Storm C, Nee J, Roser M, et al. Mild hypothermia treatment in patients resuscitated from non-shockable cardiac arrest. Emerg Med J 2012; 29(2):100–3.

56. Kory P, Fukunaga M, Mathew JP, et al. Outcomes of mild therapeutic hypothermia after in-hospital cardiac arrest. Neurocrit Care 2012;16(3):406–12.

57. Kim YM, Yim HW, Jeong SH, et al. Does therapeutic hypothermia benefit adult cardiac arrest patients presenting with non-shockable initial rhythms?: A systematic review and meta-analysis of randomized and non-randomized studies. Resuscitation 2012;83(2):188–96.

58. Field JM, Hazinski MF, Sayre MR, et al. Part 1: executive summary: 2010 American Heart Association Guidelines for Cardiopulmonary Resuscitation and Emergency Cardiovascular Care. Circulation 2010;122(18 Suppl 3):S640–56.

59. Nolan JP, Soar J, Zideman DA, et al. European Resuscitation Council Guidelines for Resuscitation 2010 Section 1. Executive summary. Resuscitation 2010;81(10):1219–76.

60. Hazinski MF, Nolan JP, Billi JE, et al. Part 1: executive summary: 2010 International Consensus on

Cardiopulmonary Resuscitation and Emergency Cardiovascular Care Science With Treatment Recommendations. Circulation 2010;122(16 Suppl 2): S250–75.

61. Goldberger ZD, Chan PS, Berg RA, et al. Duration of resuscitation efforts and survival after in-hospital cardiac arrest: an observational study. Lancet 2012;380(9852):1473–81.

62. Colbourne F, Corbett D. Delayed postischemic hypothermia: a six month survival study using behavioral and histological assessments of neuroprotection. J Neurosci 1995;15(11):7250–60.

63. Kuboyama K, Safar P, Radovsky A, et al. Delay in cooling negates the beneficial effect of mild resuscitative cerebral hypothermia after cardiac arrest in dogs: a prospective, randomized study. Crit Care Med 1993;21(9):1348–58.

64. Tomte O, Draegni T, Mangschau A, et al. A comparison of intravascular and surface cooling techniques in comatose cardiac arrest survivors. Crit Care Med 2011;39(3):443–9.

65. Gillies MA, Pratt R, Whiteley C, et al. Therapeutic hypothermia after cardiac arrest: a retrospective comparison of surface and endovascular cooling techniques. Resuscitation 2010;81(9):1117–22.

66. Heard KJ, Peberdy MA, Sayre MR, et al. A randomized controlled trial comparing the Arctic Sun to standard cooling for induction of hypothermia after cardiac arrest. Resuscitation 2010;81(1): 9–14.

67. Mayer SA, Kowalski RG, Presciutti M, et al. Clinical trial of a novel surface cooling system for fever control in neurocritical care patients. Crit Care Med 2004;32(12):2508–15.

68. Kim F, Olsufka M, Longstreth WT Jr, et al. Pilot randomized clinical trial of prehospital induction of mild hypothermia in out-of-hospital cardiac arrest patients with a rapid infusion of 4 degrees C normal saline. Circulation 2007;115(24):3064–70.

69. Kliegel A, Losert H, Sterz F, et al. Cold simple intravenous infusions preceding special endovascular cooling for faster induction of mild hypothermia after cardiac arrest–a feasibility study. Resuscitation 2005;64(3):347–51.

70. Polderman KH, Rijnsburger ER, Peerdeman SM, et al. Induction of hypothermia in patients with various types of neurologic injury with use of large volumes of ice-cold intravenous fluid. Crit Care Med 2005;33(12):2744–51.

71. Polderman KH, Herold I. Therapeutic hypothermia and controlled normothermia in the intensive care unit: practical considerations, side effects, and cooling methods. Crit Care Med 2009;37(3):1101–20.

72. Rittenberger JC, Polderman KH, Smith WS, et al. Emergency neurological life support: resuscitation following cardiac arrest. Neurocrit Care 2012; 17(Suppl 1):S21–8.

73. Lopez-de-Sa E, Rey JR, Armada E, et al. Hypothermia in comatose survivors from out-of-hospital cardiac arrest: pilot trial comparing 2 levels of target temperature. Circulation 2012;126(24):2826–33.

74. Alam HB, Rhee P, Honma K, et al. Does the rate of rewarming from profound hypothermic arrest influence the outcome in a swine model of lethal hemorrhage? J Trauma 2006;60(1):134–46.

75. Bissonnette B, Holtby HM, Davis AJ, et al. Cerebral hyperthermia in children after cardiopulmonary bypass. Anesthesiology 2000;93(3):611–8.

76. Hildebrand F, van Griensven M, Giannoudis P, et al. Effects of hypothermia and re-warming on the inflammatory response in a murine multiple hit model of trauma. Cytokine 2005;31(5):382–93.

77. Kawahara F, Kadoi Y, Saito S, et al. Slow rewarming improves jugular venous oxygen saturation during rewarming. Acta Anaesthesiol Scand 2003;47(4): 419–24.

78. Maxwell WL, Watson A, Queen R, et al. Slow, medium, or fast re-warming following post-traumatic hypothermia therapy? An ultrastructural perspective. J Neurotrauma 2005;22(8):873–84.

79. Bisschops LL, Hoedemaekers CW, Mollnes TE, et al. Rewarming after hypothermia after cardiac arrest shifts the inflammatory balance. Crit Care Med 2012;40(4):1136–42.

80. Polderman KH. Mechanisms of action, physiological effects, and complications of hypothermia. Crit Care Med 2009;37(Suppl 7):S186–202.

81. Zeiner A, Holzer M, Sterz F, et al. Hyperthermia after cardiac arrest is associated with an unfavorable neurologic outcome. Arch Intern Med 2001; 161(16):2007–12.

82. Erickson RS, Kirklin SK. Comparison of ear-based, bladder, oral, and axillary methods for core temperature measurement. Crit Care Med 1993;21(10): 1528–34.

83. Robinson J, Charlton J, Seal R, et al. Oesophageal, rectal, axillary, tympanic and pulmonary artery temperatures during cardiac surgery. Can J Anaesth 1998;45(4):317–23.

84. Akata T, Setoguchi H, Shirozu K, et al. Reliability of temperatures measured at standard monitoring sites as an index of brain temperature during deep hypothermic cardiopulmonary bypass conducted for thoracic aortic reconstruction. J Thorac Cardiovasc Surg 2007;133(6):1559–65.

85. Sessler DI. Defeating normal thermoregulatory defenses: induction of therapeutic hypothermia. Stroke 2009;40(11):e614–21.

86. De Witte J, Sessler DI. Perioperative shivering: physiology and pharmacology. Anesthesiology 2002;96(2):467–84.

87. Frank SM, Beattie C, Christopherson R, et al. Unintentional hypothermia is associated with postoperative myocardial ischemia. The Perioperative

Ischemia Randomized Anesthesia Trial Study Group. Anesthesiology 1993;78(3):468–76.

88. Frank SM, Fleisher LA, Breslow MJ, et al. Perioperative maintenance of normothermia reduces the incidence of morbid cardiac events. A randomized clinical trial. JAMA 1997;277(14):1127–34.

89. Leslie K, Sessler DI. Perioperative hypothermia in the high-risk surgical patient. Best Pract Res Clin Anaesthesiol 2003;17(4):485–98.

90. Thoresen M, Satas S, Loberg EM, et al. Twenty-four hours of mild hypothermia in unsedated newborn pigs starting after a severe global hypoxic-ischemic insult is not neuroprotective. Pediatr Res 2001;50(3):405–11.

91. Tooley JR, Satas S, Porter H, et al. Head cooling with mild systemic hypothermia in anesthetized piglets is neuroprotective. Ann Neurol 2003;53(1):65–72.

92. Oddo M, Frangos S, Maloney-Wilensky E, et al. Effect of shivering on brain tissue oxygenation during induced normothermia in patients with severe brain injury. Neurocrit Care 2010;12(1):10–6.

93. Badjatia N, Strongilis E, Gordon E, et al. Metabolic impact of shivering during therapeutic temperature modulation: the bedside shivering assessment scale. Stroke 2008;39(12):3242–7.

94. Badjatia N, Kowalski RG, Schmidt JM, et al. Predictors and clinical implications of shivering during therapeutic normothermia. Neurocrit Care 2007;6(3):186–91.

95. Wadhwa A, Sengupta P, Durrani J, et al. Magnesium sulphate only slightly reduces the shivering threshold in humans. Br J Anaesth 2005;94(6):756–62.

96. Zweifler RM, Voorhees ME, Mahmood MA, et al. Magnesium sulfate increases the rate of hypothermia via surface cooling and improves comfort. Stroke 2004;35(10):2331–4.

97. Badjatia N, Strongilis E, Prescutti M, et al. Metabolic benefits of surface counter warming during therapeutic temperature modulation. Crit Care Med 2009;37(6):1893–7.

98. Kimberger O, Ali SZ, Markstaller M, et al. Meperidine and skin surface warming additively reduce the shivering threshold: a volunteer study. Crit Care 2007;11(1):R29.

99. van Zanten AR, Polderman KH. Blowing hot and cold? Skin counter warming to prevent shivering during therapeutic cooling. Crit Care Med 2009;37(6):2106–8.

100. Frank SM, Raja SN, Bulcao CF, et al. Relative contribution of core and cutaneous temperatures to thermal comfort and autonomic responses in humans. J Appl Physiol 1999;86(5):1588–93.

101. Taniguchi Y, Lenhardt R, Sessler DI, et al. The effect of altering skin-surface cooling speeds on vasoconstriction and shivering thresholds. Anesth Analg 2011;113(3):540–4.

102. Hovdenes J, Laake JH, Aaberge L, et al. Therapeutic hypothermia after out-of-hospital cardiac arrest: experiences with patients treated with percutaneous coronary intervention and cardiogenic shock. Acta Anaesthesiol Scand 2007;51(2):137–42.

103. Oddo M, Schaller MD, Feihl F, et al. From evidence to clinical practice: effective implementation of therapeutic hypothermia to improve patient outcome after cardiac arrest. Crit Care Med 2006;34(7):1865–73.

104. Skulec R, Kovarnik T, Dostalova G, et al. Induction of mild hypothermia in cardiac arrest survivors presenting with cardiogenic shock syndrome. Acta Anaesthesiol Scand 2008;52(2):188–94.

105. Batista LM, Lima FO, Januzzi JL Jr, et al. Feasibility and safety of combined percutaneous coronary intervention and therapeutic hypothermia following cardiac arrest. Resuscitation 2010;81(4):398–403.

106. Kandzari DE, Chu A, Brodie BR, et al. Feasibility of endovascular cooling as an adjunct to primary percutaneous coronary intervention (results of the LOWTEMP pilot study). Am J Cardiol 2004;93(5):636–9.

107. Knafelj R, Radsel P, Ploj T, et al. Primary percutaneous coronary intervention and mild induced hypothermia in comatose survivors of ventricular fibrillation with ST-elevation acute myocardial infarction. Resuscitation 2007;74(2):227–34.

108. Ly HQ, Denault A, Dupuis J, et al. A pilot study: the Noninvasive Surface Cooling Thermoregulatory System for Mild Hypothermia Induction in Acute Myocardial Infarction (the NICAMI Study). Am Heart J 2005;150(5):933.

109. Maze R, Le May MR, Hibbert B, et al. The impact of therapeutic hypothermia as adjunctive therapy in a regional primary PCI program. Resuscitation 2013;84(4):460–4.

110. Nielsen N, Hovdenes J, Nilsson F, et al. Outcome, timing and adverse events in therapeutic hypothermia after out-of-hospital cardiac arrest. Acta Anaesthesiol Scand 2009;53(7):926–34.

111. Sunde K, Pytte M, Jacobsen D, et al. Implementation of a standardised treatment protocol for post resuscitation care after out-of-hospital cardiac arrest. Resuscitation 2007;73(1):29–39.

112. Wolfrum S, Pierau C, Radke PW, et al. Mild therapeutic hypothermia in patients after out-of-hospital cardiac arrest due to acute ST-segment elevation myocardial infarction undergoing immediate percutaneous coronary intervention. Crit Care Med 2008;36(6):1780–6.

113. Voipio V, Kuisma M, Alaspaa A, et al. Thrombolytic treatment of acute myocardial infarction after out-of-hospital cardiac arrest. Resuscitation 2001;49(3):251–8.

114. Weston CF, Avery P. Thrombolysis following pre-hospital cardiopulmonary resuscitation. Int J Cardiol 1992;37(2):195–8.

115. Wijdicks EF, Hijdra A, Young GB, et al. Practice parameter: prediction of outcome in comatose survivors after cardiopulmonary resuscitation (an evidence-based review): report of the Quality Standards Subcommittee of the American Academy of Neurology. Neurology 2006;67(2):203–10.

116. Levy DE, Caronna JJ, Singer BH, et al. Predicting outcome from hypoxic-ischemic coma. JAMA 1985;253(10):1420–6.

117. Fugate JE, Brinjikji W, Mandrekar JN, et al. Post-cardiac arrest mortality is declining: a study of the US National Inpatient Sample 2001 to 2009. Circulation 2012;126(5):546–50.

118. Girotra S, Nallamothu BK, Spertus JA, et al. Trends in survival after in-hospital cardiac arrest. N Engl J Med 2012;367(20):1912–20.

119. Nichol G, Thomas E, Callaway CW, et al. Regional variation in out-of-hospital cardiac arrest incidence and outcome. JAMA 2008;300(12):1423–31.

120. Reinikainen M, Oksanen T, Leppanen P, et al. Mortality in out-of-hospital cardiac arrest patients has decreased in the era of therapeutic hypothermia. Acta Anaesthesiol Scand 2012;56(1):110–5.

121. van der Wal G, Brinkman S, Bisschops LL, et al. Influence of mild therapeutic hypothermia after cardiac arrest on hospital mortality. Crit Care Med 2011;39(1):84–8.

122. Tagami T, Hirata K, Takeshige T, et al. Implementation of the fifth link of the chain of survival concept for out-of-hospital cardiac arrest. Circulation 2012;126(5):589–97.

123. Heffner AC, Pearson DA, Nussbaum ML, et al. Regionalization of post-cardiac arrest care: implementation of a cardiac resuscitation center. Am Heart J 2012;164(4):493–501.e2.

124. Jena AB, Romley JA, Newton-Cheh C, et al. Therapeutic hypothermia for cardiac arrest: real-world utilization trends and hospital mortality. J Hosp Med 2012;7(9):684–9.

125. Lick CJ, Aufderheide TP, Niskanen RA, et al. Take Heart America: a comprehensive, community-wide, systems-based approach to the treatment of cardiac arrest. Crit Care Med 2011;39(1):26–33.

126. Oksanen T, Pettilä V, Hynynen M, et al. Therapeutic hypothermia after cardiac arrest: implementation and outcome in Finnish intensive care units. Acta Anaesthesiol Scand 2007;51(7):866–71.

127. Patil S, Bhayani S, Denton JM, et al. Therapeutic hypothermia for out-of-hospital cardiac arrest: implementation in a district general hospital emergency department. Emerg Med J 2011;28(11):970–3.

128. Stub D, Bernard S, Smith K, et al. Do we need cardiac arrest centres in Australia? Intern Med J 2012;42(11):1173–9.

129. Kajino K, Iwami T, Daya M, et al. Impact of transport to critical care medical centers on outcomes after out-of-hospital cardiac arrest. Resuscitation 2010;81(5):549–54.

130. Mooney MR, Unger BT, Boland LL, et al. Therapeutic hypothermia after out-of-hospital cardiac arrest: evaluation of a regional system to increase access to cooling. Circulation 2011;124(2):206–14.

131. Roberts BW, Kilgannon JH, Mitchell JA, et al. Emergency department inter-hospital transfer for post-cardiac arrest care: initial experience with implementation of a regional cardiac resuscitation center in the United States. Resuscitation 2013;84(5):596–601.

132. Stub D, Smith K, Bray JE, et al. Hospital characteristics are associated with patient outcomes following out-of-hospital cardiac arrest. Heart 2011;97(18):1489–94.

133. Busl KM, Greer DM. Hypoxic-ischemic brain injury: pathophysiology, neuropathology and mechanisms. NeuroRehabilitation 2010;26(1):5–13.

134. Chiota NA, Freeman WD, Barrett KM. Hypoxic-Ischemic brain injury and prognosis after cardiac arrest. Continuum (Minneap Minn) 2011;17(5 Neurologic Consultation in the Hospital):1094–118.

135. Karanjia N, Geocadin RG. Post-cardiac arrest syndrome: update on brain injury management and prognostication. Curr Treat Options Neurol 2011;13(2):191–203.

136. Al Thenayan E, Savard M, Sharpe M, et al. Predictors of poor neurologic outcome after induced mild hypothermia following cardiac arrest. Neurology 2008;71(19):1535–7.

137. Cronberg T, Rundgren M, Westhall E, et al. Neuron-specific enolase correlates with other prognostic markers after cardiac arrest. Neurology 2011;77(7):623–30.

138. Rossetti AO, Oddo M, Logroscino G, et al. Prognostication after cardiac arrest and hypothermia: a prospective study. Ann Neurol 2010;67(3):301–7.

139. Rossetti AO, Urbano LA, Delodder F, et al. Prognostic value of continuous EEG monitoring during therapeutic hypothermia after cardiac arrest. Crit Care 2010;14(5):R173.

140. Rossetti AO, Oddo M, Liaudet L, et al. Predictors of awakening from postanoxic status epilepticus after therapeutic hypothermia. Neurology 2009;72(8):744–9.

141. Bouwes A, Binnekade JM, Kuiper MA, et al. Prognosis of coma after therapeutic hypothermia: a prospective cohort study. Ann Neurol 2012;71(2):206–12.

142. Leithner C, Ploner CJ, Hasper D, et al. Does hypothermia influence the predictive value of bilateral absent N20 after cardiac arrest? Neurology 2010;74(12):965–9.

143. Oksanen T, Tiainen M, Skrifvars MB, et al. Predictive power of serum NSE and OHCA score regarding 6-month neurologic outcome after out-of-hospital ventricular fibrillation and therapeutic hypothermia. Resuscitation 2009;80(2):165–70.

144. Fugate JE, Wijdicks EF, Mandrekar J, et al. Predictors of neurologic outcome in hypothermia after cardiac arrest. Ann Neurol 2010;68(6):907–14.

145. Steffen IG, Hasper D, Ploner CJ, et al. Mild therapeutic hypothermia alters neuron specific enolase as an outcome predictor after resuscitation: 97 prospective hypothermia patients compared to 133 historical non-hypothermia patients. Crit Care 2010;14(2):R69.

146. Wijman CA, Mlynash M, Caulfield AF, et al. Prognostic value of brain diffusion-weighted imaging after cardiac arrest. Ann Neurol 2009;65(4):394–402.

147. Rossetti AO, Carrera E, Oddo M. Early EEG correlates of neuronal injury after brain anoxia. Neurology 2012;78(11):796–802.

148. Fugate JE, Wijdicks EF, White RD, et al. Does therapeutic hypothermia affect time to awakening in cardiac arrest survivors? Neurology 2011;77(14):1346–50.

149. Crepeau AZ, Rabinstein AA, Fugate JE, et al. Continuous EEG in therapeutic hypothermia after cardiac arrest: prognostic and clinical value. Neurology 2013;80(4):339–44.

Ethical Issues and Palliative Care in the Cardiovascular Intensive Care Unit

Keith M. Swetz, MD, MA[a,b],*, J. Keith Mansel, MD[a,b]

KEYWORDS

- Medical ethics • Bioethics • Palliative care • Advanced heart failure • Medical technology
- End of life

KEY POINTS

- Palliative care has been shown to improve outcomes for patients in the intensive care unit (ICU), particularly in improving symptom control and satisfaction with care plans.
- Patients who are hospitalized in the ICU should have a care conference to define the goals of care within 5 days of admission, and have such meetings every 7 days during their stay in the ICU, not to discuss "withdrawal of support" but rather to focus on the complexity of multidisciplinary care.
- It is morally and ethically permissible to withhold a treatment or withdraw a treatment once started if it is not consistent with a patient's goals of care, and granting such requests is not akin to euthanasia. Such treatment includes cardiac devices such as pacemakers, defibrillators, ventricular assist devices, and total artificial hearts.
- Advance care planning can be helpful in avoiding ethical dilemmas, particularly related to issues of surrogate decision making and goals of care, when patients are critically ill and possibly approaching the end of life. Ongoing discussion and reassessment of goals is critical to patient-centered outcomes.
- There is a distinct difference between hospice and palliative care in that palliative care can be provided at any point in the continuum of illness and is not synonymous with dying or "giving up."

INTRODUCTION

Millions of Americans suffer from life-limiting, life-threatening illnesses caused by a vast array of cardiovascular maladies.[1] Although a large portion of this population suffers from advanced heart failure often related to ischemic heart disease, other congenital, electrophysiologic, and structural cardiac issues contribute to significant morbidity and mortality. Over the past few decades, there has been a relative explosion of pharmacologic and therapeutic interventions that have dramatically altered the course of many of these complicated cardiac ailments. Beyond medications, technology has advanced, providing an unfathomable array of devices that can improve symptom burden and survival for patients who previously had fatal cardiac diseases.

Funding Sources: Mayo Clinic, Department of Medicine.
Conflict of Interest: None.
a Section of Palliative Medicine, Division of General Internal Medicine, Department of Medicine, Mayo Clinic College of Medicine, Mayo Clinic, 200 First Street Southwest, Rochester, MN 55905, USA; b Program in Professionalism and Ethics, Mayo Clinic College of Medicine, Mayo Clinic, 200 First Street Southwest, Rochester, MN 55905, USA
* Corresponding author. Section of Palliative Medicine, Mayo Clinic, 200 First Street Southwest, Rochester, MN 55905.
E-mail address: swetz.keith@mayo.edu

The growth of treatment options and the associated *technological imperative* to use these treatments has essentially defined the average daily census in the modern cardiovascular intensive care unit (CICU).[2,3] The care of patients in the CICU has evolved since the days of almost certain death from cardiac illness owing to lack of effective therapies, or several weeks of close "observation" following a major acute coronary syndrome that was the norm decades earlier.

Today's CICU is a fast-paced, increasingly complex milieu where clinicians, patients, and their loved ones attempt to make the best decisions possible from a vast array of pharmacologic, surgical, and interventional therapies, each with a unique set of risks and benefits. Patients are faced with numerous decision points in situations where health is unstable and emotions and stakes are high, which can lead to a host of ethical conundrums. All of this occurs against a background of uncertainty, particularly regarding our ability to accurately prognosticate in these complex situations with therapies that are ever evolving.

Despite major successes regarding survival and length of stay of patients in the CICU, this remains an area where ethical challenges are frequently encountered and where palliative care opportunities remain plentiful. This article presents an overview of some of the ethical and palliative care issues encountered in the CICU, with recommendations for initial approaches to these issues and consideration of when specialist involvement by an ethics or palliative medicine consultation may be warranted.

ETHICAL ISSUES IN THE CICU

As discussed in the introduction, there are countless treatments available in the setting of advanced cardiac illnesses. Indeed, the topics covered throughout in this issue of *Cardiology Clinics* discuss many of these technological triumphs. In its most basic sense, medical ethics strives to go beyond the question of what we *can* do in a clinical situation, and rather seeks solutions to the questions of what we *should* do. As there may be varying competing ideals about what the goals of medicine are and how those can be best achieved, there may be inherent tension created out of a desire to satisfy those competing ideals.

Beauchamp and Childress[4] are credited with a widely used approach to ethical issues known as principlism or the 4-principle approach, whereby each of the benefits in a situation is evaluated. Their approach focuses on consideration of

beneficence (our desire to do good for the patients), nonmaleficence (our desire to avoid harming patients), respect for the patient's autonomy, and an evaluation of issues of justice in how care is provided. As one can imagine, care in the CICU often pits many of these ideals against one another.

Consider the following case vignette. An 81-year-old man is admitted to the CICU with high-grade heart block and is being considered for implantation of a permanent implantable pacemaker. Telemetry confirms the finding and the patient's heart rate can only be sufficiently augmented by use of transvenous pacing, suggesting the need for an implantable device. The patient's history is notable for advanced dementia whereby he lives in a care facility and can speak only a few words, only intermittently recognizes his 2 daughters, and does not participate in activities of daily living. Both daughters are the patient's duly appointed surrogate decision makers by an advance directive if the patient lacks capacity. What should the next step be?

This situation, or a similar one, may be very familiar to the reader. Several aspects of the case could be in conflict and need to be considered before a course of action can be decided upon. Determining what is "best" for the patient, what may help or harm the patient, and what quality of life exists for this patient are questions that consider beneficence and nonmaleficence. In considering autonomy, one may ask questions regarding whether the patient has the capacity to make a decision, who the surrogate decision maker should be if the patient lacks decision-making capacity, and how to approach situations whereby surrogates are in conflict with each other.

Justice, however, involve a more global and society-wide approach to ethical issues. Questioning whether placement of the pacemaker is fair and equitable in this situation does not affect whether it is fair and equitable for *this* patient to receive a device. Rather, such questions should be posed at a societal level to determine if certain criteria should be in place that guide whether the pacemaker is fair and equitable across the medical landscape. This point is important to consider because justice issues are often invoked at the bedside, although clinicians should not consider these resource utilization issues in the context of an isolated patient encounter.

This case vignette represents one example of the clinical challenges encountered in the CICU. While the issues presented do illustrate complexity in medical decision making and the role of technology in patient care, this case may fall on the side of jejune relative to cases encountered in the modern CICU. Pacemakers and implantable cardioverter-defibrillators represent technology that has, in essence, become the standard of care for many patients with cardiac disease who meet set criteria. Some may question whether there is a moral obligation to treat this patient with a life-sustaining treatment if it is available. It has been largely decided that patients maintain the right to refuse medical treatment for which the benefits of the treatment outweigh the burdens (**Table 1**). This right to refuse treatment applies not only to withholding medical therapies but also to withdrawing such therapies if they no longer meet the patient's goals of care. This issue is discussed later in this article.

Lastly, many challenging encounters involve the use of technology with increasing cost and burden to the patient and caregiver (eg, mechanical circulatory support or renal replacement therapy), and often occur in the setting of multiple medical morbidities, uncertainty or lack of clarity regarding prognosis, and other psychosocial, financial, cultural, and religious challenges. Indeed, prognosis may vary widely and can be challenging to predict, particularly in diseases such as advanced heart failure that are punctuated by recurrent exacerbations, as opposed to other organ-failure syndromes or cancer that may have a more predictable decline (**Fig. 1**). In these situations, involvement of an ethics or palliative medicine consultant may be helpful in nuancing these challenges, particularly when they involve end-of-life decision making.

ADVANCE CARE PLANNING AND SHARED DECISION MAKING

The Patient Self-Determination Act of 1991 sought to solidify a patient's ability to name a surrogate decision maker and to complete advance directive documents, although the benefit of such documents has been questioned.[5] These documents seek to allow patients to consider potential future health care situations but, unfortunately, patients may still struggle with making decisions "in the moment."[5] The American Heart Association (AHA) released a scientific statement in 2012 focusing on the challenges and opportunities for promotion of decision making in advanced heart failure.[6] This document expertly outlines key approaches to promoting patient-centered outcomes.[6]

The AHA guidelines emphasize to clinicians the need to consider all outcomes relevant to an individual patient to promote patient autonomy and maximum good, while minimizing harm to patients. It is noteworthy that the benefits to a given patient go beyond the survival benefit a treatment may promote. Quality of life and the costs and benefits to patients may be equally or more important than survival benefit, and these aspects must be explored when clinicians seek informed consent from patients and their surrogates.[6] A clinician's understanding of how survival, quality of life, and benefits/burdens of treatment affect why patients and surrogates make the decisions that they do is important for considering another often cited ethical issue in the CICU—futility—which is discussed in the next section.

Table 1
Spectrum of ethical care at the end of life

	Withhold LST	Withdraw LST	Palliative Sedation	Physician Aid in Dying	Euthanasia
Cause of death	Underlying disease	Underlying disease	Underlying disease[a]	Intervention prescribed by physician and used by patient	Intervention used by physician
Intent/goal of intervention	Avoid burdensome intervention	Remove burdensome intervention	Relieve symptoms	Termination of patient's life	Termination of patient's life
Legal?	Yes[b]	Yes[b]	Yes	Limited by jurisdiction[c]	No

Abbreviation: LST, life-sustaining treatment.
[a] Note "double effect."
[b] Several states limit the power of surrogate decision makers regarding LSTs.
[c] Legal only in states of Oregon, Washington, Montana, and Vermont in the United States (other states exploring).
Adapted from Olsen ML, Swetz KM, Mueller PS. Ethical decision making with end-of-life care: palliative sedation and withholding or withdrawing life-sustaining treatments. Mayo Clin Proc 2010;85(10):952; with permission.

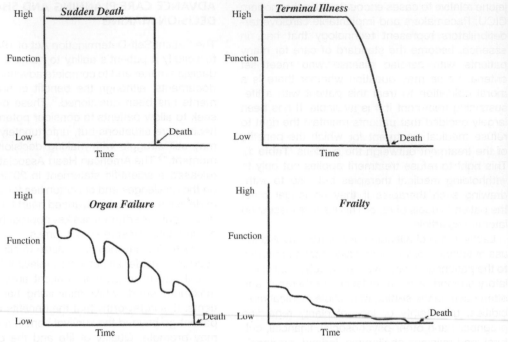

Fig. 1. Proposed trajectories of patients approaching the end of life. (*From* Lunney JR, Lynn J, Hogan C. Profiles of older Medicare decedents. J Am Geriatr Soc 2002;50(6):1109; with permission.)

FUTILITY

The term "futility" is often clinically invoked when a seriously ill patient has a low likelihood of a meaningful recovery. What defines recovery and what the goals of care are vary from patient to patient. The dictionary definition of the term "futile" is "incapable of producing any result; ineffective; useless; not successful,"[7] and in exploring this definition one may note that it is rarely, if ever, a maxim.

Situations that invoke questions about futility are ubiquitous in the CICU. Chronic critical illness has resulted from a dramatic improvement in health care delivery, particularly technology and therapeutic options, most notably over the past half century. Before the development of mechanical circulatory support, ventilators, hemodialysis, and so forth, patients would die of advanced organ-system or multiorgan system failure not compatible with survival. However, patients can survive for extended and indefinite (but not infinite) time frames through heroic measures, which can be of great cost (25% of Medicare dollars are spent in the last year of life).[8]

Furthermore, beyond costs, clinicians, nurses, and others may experience moral distress,[9] and question whether they are showing beneficence toward patients or violating nonmalificence. Clinicians may question whether a plan of care is contributing to a successful outcome, what an accurate prognosis might be and whether everyone appreciates it, or whether it is moral or ethical to continue to offer aggressive measures with limited gains.

Jurisdictions, such as the state of Texas, have passed legislation that operationalizes the definition of "futility" and allows for health care providers, through a due-process approach, to withdraw life-sustaining measures if they are not meeting set medical objectives.[10] Hospitals are essential, given the right to establish "futility" policies to determine if appropriate care is being given and if that care should be stopped, which is not the norm across the current American medical landscape.

It is well recognized that physicians are not obligated to provide nonbeneficial treatments, with a simple example being the right to refuse a request of antibiotics for a viral syndrome.[11,12] Similarly, the Texas statute places limits on requests for treatments that are unlikely to be beneficial. Schneiderman and colleagues[13] contend that physicians "can judge a treatment to be futile and are entitled to withhold a procedure on this basis" alone, and add that if experientially a treatment has worked (or not) in the past 100 times it has been tried, a given physician should have an idea whether a treatment is likely to be beneficial. Although more widespread statutes support clinicians in withholding provisions such as cardiopulmonary resuscitation if judged to be nonbeneficial,[14] the courts outside of Texas have ruled in other cases that measures of disputed efficacy should not be stopped unilaterally.[15,16]

It is often helpful to consider the concept of futility in 3 major domains: physiologic, quantitative, and qualitative.[17] Physiologic futility examines whether a treatment or technology is efficacious in meeting its intended purpose on a given patient. Common examples of whether a treatment is physiologically meeting its goal include if a vasopressor is keeping blood pressure stable, if dialysis is adequately replacing renal function, or if a ventricular assist is supporting cardiac output and reversing cardiogenic shock. However, the quantitative and qualitative aspects of "futility" are much more difficult for a clinician to parse out, as they harbor considerable components of value judgments.[17] Qualitative futility is only met if a treatment is not allowing a patient to live his or her life according to his or her standards and goals of care.

Using the case example discussed earlier, defining what "the value of a life" is (or is not) is not something to be determined clinically, or by how the last 100 patients responded in a given situation. These authors contend that it is a sacred, individual responsibility of clinicians to carry out their fiduciary responsibility to the patient, to determine if a treatment is meeting a patient's goals of care. Life in the intensive care unit (ICU) may not be desirable for the majority of society, but this is a value judgment, whether or not the quality of life is acceptable. If life is sacred and valued at any cost for a given patient, then 6 months in the ICU may be perfectly in concordance with a patient's goals of care.

Similarly, quantitative futility is also value laden. How much time one "gets" out of a treatment is variable, and to gain 1 day, 1 week, 1 month, or 1 year of life under any circumstance may allow a patient to meet the goals of care: one more discussion to be had, a family event to attend, or likewise. These 3 aspects of futility are well summarized by Edmund Pellegrino's[18,19] moral analysis of withdrawal of life-sustaining treatments: the efficacy of a treatment is for clinicians to assess and comment on, but the burdens and benefits of a treatment (in terms of its quantitative or qualitative goals) is in the purview of the patient.

To proceed with a due-process futility policy such as Texas's law prioritizes a primary focus on the physiologic efficacy of a treatment, which may lead to an incomplete understanding of the patient, his or her family, and their world view. Pellegrino asserts that a definition of futility "must be a joint determination of the physician and patient or surrogate, and that futility is a prudential judgment based on our best, but fallible, assessment of the beneficial clinical outcome versus the burden of a treatment."[20]

Given the complexity of these situations, one may wonder whether it is helpful to consider if a treatment is "futile." Nevertheless, if providers are considering a treatment as potentially being futile, this may be a signal to avoid using such value-laden terms and instead explore a patient's goals of care in a meaningful fashion.[19]

INTERFACE OF ETHICS AND CARE AT THE END OF LIFE

As discussed thus far, there is often substantial overlap between ethical issues at the end of life in the CICU and if and when palliative care may be appropriate. Ethics and palliative care consultants can be helpful in cases where there is lack of clarity regarding goals of care or the best way to achieve symptom control. The following sections discuss what palliative care is, how it is delivered, and how it may be beneficial to patients in the CICU.

WHAT IS PALLIATIVE CARE?

Palliative care (from the Latin word *palliare*, "to cloak") is a domain of health care that in its simplest definition focuses on the prevention and relief of suffering. Palliative medicine uses an interdisciplinary team approach (including physicians, mid-level providers, nurses, social workers, pharmacists, chaplains, and other allied health professionals) to focus on patients with life-limiting medical conditions with symptom burden. The palliative care approach is a holistic one that focuses on the physical, spiritual, emotional, and social distress experienced by patients and their loved ones. The concepts of palliative care are often presented along with disease-specific therapy, and such therapies are ramped up when less effective disease-targeted treatments are available (**Fig. 2**).

The most recent advances in palliative care date to the mid-twentieth century and John Bonica's first textbook of pain medicine published in 1953.[21] This interest in alleviation in suffering coincided with the emergence of Dame Cicely Saunders, a former nurse and social worker who later returned to medical school and opened the world's first modern hospice at Saint Christopher's in South London in 1967, and who is considered the founder of the modern hospice movement. Dr Balfour Mount coined the term "Palliative Care" in 1974. The most recent definition of

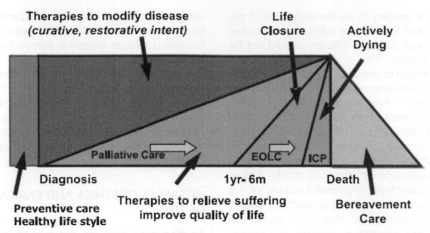

Fig. 2. Care across a patient's life span. EOLC, end-of-life care; ICP, integrated care pathway. (*From* Macaden SC. Moving toward a national policy on palliative and end of life care. Indian J Palliat Care 2011;17(Suppl):S42–4; with permission.)

palliative care is provided from the World Health Organization:

Palliative Care is an approach that improves the quality of life of patients and their families facing the problems associated with life-threatening illness, through the prevention and relief of suffering by means of early identification and impeccable assessment and treatment of pain and other problems, physical, psychosocial, and spiritual.[22]

Grounded in the definition, one can consider the role that palliative medicine may play in the ICU. As there is a growing body of literature regarding palliative care in the ICU in general, these data are presented for consideration of how the approach might work in the CICU.

WHY PALLIATIVE CARE IN THE ICU AND HOW CAN IT RELATE TO CARE IN THE CICU?

The topic of providing palliative care to patients requiring ICU-level care is a timely topic that has engaged the interest of both the medical profession and the lay public. Recent data suggest that more than 20% of Americans who die each year (approximately 500,000 people annually) die in, or shortly after, ICU care.[23] In addition, there are approximately 100,000 ICU survivors each year who suffer heavy symptom burdens on a chronic basis.[23]

The role of palliative care in the ICU is not only to provide symptom management at life's end, but also to help align the patient's goals and values with the clinical realties and to provide guidance and support for both patients and families. Most would agree that patients and families often desire both active treatment and concurrent relief of symptoms, but fewer realize that palliative care and critical care are often mutually enhancing rather than exclusive.

Other reasons to provide palliative care in the ICU include difficulties with prognostication and alignment of desired goals with realistic possibilities regarding clinical outcomes. Indeed, studies[24–27] have defined gaps in palliative care and the care of critically ill patients in the ICU, including the following:

- Untreated pain and other symptoms
- Unmet needs for care of families and loved ones
- Inadequate communication
- Conflict resolution among clinicians, patients, and families
- Divergence of treatment goals from patients and family preferences
- Inefficient resource utilization
- Clinician "moral distress" and burnout

In addition to potential benefits conferred to clinicians, patients, and families, resource utilization and cost savings may be associated with palliative care consultation in the ICU. Studies have documented reduced length of stay and up to $7700 reduced cost for patients receiving palliative care consultation while in the ICU.[28] Most importantly, in times when concerns over rationing and "death panels" are often invoked, it is crucial that these palliative care benefits have occurred without any documented increase in mortality.[28]

Successful communication between clinicians and families is often challenging in the care of critically ill patients. It is often noted that both patients and families have an inadequate understanding of the plan of care, and physicians often have limited time to reflectively listen and provide feedback.

Unfortunately, care conferences or family meetings are not timely, if they occur at all. To help strengthen the clinical care of patients in the ICU and further improve communication, a "Care and Communication Bundle," which includes 9 core Palliative Care Quality Measures, has been developed (Table 2).[29] These items provide a time frame within which clinicians should approach key palliative care–related elements in the ICU. How these measures should be tracked and how services could be provided in the CICU is discussed next.

STRUCTURING PALLIATIVE CARE IN THE CICU

Palliative care teams traditionally have participated as integrated or consultative roles in the ICU.[30] Both the integrated and consultative functions have advantages and disadvantages, and should not be considered mutually exclusive. The consultative role provided by a palliative care consulting service can provide expert skills using an interdisciplinary team, and provide continuity and transitions during and after ICU discharge. This type of model, however, does require increases in staffing and other resources needed for an interdisciplinary team. In addition, some

Table 2 Palliative care quality measures and goals for ICU care (Care and Communication Bundle measures)	
Goal of Meeting Target on or Before Listed Day of ICU Admission	**Care and Communication Bundle Measures**
Day 1	Identify medical decision maker Address advance directive status Address cardiopulmonary resuscitation status Distribute information leaflet to family Assess pain and other symptoms regularly Manage pain optimally
Day 3	Offer social work support Offer spiritual support
Day 5	Interdisciplinary family meeting

Data from Nelson JE, Mulkerin CM, Adams LL, et al. Improving comfort and communication in the ICU: a practical new tool for palliative care performance measurement and feedback. Qual Saf Health Care 2006;15(4): 264–71.

cardiovascular and critical care specialists in the CICU may feel comfortable in their ability to provide palliative care. In this situation the role of the palliative care clinician may be less well defined, which can lead to fragmentation of care and suboptimal communication.

Alternatively, an integrated model allows the CICU team to provide palliative care services as part of the daily care of patients. Consultation is not required, as palliative care services are embedded as a core principle of the CICU care. However, this can require a significant time commitment from the cardiology and critical care physicians, as well as a need for increased and ongoing education regarding skills and knowledge of palliative care. With increasing responsibilities being placed on clinicians, the resources needed for a true interdisciplinary team may be lacking in this model.

Recently a more sustainable combined model of palliative care has been described that may be applied to the CICU.[31] Under this model, primary palliative care such as basic management of symptoms along with discussions regarding values, goals, preferences, and prognosis are expectations of the primary CICU team. Specialty palliative care consultation could be requested from the palliative care interdisciplinary team in matters of refractory symptoms, conflict resolution, and differences regarding goals of care and care plans. This model may be more feasible across hospital settings with variable resources.

A recent study evaluated the occurrence of a short meeting each morning between a critical care fellow and a palliative care fellow. Potentially this seems to be a way of moving forward and providing a consultative and/or integrated palliative care approach that can be individualized to each patient's needs.[32]

BARRIERS TO PALLIATIVE CARE IN THE CICU

One of the most significant barriers to providing palliative care in the CICU is the lack of understanding among patients, families, and clinicians as to the role of palliative care in the ICU. Too often, the perception of palliative care is a narrow one that views the role of palliative care as synonymous with hospice care or "giving up." When palliative care is seen as only providing end-of-life care and comfort care for patients, opportunities are missed to improve communication and clarify goals and values of patients, while aligning these with a realistic plan of care. There continues to be a perception in segments of the lay public and in the medical community that palliative care and intensive care are exclusive. Much has been done in the last 2 decades to break down some of these barriers, but much is yet to be accomplished in the realms of education and research.

Care in the ICU can be fragmented as the pace and turnaround of care continues to increase. Care transitions occur frequently, and there is often inadequate time for interdisciplinary care conferences, family meetings, and prolonged discussions on goals of care. Very often there are many specialty teams involved in the care of these patients, and coordinating not only care but also communication across the disciplines can be challenging.

Efforts to break down barriers to palliative care in the ICU are under way; specifically, the Center to Advance Palliative Care initiative called the IPALL-ICU. The IPALL-ICU program provides formalized support to clinicians and administrators in the form of educational resources and strategies, with detailed initiatives aimed at promoting high-quality palliative care in the ICU. A recent educational forum for palliative care and critical care physicians defined concrete ways to ensure support and comfort for patients and families in the ICU.[33] Education for the lay public outlining the role of palliative care will be essential, and has been endorsed as a way of enhancing care for all critically ill patients.[33]

COMMUNICATION ISSUES IN THE CICU

Effective communication with patients, their families, and care providers is an essential component of palliative care in the ICU, and is the foundation on which optimal care is provided in this setting. The CICU can be a bewildering and frightening place for both patients and their loved ones. Many families have never experienced a critically ill family member, and the initial interaction with their loved one who appears entangled in tubes and catheters can be unsettling.

Communication is a critical part of the Care and Communication Bundle when providing palliative care in the ICU, and part of this bundle emphasizes the importance of an interdisciplinary family care conference to be held by day 5 of the ICU stay.[29] Not infrequently, the palliative care team is asked to participate in or facilitate an interdisciplinary family conference, which may be used to establish goals of care and also to discuss the patient's clinical status and prognosis. It is important that all clinicians involved come prepared when meeting with families and patients. A pre-meeting, or session before the main meeting, is recommended with involved care providers to allow clinicians to air any concerns or disagreement before being in the presence of the patient or family members.

Several models have been proposed as guides for conducting goals-of-care discussions.[34,35] In general, it is helpful for the palliative care team to introduce themselves and explain the reason they have been consulted. Often discussions are held with family members or surrogates, as critically ill patients may not be able to communicate. It may be helpful to set the scene by way of introduction to learn something about the patient's personal background as well as current clinical status. Open-ended questions such as "tell me about your loved one" or "how long have you been married?" can serve as an introduction and allow time to put the family at ease.

It is usually helpful to ask permission to conduct an interview to glean some idea from the patient and/or the family regarding how they would like to receive their information. Some patients prefer to have exquisite details explained, whereas others like to have a larger overview of their overall clinical status. Once this invitation has been issued, it is often helpful to learn from the patient and/or family how they understand their medical situation. Not uncommonly, patients and loved ones may respond with emotion. It is important for the clinician to respond in a respectful, understanding, and empathic way. Several different formats have been developed that can help guide the treating physician to respond appropriately to emotion.

Before a family meeting is held, it is helpful for all the caregivers involved to meet before the discussion with the family. Pertinent review of the medical history, clinical status, prognosis, and clinical options available are all issues that should be given high priority for the clinicians to discuss. Knowledge of the patient's decision-making capacity, review of an advance directive (if one exists), and any potential surrogate decision makers should be outlined ahead of time. If there have been prior meetings or if there are psychosocial issues outstanding (eg, potential family conflict), all should be made aware of such before entering the family meeting. The setting should be nonthreatening, and the meeting conducted in a private environment with interruptions minimized. It is important after the meeting that the teams debrief, reiterate the steps of the family encounter, and discuss processes that need to be undertaken to move forward.

It should be pointed out that the ultimate goal of a patient and family conference is not only to establish a do-not-resuscitate status or to obtain a withdrawal of aggressive care, although this may well be an important part of the conversation. It is often most important to define the patient's values and goals and align this in a shared decision-making process. Depending on the precise clinical situation, it is often appropriate for the treating clinicians to make a recommendation to the family on the appropriate next steps in care. Sometimes this does refer specifically to recommendations of a change in resuscitation status, but it also might be in reference to whether an invasive treatment strategy is recommended in respect of the patient's stated goals of care.

Finally, most interventions in the CICU should be presented to patients and families as time-limited trials rather than indefinite and irreversible options. Although an open-ended discussion can be a useful communication tool, an open-ended plan of care can leave families confused and can lead to conflict when the clinical outcomes do not match the desired outcome of the patient and family.

SPIRITUAL AND EMOTIONAL SUPPORT OF PATIENTS AND FAMILIES

A critical illness not only affects patients' clinical and physiologic status, it may also affect the emotional, social, and spiritual needs of patients and their families. Social and spiritual support should be offered to patients and families and is part of the Care and Communication bundle previously mentioned. Bereavement is a normal process, and it is imperative for clinicians to appreciate this.[36] Empathic responses and open listening are meaningful to families and loved ones during a time of great uncertainty. Clinicians should not hesitate to ask for help from chaplains, social workers, counselors, and others that can offer assistance. Grief in the CICU can be especially challenging because a death is sometimes quick and unexpected, and a broad support system may be needed to meet the needs of the bereaving family members.

PALLIATIVE SEDATION

Palliative sedation is defined as the "use of a sedative medication to reduce patient awareness of distressing and intractable symptoms that are insufficiently controlled by symptom-specific therapies."[37] Though controversial within some circles when confused with physician aid in dying or euthanasia, the American Academy of Hospice and Palliative Medicine has a position paper on palliative sedation supporting its use, as do many critical care organizations.

Three major factors are commonly considered when evaluating the ethical permissibility of palliative sedation.[38] First, the intent of use of pain medication or sedation should be clearly articulated. Whether it is to render a patient less pain but be able to still interact, or to be pain free, at any point across the spectrum the intent should be explicit. It is important that the level of sedation should be proportionate to the patient's level of distress, and alertness be preserved as much as possible.

Next, the medications selected should be proportional to the patient's tolerance and previous requirements. For example, 10 mg per hour of morphine may be completely appropriate for some patients (proportionate), but may essentially be lethal if considered as a starting point for an opioid-naïve patient.

Third, the goal of palliative sedation should be to provide comfort and relief of symptoms that has been refractory to other therapies. The marker of a successful intervention is that one provides the patient with appropriate comfort. The possibility that palliative sedation might hasten death as an unintended consequence does exist; however, some studies have shown that palliative sedation is actually not associated with hastening death when the above mentioned criteria are followed.[39,40]

The intent of palliative sedation should always be the alleviation of suffering, using appropriate medications with explicitly stated goals. Palliative sedation may occasionally be useful in CICU patients, including those with unremitting dyspnea, delirium, or pain. Opioid infusions alone are often not sufficient, and are often combined with sedative drugs. For opioid-naïve patients, low-dose fentanyl may be reasonable, but for patients with more tolerance to opioids the use of hydromorphone, morphine, or methadone may be required. Benzodiazepines, such as midazolam or lorazepam, are usually the first-line drugs for sedation. In the CICU, clinicians may be more comfortable with dexmedetomidine or propofol, which often are reasonable alternatives.

WITHDRAWAL OF LIFE-SUSTAINING TREATMENTS

Despite the arsenal of advanced, life-prolonging therapies commonly available in the CICU, patients or their surrogate decision makers may decide that such therapies are no longer concordant with their goals of care. As mentioned earlier, patients have the right to request to refuse therapy or request that it be discontinued, and that neither of these is akin to physician aid in dying or euthanasia. However, how patients live and die with or without such interventions can vary, and this point warrants consideration.

Mechanical Ventilation

The discontinuation of a mechanical ventilator is commonly carried out in the CICU. Often, patients can survive this event as they are not dependent on the ventilator; however, the ventilator is often withdrawn as the penultimate step in initiating comfort-directed care only. Weaning of a ventilator may be so commonplace in the CICU that the impact of withdrawing such a therapy or managing symptoms in an anticipatory fashion may be second nature. Nevertheless, the authors believe it is important to have a protocol to systematize the process but also to allow for individual needs of patients and their loved ones (eg, whether family is or is not present, exact location of ventilator withdrawal).[41,42] Symptoms of dyspnea and pain should be managed in an anticipatory fashion with opioids and benzodiazepines (in a proportionate fashion, as discussed in the Palliative Sedation section).[43] Suctioning of the patient before withdrawal of the endotracheal tube is reasonable, but ongoing deep suctioning is often not helpful for secretion management and is not routinely recommended. Anticholinergic agents such as glycopyrrolate or scopolamine are commonly used to assist with secretion management. Although these may be helpful for some patients on a case-by-case basis, there has been varied efficacy noted when studied systematically.[44]

Mechanical Circulatory Support and Permanent Pacemakers

Patients may survive for a significant time after a mechanical ventilator is withdrawn, but patients who are on mechanical circulatory support or who are pacemaker dependent and have such therapies discontinued often die quickly. Although this may "feel different" to the provider, the most common and mainstream ethical-legal arguments are such that withdrawal of either mechanical circulatory support[6,45] or pacemakers[46] is analogous to withdrawal of any life-sustaining treatment, in that the person dies of the underlying disease process (not the withdrawal of the treatment). Ethical analysis of how quickly the person dies after treatment is withdrawn (hours or days), how long the person has been treated with the therapy (days or years), whether the therapy is continuous (as with some pacemakers) or intermittent (like hemodialysis), and whether the therapy is internal or external to the patient, are all factors that are not morally decisive in swaying the ethical-legal permissibility of discontinuing such therapies.[47,48]

From a practical perspective, discontinuation of such therapies should be carried out by persons who are comfortable with the logistics, and in assuring patient comfort and supporting the loved ones present. Questions of whether the patient will develop symptoms of acute heart failure have

not been definitively answered, and truly vary on a case-by-case basis. It is recommended that opioids, benzodiazepines, and anticholinergic agents be available in case the patient experiences symptoms when therapies are discontinued,[6,49] and that standard procedure is followed to minimize potential alarms or noises that can potentially be distressing to patients or families.[49]

Lastly, it is important to recognize that individual providers may not have beliefs that are consistent with the mainstream consensus of the ethical and legal permissibility of withdrawing pacemaker or mechanical circulatory support in a patient who is dependent on such therapy. It is important to respect a provider's right to conscientiously object to providing such care if it is not consistent with his or her moral, cultural, spiritual, or religious preferences.[6,46] In such situations, consultation with ethics services and colleagues within one's division is recommended to arrange for how the patient's care will be provided without significant interruption.

SUMMARY

The CICU is an impressive location for care in the health care system, where patients can receive high-intensity care that can rescue them from the clutches of death. Unfortunately, situations can be encountered whereby ethical or end-of-life decisions remain pervasive despite the best medical efforts. The role of the palliative care team in the care of patients in the CICU is an evolving concept, and the authors are hopeful that this review provides a practical overview of the potential for excellence in the care of patients in the CICU.

REFERENCES

1. Go AS, Mozaffarian D, Roger VL, et al. Heart disease and stroke statistics—2013 update: a report from the American Heart Association. Circulation 2013;127(1):e6–245.
2. Kaufman SR. Making longevity in an aging society: linking Medicare policy and the new ethical field. Perspect Biol Med 2010;53(3):407–24.
3. Kaufman SR, Shim JK, Russ AJ. Revisiting the biomedicalization of aging: clinical trends and ethical challenges. Gerontologist 2004;44(6):731–8.
4. Beauchamp TL, Childress JF. Principles of biomedical ethics. 7th edition. New York: Oxford U P; 2012.
5. Sudore RL, Fried TR. Redefining the "planning" in advance care planning: preparing for end-of-life decision making. Ann Intern Med 2010;153(4):256–61.
6. Allen LA, Stevenson LW, Grady KL, et al. Decision making in advanced heart failure: a scientific

statement from the American Heart Association. Circulation 2012;125(15):1928–52.

7. Dictionary.com. Available at: http://dictionary.reference.com/browse/futile. Accessed December 16, 2011.

8. Riley G, Lubitz J. Long-term trends in Medicare payments in the last year of life. Health Serv Res 2010;42(2):565–76.

9. Mobley MJ, Rady MY, Verheijde JL, et al. The relationship between moral distress and perception of futile care in the critical care unit. Intensive Crit Care Nurs 2007;23(5):256–63.

10. Tex. Health & Safety Code, Sec. 166.046. Procedure if not effectuating a directive or treatment decision. Available at: http://www.statutes.legis.state.tx.us/SOTWDocs/HS/htm/HS.166.htm#166.046. Accessed August 24, 2013.

11. American Medical Association. Code of medical ethics: current opinions with annotations. 2010-2011 ed.

12. Angell M. The case of Helga Wanglie. A new kind of "right to die" case. N Engl J Med 1991;325(7):511–2.

13. Schneiderman LJ, Jecker NS, Jonsen AR. Medical futility: its meaning and ethical implications. Ann Intern Med 1990;112(12):949–54.

14. Gilgunn v. Massachusetts General Hospital. Suffolk County Superior Court (42); 1995.

15. In Re the conservatorship of Helga M. Wanglie, No. PX-91-283, District Probate Division, 4th Judicial district of the County of Hennepin, State of Minnesota. 6th ed.

16. Betancourt v. Trinitas. Superior Court of New Jersey, A-3849-08T2; 1 A.3d 823 (N.J.Super.A.D. 2010); 2010.

17. Youngner SJ. Who defines futility? JAMA 1988;260(14):2094–5.

18. Pellegrino ED. Decisions to withdraw life-sustaining treatment: a moral algorithm. JAMA 2000;283(8):1065–7.

19. Pellegrino ED. Futility in medical decisions: the word and the concept. HEC Forum 2005;17(4):308–18.

20. Pellegrino ED. Decision at the end of life: the use and abuse of the concept of futility. In: De Dios J, Correa V, Sgreccia E, editors. The dignity of the dying person: Proceeding of the Fifth Assembly of the Pontifical Academy for Life. Vatican City: Libreria Editrice Vaticana; 1999. p. 219–41.

21. Bonica JJ. The management of pain: with special emphasis on the use of analgesic block in diagnosis, prognosis, and therapy. Philadelphia: Lea & Febiger ; 1953.

22. Sepulveda C, Marlin A, Yoshida T, et al. Palliative care: the World Health Organization's global perspective. J Pain Symptom Manage 2002;24(2):91–6.

23. Angus DC, Barnato AE, Linde-Zwirble WT, et al. Use of intensive care at the end of life in the United States: an epidemiologic study. Crit Care Med 2004;32(3):638–43.

24. Azoulay E, Pochard F. Meeting the needs of intensive care unit patients' family members: beyond satisfaction. Crit Care Med 2002;30(9):2171.

25. Campbell ML, Guzman JA. Impact of a proactive approach to improve end-of-life care in a medical ICU. Chest 2003;123(1):266–71.

26. Erdek MA, Pronovost PJ. Improving assessment and treatment of pain in the critically ill. Int J Qual Health Care 2004;16(1):59–64.

27. Lilly CM, De Meo DL, Sonna LA, et al. An intensive communication intervention for the critically ill. Am J Med 2000;109(6):469–75.

28. Morrison RS, Penrod JD, Cassel JB, et al. Cost savings associated with US hospital palliative care consultation programs. Arch Intern Med 2008;168(16):1783–90.

29. Nelson JE, Mulkerin CM, Adams LL, et al. Improving comfort and communication in the ICU: a practical new tool for palliative care performance measurement and feedback. Qual Saf Health Care 2006;15(4):264–71.

30. Nelson JE, Bassett R, Boss RD, et al. Models for structuring a clinical initiative to enhance palliative care in the intensive care unit: a report from the IPAL-ICU Project (Improving Palliative Care in the ICU). Crit Care Med 2010;38(9):1765–72.

31. Quill TE, Abernethy AP. Generalist plus specialist palliative care—creating a more sustainable model. N Engl J Med 2013;368(13):1173–5.

32. Villarreal D, Restrepo MI, Healy J, et al. A model for increasing palliative care in the intensive care unit: enhancing interprofessional consultation rates and communication. J Pain Symptom Manage 2011;42(5):676–9.

33. Nelson JE, Azoulay E, Curtis JR, et al. Palliative care in the ICU. J Palliat Med 2012;15(2):168–74.

34. Back AL, Arnold RM, Baile WF, et al. Approaching difficult communication tasks in oncology. CA Cancer J Clin 2005;55(3):164–77.

35. Tulsky JA. Beyond advance directives: importance of communication skills at the end of life. JAMA 2005;294(3):359–65.

36. Markowitz AJ, Rabow MW. Caring for bereaved patients: "All the doctors just suddenly go". JAMA 2002;287(7):882.

37. Elsayem A, Curry E, Boohene J, et al. Use of palliative sedation for intractable symptoms in the palliative care unit of a comprehensive cancer center. Support Care Cancer 2009;17(1):53–9.

38. Olsen ML, Swetz KM, Mueller PS. Ethical decision making with end-of-life care: palliative sedation and withholding or withdrawing life-sustaining treatments. Mayo Clin Proc 2010;85(10):949–54.

39. Maltoni M, Pittureri C, Scarpi E, et al. Palliative sedation therapy does not hasten death: results from a

prospective multicenter study. Ann Oncol 2009; 20(7):1163–9.

40. Maltoni M, Scarpi E, Rosati M, et al. Palliative sedation in end-of-life care and survival: a systematic review. J Clin Oncol 2012;30(12):1378–83.

41. von Gunten C, Weissman DE. Information for patients and families about ventilator withdrawal. J Palliat Med 2003;6(5):775–6.

42. von Gunten C, Weissman DE. Ventilator withdrawal protocol. J Palliat Med 2003;6(5):773–4.

43. Von Gunten C, Weissman DE. Symptom control for ventilator withdrawal in the dying patient. J Palliat Med 2003;6(5):774–5.

44. Wee B, Hillier R. Interventions for noisy breathing in patients near to death. Cochrane Database Syst Rev 2008;(1):CD005177.

45. Mueller PS, Swetz KM, Freeman MR, et al. Ethical analysis of withdrawing ventricular assist device support. Mayo Clin Proc 2010;85(9):791–7.

46. Lampert R, Hayes DL, Annas GJ, et al. HRS expert consensus statement on the management of Cardiovascular Implantable Electronic Devices (CIEDs) in patients nearing end of life or requesting withdrawal of therapy. Heart Rhythm 2010;7(7):1008–26.

47. Sulmasy DP. Killing and allowing to die: another look. J Law Med Ethics 1998;26(1):55–64, 54.

48. Sulmasy DP. Within you/without you: biotechnology, ontology, and ethics. J Gen Intern Med 2008; 23(Suppl 1):69–72.

49. Gafford EF, Luckhardt AJ, Swetz KM. Deactivation of a left ventricular assist device at the end of life #269. J Palliat Med 2013;16(8):980–2.

Index

Note: Page numbers of article titles are in **boldface** type.

Cardiol Clin 31 (2013) 669–675
http://dx.doi.org/10.1016/S0733-8651(13)00106-9
0733-8651/13/$ – see front matter © 2013 Elsevier Inc. All rights reserved.

United States Postal Service

Statement of Ownership, Management, and Circulation
(All Periodicals Publications Except Requestor Publications)

1. Publication Title	2. Publication Number	3. Filing Date
Cardiology Clinics	0 0 0 - 7 0 1	9/14/13

4. Issue Frequency	5. Number of Issues Published Annually	6. Annual Subscription Price
Feb, May, Aug, Nov	4	$305.00

7. Complete Mailing Address of Known Office of Publication (Not printer) (Street, city, county, state, and ZIP+4®)

Elsevier Inc.
360 Park Avenue South
New York, NY 10010-1710

Contact Person
Stephen R. Bushing
Telephone (Include area code)
215-239-3688

8. Complete Mailing Address of Headquarters or General Business Office of Publisher (Not printer)

Elsevier Inc., 360 Park Avenue South, New York, NY 10010-1710

9. Full Names and Complete Mailing Addresses of Publisher, Editor, and Managing Editor (Do not leave blank)

Publisher (Name and complete mailing address)

Linda Belfus, Elsevier, Inc., 1600 John F. Kennedy Blvd. Suite 1800, Philadelphia, PA 19103-2899

Editor (Name and complete mailing address)

Barbara Cohen-Kligerman, Elsevier, Inc., 1600 John F. Kennedy Blvd. Suite 1800, Philadelphia, PA 19103-2899

Managing Editor (Name and complete mailing address)

Barbara Cohen-Kligerman, Elsevier, Inc., 1600 John F. Kennedy Blvd. Suite 1800, Philadelphia, PA 19103-2899

10. Owner (Do not leave blank. If the publication is owned by a corporation, give the name and address of the corporation immediately followed by the names and addresses of all stockholders owning or holding 1 percent or more of the total amount of stock. If not owned by a corporation, give the names and addresses of the individual owners. If owned by a partnership or other unincorporated firm, give its name and address as well as those of each individual owner. If the publication is published by a nonprofit organization, give its name and address.)

Full Name	Complete Mailing Address
Wholly owned subsidiary of	1600 John F. Kennedy Blvd., Ste. 1800
Reed/Elsevier, US holdings	Philadelphia, PA 19103-2899

11. Known Bondholders, Mortgagees, and Other Security Holders Owning or Holding 1 Percent or More of Total Amount of Bonds, Mortgages, or Other Securities. If none, check box ☐ None

Full Name	Complete Mailing Address
N/A	

12. Tax Status (For completion by nonprofit organizations authorized to mail at nonprofit rates) (Check one)
The purpose, function, and nonprofit status of this organization and the exempt status for federal income tax purposes:
☐ Has Not Changed During Preceding 12 Months
☐ Has Changed During Preceding 12 Months (Publisher must submit explanation of change with this statement)

PS Form **3526**, September 2007 (Page 1 of 3 (Instructions Page 3)) PSN 7530-01-000-9931 PRIVACY NOTICE: See our Privacy policy in www.usps.com

---

13. Publication Title	14. Issue Date for Circulation Data Below
Cardiology Clinics	August 2013

15. Extent and Nature of Circulation			Average No. Copies Each Issue During Preceding 12 Months	No. Copies of Single Issue Published Nearest to Filing Date
a. Total Number of Copies (Net press run)			703	620
b. Paid Circulation (By Mail and Outside the Mail)	(1)	Mailed Outside-County Paid Subscriptions Stated on PS Form 3541. (Include paid distribution above nominal rate, advertiser's proof copies, and exchange copies)	337	302
	(2)	Mailed In-County Paid Subscriptions Stated on PS Form 3541 (Include paid distribution above nominal rate, advertiser's proof copies, and exchange copies)		
	(3)	Paid Distribution Outside the Mails Including Sales Through Dealers and Carriers, Street Vendors, Counter Sales, and Other Paid Distribution Outside USPS®	155	138
	(4)	Paid Distribution by Other Classes Mailed Through the USPS (e.g. First-Class Mail®)		
c. Total Paid Distribution (Sum of 15b (1), (2), (3), and (4))			492	440
d. Free or Nominal Rate Distribution (By Mail and Outside the Mail)	(1)	Free or Nominal Rate Outside-County Copies Included on PS Form 3541	53	33
	(2)	Free or Nominal Rate In-County Copies Included on PS Form 3541		
	(3)	Free or Nominal Rate Copies Mailed at Other Classes Through the USPS (e.g. First-Class Mail)		
	(4)	Free or Nominal Rate Distribution Outside the Mail (Carriers or other means)		
e. Total Free or Nominal Rate Distribution (Sum of 15d (1), (2), (3) and (4))			53	33
f. Total Distribution (Sum of 15c and 15e)			545	473
g. Copies not Distributed (See instructions to publishers #4 (page #3))			158	147
h. Total (Sum of 15f and g)			703	620
i. Percent Paid (15c divided by 15f times 100)			90.28%	93.02%

16. Publication of Statement of Ownership

☐ If the publication is a general publication, publication of this statement is required. Will be printed in the November 2013 issue of this publication.   ☐ Publication not required

17. Signature and Title of Editor, Publisher, Business Manager, or Owner	Date
[signature] Stephen R. Bushing – Inventory Distribution Coordinator	September 14/2013

I certify that all information furnished on this form is true and complete. I understand that anyone who furnishes false or misleading information on this form or who omits material or information requested on the form may be subject to criminal sanctions (including fines and imprisonment) and/or civil sanctions (including civil penalties).

PS Form **3526**, September 2007 (Page 2 of 3)